The American Institute for
Preventive Medicine's

SELF-CARE

Your Family Guide to Symptoms and How to Treat Them

Don R. Powell, Ph.D.

≡People's Medical Society®

Allentown, Pennsylvania

A note to the reader: This book is not intended as a comprehensive guide to health care, nor should you substitute the information it contains for expert medical advice or treatment. The information is designed to help you make informed choices about your health. If, while under a doctor's care, you receive advice that is contrary to this book, follow his or her advice instead. If the problem you are reading about doesn't go away after a reasonable amount of time, you should see or call your doctor.

Many of the designations used by manufacturers and sellers to distinguish their products are claimed as trademarks. Where those designations appear in this book and the People's Medical Society was aware of a trademark claim, the designations have been printed in initial capital letters (e.g., Advil).

Library of Congress Cataloging-in-Publication Data

Powell, Don R.
   [Self-care]
   The American Institute for Preventive Medicine's Self-care : your family guide to symptoms and how to treat them / Don R. Powell.
     p. cm.
   Includes index.
   ISBN 1-882606-24-8 (hardcover). —
ISBN 1-882606-50-7 (trade paper)
   1. Medicine, Popular. 2. Self-care, Health.
3. Symptomatology. I. American Institute for Preventive Medicine. II. Title.
RC81.P844   1996
616—dc20   95-34190
                              CIP

1 2 3 4 5 6 7 8 9 0
First printing, February 1996

Telephone Numbers and Information

Emergency Telephone Numbers

Emergency Medical Service (EMS): _____

Fire: _____

Police: _____

Poison Control Center: _____

Crisis Intervention Center: _____

Suicide Prevention Center: _____

Pharmacy: _____

24-Hour Pharmacy: _____

Hospital: _____

Health Care Professionals

Physicians:

Name	Specialty	Telephone Number
_____	_____	_____
_____	_____	_____
_____	_____	_____
_____	_____	_____

Dentist: _____

Employee Assistance Program (EAP): _____

Health Insurance Company Information

Company: _____

Address: _____

Phone Number: _____

Policyholder's Name: _____

Policy Number: _____

Social Security Number: _____

CONTENTS

SECTION III

MAJOR MEDICAL CONDITIONS 193

SECTION IV

EMERGENCY PROCEDURES AND CONDITIONS 225

ACKNOWLEDGMENTS

The material in *Self-Care* went through an extensive editing and fact-checking process in order to ensure medical accuracy and present the latest medical research. We are indebted to the following physicians and other health professionals who served on our clinical review team.

Charles B. Arnold, M.D., M.P.H., Medical Director, Medical Relations, Metropolitan Life Insurance Company, New York, New York

Jeffrey D. Band, M.D., Corporate Epidemiologist, Chief of Infectious Diseases and Medical Director, InterHealth: Health Care for International Travelers, William Beaumont Hospital, Royal Oak, Michigan

Ronald Berris, D.D.S., Team Dentist, Detroit Pistons basketball team, and Family Dentistry, West Bloomfield, Michigan

Dwight L. Blackburn, M.D., Associate Medical Director, Blue Cross/Blue Shield of Kentucky, Louisville, Kentucky

Dennis I. Blender, Ph.D., Psychologist, Plante Moran, Southfield, Michigan

Joyce Brownson-Booth, M.A., Director of Training, American Institute for Preventive Medicine, Dallas, Texas

Marilyn Citron, M.S., M.A., Creative Consultant and Medical Writer, Birmingham, Michigan

Lynn DeGrande, A.C.S.W., CEAP, DeGrande & Associates, and Senior Consultant, General Motors Employee Assistance Program, Detroit, Michigan

Frances B. DeHart, R.N. B.S.N., Director, Health Styles Corporate Health Risk Management, Greenville Hospital System, Greenville, South Carolina

Jacquelyn B. Elmers, Manager, Graphic Design, American Institute for Preventive Medicine, Farmington Hills, Michigan

Peter Fass, M.D., Medical Director, KeyCorp, Albany, New York

Kathy Foltner, M.A., CCC-A, Certified Audiologist, and President, Audio-Vestibular Testing Center, Okemos, Michigan

Robin Foust, Director, Product and Marketing Development, Health Management Corporation, Richmond, Virginia

Elaine Frank, M.Ed., R.D., Vice President, American Institute for Preventive Medicine, Farmington Hills, Michigan

Barry A. Franklin, Ph.D., Director, Cardiac Rehabilitation and Exercise Laboratories, William Beaumont Hospital, Royal Oak, Michigan

Dwight D. Gaal, M.A., Director, Health Promotion, Bon Secours Hospital, Grosse Pointe, Michigan

Abe Gershonowicz, D.D.S., Family Dentistry, Sterling Heights, Michigan

Donald Hayes, M.D., Medical Director, Sara Lee Corporation, Winston-Salem, North Carolina

William Hettler, M.D., Director, University Health Service, University of Wisconsin, Stevens Point, Wisconsin

Ronald Holmes, M.D., Co-Director, Division of General Pediatrics, Clinical Associate Professor of Pediatrics, Department of Pediatrics, University of Michigan Medical Center, Ann Arbor, Michigan

Susan Hoover, M.S., Director, Corporate/Community Services, Florida Hospital, Orlando, Florida

Susan Horton, M.P.H., Director of Health Directions, Lexington Medical Center, West Columbia, South Carolina

Jeanette Karwan, R.D., Director, Product Development, American Institute for Preventive Medicine, Farmington Hills, Michigan

Amy Kentera, M.P.H., Senior Vice President, Network Systems, Preferred Health Care, Wilton, Connecticut

Ronald D. Kerwin, M.D., Clinical Instructor, Department of Dermatology, Wayne State University School of Medicine, and Staff Physician, Crittenton Hospital, Rochester, Michigan, and Sinai Hospital, Detroit, Michigan

James Kohlenberg, M.D., Internal Medicine, John R. Medical Clinic, Madison Heights, Michigan

Melvin Korobkin, M.D., Professor of Radiology, University of Michigan Medical School, Ann Arbor, Michigan

SECTION I

WISE MEDICAL CONSUMERISM

About This Section

Section I helps you learn to be a wise medical consumer.

- Chapters 1 through 6 give many tips and guidelines to help you use the health care system wisely.
- Chapter 7 offers information on what you should do about basic dental health.
- Chapter 8 lists common mental health problems and reasons to seek help for them.
- Ways to stay well and prevent disease are presented in Chapter 9.

This section combines important information and a commonsense approach to make it easier for you and your family to take responsibility for your own health and well-being.

CHAPTER 1

YOU AND YOUR DOCTOR

Choosing a Doctor

Selecting a doctor takes great care. These guidelines can help:

- Find out if the doctor accepts your health insurance. If you belong to a health maintenance organization (HMO), you will need to go to participating doctors. You may be able to choose among many doctors within the plan.
- Ask relatives and friends for recommendations. A "good reputation" means a lot.
- Check with the local medical society. You can specify what type of doctor you are looking for by location, sex, specialty and age.
- Look for a doctor you can relate to and who meets your expectations of how medical decisions are made (the doctor alone, you alone, you and the doctor together).
- Call the American Board of Medical Specialties at 800-776-2378 to find out if the doctor is "board certified" or "board eligible," and the board or boards under which the physician has received certification. "Board certified" means that he or she has two or more years of training in a specialty after graduation from medical school and has passed a national examination. "Board eligible" means that the training has been completed, but not the exam. The local medical society can provide this information, but remember, these credentials do not guarantee that a doctor is competent.
- Interview several doctors before you decide on the one you want. Find out if you agree with his or her general health philosophies and treatment approaches.

- Ask about office hours, staffing and fees and ask whether the doctor makes house calls. Find out how long you must wait for an appointment.
- Ask about the office policy regarding payment—whether you must pay for your visit at that time or whether you can be billed and pay later.
- Find out if the doctor is alone or in a group practice. If alone, ask what other doctors serve as backups.
- Find out which hospital the doctor sends patients to and if your health insurance plan is accepted there.

Finding the right doctor is a big part of being a wise medical consumer. Look for a doctor who:

- Is competent and can care for all your general health needs, or can refer you to other appropriate health care providers for any special health needs
- You feel comfortable with
- You trust

Doctors and Their Specialties

The most common specialists and what they do are:

Allergist - Diagnoses and treats allergies

Anesthesiologist - Administers anesthetics that are used during surgery

Cardiologist - Diagnoses and treats problems of the heart and blood vessels

Dermatologist - Diagnoses and treats diseases and problems of the skin

Emergency Medicine - Specializes in rapid recognition and treatment of trauma or acute illness

Endocrinologist - Diagnoses disorders of internal glands such as the thyroid and adrenal glands

Family practitioner - Provides total health care of the individual and the family. Scope is not limited by age, sex or organ system.

Gastroenterologist - Diagnoses and treats disorders of the digestive tract: stomach, bowels, liver, gallbladder and related organs

Gynecologist - Diagnoses and treats disorders of the female reproductive system

Internist - Diagnoses and treats diseases, especially those of adults

Nephrologist - Diagnoses and treats diseases and problems of the kidneys

Neurologist - Diagnoses and treats disorders of the nervous system

Obstetrician - Provides care and treatment of females during pregnancy, labor and delivery, and six weeks after delivery

Oncologist - Diagnoses and treats all types of cancer and other types of benign and malignant tumors

Ophthalmologist - Diagnoses, monitors and treats vision problems and other disorders of the eye, and prescribes prescription lenses

Orthopedist - Diagnoses and treats skeletal injuries and diseases of the bones and muscles

Otolaryngologist - Diagnoses and treats disorders that affect the ears, respiratory and upper alimentary systems (in general, the head and neck)

Pathologist - Examines and diagnoses organs, tissues and body fluids

Pediatrician - Diagnoses and treats the physical, emotional and social problems of children

Physiatrist - Provides physical and rehabilitative treatment of muscle and bone disorders

Psychiatrist - Treats and prevents mental, emotional and/or behavioral disorders

Radiologist - Uses X-rays and radiant energy for diagnosis and treatment of disease

Urologist - Diagnoses and treats diseases of the urinary or urogenital tract

Calling Your Doctor Checklist

There will be times when you must call your doctor or other health care provider. Find these things out in advance:
- When is the best time to call?
- What is the doctor's rule for returning calls?
- Who should you speak with (physician's assistant, nurse, etc.) if the doctor can't come to the phone?
- What is the phone number for emergency calls or calls when the office is closed?
- Who can you call if your doctor is out of town?

When you reach your doctor or other health care provider by phone, be prepared to:
- Get to the point of your call quickly, especially if you've phoned after hours. (Have someone else call the doctor for you if you are unable to talk.)
- Define your problems and symptoms. Write these down and keep them by the telephone so you can report them quickly and completely.
- Report results of self-tests and things you have been keeping track of, such as a temperature of 101°F for two days, diarrhea that has lasted for 48 hours, and so on.
- Ask the doctor what you should do. Write it down.
- Have your pharmacist's phone number handy in case the doctor needs to prescribe medicine.
- Ask if and when you should call back, or if you should come to the office.
- Ask what things might occur that would require you to go to the emergency room.
- Thank the doctor for talking to you on the telephone.

Making the Most of a Doctor Visit

Patients often feel rushed or uneasy at the doctor's office. And when you're sick, there is a tendency to feel vulnerable and passive. Plan ahead of time what you want to discuss with the doctor. Write it down and take it with you. Be prepared to talk about your current problems, symptoms and needs. Also be able to state your medical history.

What Your Doctor Should Know About You

Aside from a general health history, it is important that your doctor know about the following:

Dietary habits - Are you a frequent junk-food eater? Are you especially fond of cheesecake, sour cream or other fatty foods?

Your occupation - Do you work in a high-stress job? Are you exposed to nickel, nuclear power radiation or other toxic substances?

Sleep habits - Do you frequently awaken before dawn or have problems getting to sleep?

Family problems - Are you currently going through a divorce or having problems with a family member?

Lifestyle - Do you get any exercise?

Stress - Do you work in a hectic environment? Are you dealing with any major problems?

Health attitude - Are you serious about quitting smoking, getting more exercise or eating better?

History of family illness - Does heart disease, high blood pressure, diabetes, kidney problems or cancer run in your family?

Major life events - Have you recently retired from work?

Living arrangements - Do you live alone?

Doctor-Patient Communication

Communication is a two-way process. Listening as well as speaking to one another is something both doctor and patient must work on together. Being honest and open with each other is also important. The more honest you are, the better your doctor can help you. You can make the most of your doctor-patient communication with these suggestions:

- Plan ahead of time what you will say to your doctor about your problem. Your observations about a health problem can be invaluable in making a diagnosis.
- Repeat in your own words what the doctor has told you. Use simple phrases like "Do I hear you say that . . . ?" or "My understanding of the problem is . . . ."
- Take notes on what is wrong and what you need to do.
- If you are confused by medical terms, ask for simple definitions. There is no need to be embarrassed by this. When a medication is prescribed, ask about its possible side effects, its effectiveness and how long it must be taken. If your doctor discusses surgery, ask about alternatives, risks and a second opinion.
- Be frank with the doctor if any part of the office visit is annoying, such as lengthy waiting time or discourteous staff. Be tactful, but honest.
- Don't be afraid to voice your fears about what you've heard. The doctor may be able to clarify any misconceptions.
- Discuss any self-care practices you've used that have relieved symptoms.
- Find out the best time to call your doctor if you have any questions after you leave the office.

Rating Your Doctor

In order to feel good about your medical care, you should feel good about your doctor, too. Ask yourself the following questions to evaluate your physician:

- Does your doctor listen to you and answer all your questions about the causes and treatment of your medical problems, or is he or she vague, impatient or unwilling to answer?
- Are you comfortable with your doctor? Can you openly discuss your feelings and talk about personal concerns, including sexual and emotional problems?
- Does your doctor take a thorough history, asking about past physical and emotional problems, family medical history, medications you are taking and other matters affecting your health?
- Does your doctor address the root causes of your medical problems or simply prescribe drugs to treat the symptoms?
- Are you satisfied with the doctor's stand-in when he or she is unavailable?
- Do you feel at ease asking your doctor questions that may sound "silly"?
- Does your doctor explain things in simple terms?
- Is the office staff friendly? Do they listen to you?
- Does your doctor answer your telephone calls promptly?
- Are you generally kept waiting for a long time when you have an appointment?
- Does the doctor have hospital privileges at a respected hospital?

If you are not satisfied with your answers to these questions, discuss your concerns with your doctor. If after this discussion you are still not satisfied, consider looking for another doctor.

CHAPTER 2

MEDICAL EXAMS AND TESTS

Having a Routine Checkup

The routine physical exam in a doctor's office or at a health clinic is a way to determine the state of your health. It also allows you to ask your doctor questions and to benefit from finding out if you have a health problem you didn't know about. Some diseases like high blood pressure and some cancers may not have any symptoms in the early stages. Tests your doctor does can help detect these. Check the chart on page 17 for when health tests and checkups are recommended.

The basic parts of a checkup are:
- A complete medical history (questions on family health history, previous illness, emotional well-being)
- A check of how well body organs are functioning (eyes, ears, heart, skin, bowels, etc.)
- A check of the vital signs (blood pressure, pulse, breathing rate, temperature)
- Actual body examination (listening, thumping and looking at specific body parts)
- Routine diagnostic tests (blood tests, X-rays, etc.)
- A check of specific health concerns

Tests and What They Are For

Blood pressure test - Checks two kinds of pressure within the blood vessels. The higher number (systolic) gauges the pressure when your heart is pumping and the lower number (diastolic) represents the pressure between heartbeats. High blood pressure is a symptomless disease that can lead to a heart attack and/or a stroke.

Vision - Checks for marked changes or degeneration of eye functioning

Pap smear - Is used to detect the early signs of cervical cancer, uterine cancer and herpes

Mammography - An X-ray that detects breast tumors or problems

Professional breast exam - An exam by a physician or nurse to check the breasts for signs of abnormalities

Digital rectal exam - Checks for early signs of colorectal and/or prostate abnormalities, including cancer

Stool blood test - Checks for early signs of colorectal abnormalities, including cancer

Sigmoidoscopy - Checks for early signs of colorectal abnormalities, including cancer

Cholesterol blood test - Checks the levels of fatty deposits (cholesterol) in the blood. High cholesterol levels are linked to heart disease.

Glaucoma screening - Checks for increased pressure within the eye. Glaucoma can result in blindness if not treated.

Common Health Tests and How Often to Have Them

AGES		20-29	30-39	40-49	50+
Physical exam		Every 2-3 years	Every 2-3 years	Every 2-3 years	Every 1-2 years
Blood pressure		Every 1-2 years	Every 1-2 years	Every 1-2 years	Every 1-2 years
Vision		Every 3-5 years	Every 3-5 years	Every 3-5 years	Every 2-3 years
Pap smear[1]	**W**	Every 2-3 years	Every 2-3 years	Every 2-3 years	Every 2-3 years
Mammography[2]	**O**				Every year
Breast self-exam*	**M** **E**	Monthly	Monthly	Monthly	Monthly
Professional breast exam	**N**			Every year	Every year
Testicular self-exam*		Discuss with your doctor	Discuss with your doctor	Discuss with your doctor	Discuss with your doctor
Digital rectal exam				Discuss with your doctor	Discuss with your doctor
Stool blood test					Discuss with your doctor
Sigmoidoscopy					Every 3-5 years
Cholesterol blood test[3]		Every 3-5 years	Every 3-5 years	Every 3-5 years	Every 3-5 years
Glaucoma screening[4]					Every 2-3 years
Regular dental checkup		Every year	Every year	Every year	Every year

Legend: ■ Every year | ▥ Every 1-2 years | ▦ Every 2-3 years | ▧ Every 3-5 years

Note: Recommendations for routine medical exams may vary. These apply only to healthy people who do not have symptoms of illnesses. If you have an increased risk of a particular illness, testing may need to be done sooner or more often. Extra tests may also need to be done. Follow your doctor's advice. Also, check with your insurance company to see if and when tests are covered.

[1] Pap smears should start at age 18 or under age 18 if sexual activity has begun. They should be given every year until tests are normal three years in a row. Thereafter, Pap smears should be given at least every three years. *(Note: The American College of Obstetricians and Gynecologists recommends an annual Pap smear.)*

[2] As recommended by the National Cancer Institute. Check with your doctor for his or her recommendations.

[3] The National Cholesterol Education Program recommends that a blood cholesterol test be given at least once every five years and that high-density lipoprotein (HDL) be part of the initial cholesterol testing.

[4] Glaucoma screening is recommended earlier for African Americans. It should be done every two to three years between the ages of 40 and 49.

* *Ask your doctor or call the Cancer Information Service at 800-4-CANCER (800-422-6237) for a step-by-step self-examination guide.*

Sources: American Cancer Society; National Cancer Institute; American Academy of Physicians; the report of the U.S. Preventive Task Force's Guide to Clinical Services; and the National Heart, Lung and Blood Institute.

Immunization Schedule

	IMMUNIZATIONS					WHEN & WHERE			
Age	**Hepatitis B (HB)**	**Oral Polio (OPV)**	**Diphtheria Tetanus Pertussis DTP**	***H. influenzae type b* (Hib)[2]**	**Measles Mumps Rubella (MMR)[3]**	**Name**	**Name**	**Name**	**Name**
Birth	HB Birth-2 mos.								
2 mos.	HB 2-4 mos.	OPV	DTP	Hib					
4 mos.		OPV	DTP	Hib					
6 mos.	HB 6-18 mos.	OPV 6-18 mos.	DTP	Hib					
12-15 mos.			DTP 12-18 mos.	Hib	MMR				
4-6 years		OPV	DTP		MMR[3]				
11-16 years			T(d)[1] & every 10 yrs. thereafter						

Recommendations through age 16 were approved by the Advisory Committee on Immunization Practice (ACIP), the American Academy of Pediatrics (AAP) and the American Academy of Family Physicians (AAFP), January 1995.

[1] Tetanus and diphtheria without pertussis.

[2] *H. influenzae type b* protects against several diseases, most notably meningitis. Shown is one schedule for Hib using one type of the vaccine. An alternate time schedule of 2, 4 and 12-15 months can be followed using a different form of the vaccine. Persons over 5 years of age are not given this vaccination unless sickle-cell anemia or problems with the spleen are present.

[3] The second dose of MMR vaccine should be given EITHER at 4-6 years OR at 11-12 years of age, depending on state school requirements.

ADULT IMMUNIZATIONS			
T(d)[1]	**Tuberculin Tests**	**Influenza Vaccine (A&B)[4]**	**Pneumo-coccal Vaccine[5]**
Every 10 years after 11-16 yrs. of age	Upon Exposure	Annually After 65 Years	Once at 65 Years

[4] Influenza vaccine may be recommended sooner than age 65 if you have a chronic medical condition such as diabetes, heart and/or respiratory diseases. Check with your doctor.

[5] Pneumococcal vaccine may be recommended sooner than age 65 if you have conditions that increase the risk of pneumonia such as chronic heart or lung disease, sickle-cell disease, diabetes, Hodgkin's disease or other conditions associated with a suppressed immune system.

Note: Check with your doctor or health department about a new vaccine for chicken pox.

Source: Centers for Disease Control and Prevention.

Home Medical Tests

Medical self-testing kits are easy to use, relatively inexpensive and readily available. They can be used without a visit to the doctor, so it's no wonder Americans in ever-increasing numbers are buying them—and spending over $500 million annually in the process. Home tests can offer you a sense of self-reliance that can assist, though not take the place of, the service of your doctor.

While some 150 different medical self-testing kits exist, they generally can be grouped into two categories:

- Those that diagnose when conditions are or are not present. These include the popular self-testing kits for pregnancy and kits that test for blood in the stool.
- Those that monitor an ongoing condition. These include glucose testing for diabetes and blood pressure kits for high blood pressure.

The U.S. Public Health Service and the Food and Drug Administration (FDA) offer some suggestions for safe and proper use of self-testing kits. (Each of these does not necessarily apply to all tests.):

- For test kits that contain chemicals, note the expiration date. Beyond that date, chemicals may lose potency and affect results. Don't buy or use a test kit after the expiration date.
- Check whether the product needs protection from heat or cold. If so, don't leave it in the car trunk or by a sunny window on the trip home. At home, follow storage directions. Study the package insert. First, read it through to get a general idea of how to perform the test. Then go back and review the instructions and diagrams until you fully understand each step.
- Be sure you understand what the test is intended to do and what its limitations may be. Remember, the tests are not 100-percent accurate.
- If the test results rely on color comparison and you're color-blind, be sure someone who is not color-blind helps you interpret the results.
- Note special precautions, such as avoiding physical activity or certain foods and drugs before testing.
- Follow instructions exactly, including the specimen collection process, if that is a part of the test. Sequence is important.
- Don't skip a step.
- When collecting a urine specimen (unless you use a container from a kit), wash the container thoroughly and rinse out all soap traces, preferably with distilled water.
- When a step is timed, be precise. Use a stopwatch or at least a watch with a second hand.
- Note what you should do if the results are positive, negative or unclear.
- If something isn't clear, don't guess. Consult a pharmacist or other health professional or check the package for a toll-free number to call for more information.
- Keep accurate records of results.
- As with medications, keep test kits that contain chemicals out of the reach of children. Throw away used test materials as directed.
- Any malfunction of a self-test should be reported to the manufacturer or to the FDA through the agency's reporting system at the U.S. Pharmacopeia (USP). To report a problem to the pharmacopeia, write to: USP, Practitioner's Reporting Network, 12601 Twinbrook Parkway, Rockville, MD 20852. The network may also be called toll-free at 800-638-6725.

CHAPTER 3

MEDICATIONS

Before Taking Medications

Medications are powerful and can be harmful if not used properly. These tips will help reduce medication-related problems:

- Ask your doctor to not only tell you what a medicine is for, but ask him or her to write it down, too. If not, you might forget what the doctor says, especially if you're taking more than one medicine at a time. Your doctor should also tell you when to take it, for how long and if it should be taken in a special way (e.g., with food or plenty of water).
- Use the same pharmacy to buy prescriptions as well as over-the-counter (OTC) medications. This way, a complete record of your medicines can be kept in one place. This is especially important if more than one doctor has been writing your prescriptions. Your pharmacist can also spot possible harmful combinations of medicines.
- Tell your doctor and have him or her record all medicines you take. This includes OTC items like vitamins, aspirin and laxatives, as well as any medicine another doctor has prescribed.
- Ask your pharmacist to clearly mark each vial with all necessary instructions.
- Always keep medicines in their original containers.
- Let your doctor know about your past reactions to certain medicines. Tolerance levels may change with age. For instance, as some people age, they may show greater sensitivity to some medications such as painkillers or tranquilizers.

- Ask about the possible side effects of a medication. If you do experience some, don't stop taking it, but instead call your physician immediately. Often, just a change in dosage is all that is needed.
- Never take someone else's medication.
- Throw away all medications that have expired.
- Try to reduce the need for medications such as sleeping pills or laxatives. For example, a hot bath and a glass of milk might help you sleep at night. Changing your diet to increase fiber intake might effectively substitute for a laxative. Even cutting down on salt and losing weight might lower blood pressure, avoiding the need for medication. Check with your doctor for nonmedical alternatives.
- Don't stop taking prescription medications even if you feel better. Check with your doctor first.

Understanding a Prescription

If you can't understand your doctor's prescription, much less read his or her handwriting, the following information will be helpful. Listed are frequently used abbreviations that are meant to give directions to both the pharmacist filling the prescription and to the patient taking the medication:

ad lib. - Freely, as needed

a.c. - Before meals

b.i.d. - Twice a day

caps - Capsule

gtt. - Drops

h.s. - At bedtime

p.c. - After meals

p.o. - By mouth

p.r.n. - As needed

q.4.h. - Every four hours

q.d. - Daily

q.i.d. - Four times a day

q.o.d. - Every other day

t.i.d. - Three times a day

Ut dict., UD - As directed

Questions to Ask About Medications

Make sure you get clear answers to these questions before you take any medications:

- What is the name of the medication?

- What will it do?

- When should it be taken?

- How long should it be taken?

- Are there side effects?

- Should I take it with meals?

- Is there a generic equivalent?

- Will it interfere with other medicines I am taking?

- Should I stop taking it if I feel better?

- Is there anything I should avoid while taking it (e.g., alcohol and sunlight)?

Medication Matchup

Categories of medicines and what they do are:

Amphetamines - Stimulants that affect the central nervous system

Analgesics - Pain relievers such as aspirin

Antacids - Medications to relieve heartburn and indigestion by neutralizing stomach acid

Antibiotics - Medications to treat infection (usually bacterial)

Antiemetics - Medications to treat nausea and vomiting

Antihistamines - Medications used to treat colds or allergic reactions

Barbiturates - Sleep inducers

Decongestants - Medications to reduce swollen mucous membranes in the nose and sinuses

Diuretics - Medications to lower blood pressure by increasing the flow of urine

Laxatives - Medications to treat constipation

Muscle Relaxants - Medications to relieve muscle spasms

Narcotics - Painkillers and sleep inducers that can be addictive

Sedatives - Calming agents, tranquilizers or sleep inducers

Other medicine-related terms:

Antiseptics - Chemicals used to destroy harmful germs

Buffered - Indicates antacids have been added to protect stomach lining

Elixir - A liquid form of medicine that is usually pleasant tasting

Generic - The name of a drug available to be used by each drug manufacturer; often used to mean a less-expensive equivalent of a brand-name drug

Seven Golden Rules of Prescriptions

Popping that pill into your mouth or spooning down that elixir may be hazardous to your health if you don't observe some basic rules:

- Report adverse reactions, especially unexpected side effects, to your physician. Not everyone responds to medication in the same manner.
- Because two or more medications taken within a 24-hour period may interact negatively, tell your doctor about all medications you are taking. One medicine may slow down or speed up the effect of the other. If you don't know which medications you are taking, bring them (in their original containers) to your doctor for review.
- Ask your pharmacist about food and drug interactions. Some foods may affect the rate at which a medication works, or may prevent it from working at all. Some combinations may have even more dangerous consequences. For example, when MAO inhibitors (prescription drugs used to treat depression) are consumed with cheese and other foods containing tyramine, dangerously elevated blood pressure levels may result.
- If you are having laboratory tests performed, be sure to inform the physician of all medications, including nutritional supplements, you have been taking. Certain test results can be influenced. If you have administered a medical self-test, ask your pharmacist about possible drug influence.
- Don't drink alcohol while on a medication if you don't know the resulting effect. Regular alcohol use can speed up the metabolism of certain medications, reducing their intended effectiveness. When alcohol is present in the system, other medications such as sedatives can become deadly.
- Always ask your physician if a generic equivalent would be okay to use. Generics are usually less expensive than the brand-name versions and may be equally effective. There are certain situations in which a specific brand of medication may be required in order to ensure a consistent effect. This is particularly important with medications for the heart and lung, and for hormonal disorders.
- Tell your doctor if:
  - You've ever experienced an allergic reaction, and to what
  - You are pregnant or breast-feeding
  - Another doctor is also treating you
  - You have diabetes or kidney or liver disease
  - You're regularly taking vitamins, birth control pills, insulin or other medications
  - You use alcohol, tobacco or illegal ("street") drugs

Over-the-Counter Medications

Taken by millions of people, over-the-counter (OTC) drugs are widely advertised in magazines and on TV. Generally less potent than prescription drugs, they can be taken without the authorization of a doctor. Ask these questions before buying an OTC drug:

- Am I trying to cover up symptoms that need to be evaluated by a doctor?
- Will continued use cause new problems (dependency on laxatives or sleeping pills, for example)?
- Are there unwanted side effects from these drugs (e.g., increased blood pressure, dizziness, headaches, rashes)?
- Do I already have a similar product at home?

Often, reading the package labels, looking up the name of the drug in the *Physician's Desk Reference for Nonprescription Drugs* or asking the pharmacist can help you answer these questions. Keep in mind that when taken in large quantities, an OTC drug might equal the dose of a medicine that is available only by prescription. If you are unsure whether a particular OTC medication will help or harm you, call and check with your doctor before you purchase it.

Overhauling Your Medicine Cabinet

Who knows what mysterious bottles lurk on the shelves of your bathroom medicine cabinet? If it has been more than a year since you last housecleaned your cabinet, it's certainly time to take inventory. Here's how:

- Take out the entire contents of the medicine cabinet and get some clear idea of what you really need to keep.
- Check expiration dates. Throw out all out-dated medicine. If you're uncertain about a particular item, call your pharmacist and ask what the shelf life is.
- Are all medications in original containers and labeled clearly? If not, into the trash they go. It's dangerous to store medicines in anything but their original containers. Some medicines come in tinted glass, for example, because exposure to light may cause them to deteriorate.
- Discard old tubes of cream that have hardened or cracked. Throw out any liquid medicines that now appear cloudy or filmy.
- If there are children in the house, every medication is a potential poison. Discard all unnecessary medications by flushing them down the toilet, and keep all others locked in a high cabinet, well out of children's reach.
- Keep a container of syrup of ipecac handy in case of accidental poisoning. Call the poison control center before giving syrup of ipecac.

CHAPTER 4

HOSPITALS AND SURGERY

Ambulatory Surgery

Can you have surgery without being admitted to a hospital? Yes, and it's recommended in many cases. Ambulatory surgery can be done on an outpatient basis at a hospital or at facilities that perform outpatient surgeries. Procedures that best qualify for ambulatory centers:
• Do not require opening a primary body section like the chest or skull
• Do not require blood transfusions
• Require very little or no general anesthesia
• Do not require specialized postoperative care
• Do not require hours on the operating table
• Pose little risk of complication or additional surgery

The most common types of surgeries performed in an ambulatory care center include:
• Hernia repair
• Some plastic surgeries
• Tubal ligation
• Dilation and curettage (D&C)
• Breast biopsy
• Tonsillectomy
• Cataract removal
• Adenoidectomy
• Orthopedic procedures (e.g., setting a broken bone)
• Cystoscopy
• Varicose vein surgery
• Glaucoma procedures

There are several important advantages of ambulatory, or outpatient, surgery:
• Hospitalization poses the risk of exposure to infection and may also keep patients bed-ridden longer than is necessary.
• Ambulatory surgery gets you in and out quickly.

• The patient has a good deal of choice as to when the surgery will occur. The surgeries are scheduled by appointment for patient convenience.
• Most people prefer healing at home in their own beds to staying in a hospital. Familiar surroundings and the comforts of home can be a more conducive environment in which to heal than the hectic atmosphere of many hospitals.
• Medical bills are much lower if you don't have to stay in a hospital overnight.

Things to consider:
• Many procedures require special preparation before the procedure. Follow your doctor's orders exactly.
• You may need someone to drive you home and stay with you as you recover.
• Do not bring valuables with you when you are admitted to the hospital.

Hospital Admissions

The golden rule here is to take care of as much as you can *before* being admitted. Ask the following questions:
• Is it possible to have the needed forms mailed to your home prior to being admitted so that you can have the opportunity for careful review? Can you be preadmitted over the telephone?
• Is your insurance coverage well understood both by the billing department and yourself?
• Can you reserve a private or semiprivate room with your coverage?
• What identification will you need to have?
• Do you require special food preparations?

Medical Prefixes and Suffixes

Sometimes medical words require a "translation" into lay terms. The following word beginnings and endings may help clarify the meanings of some medical terms:

Prefix	Definition	Example
angio-	blood vessels	angioplasty
arthro-	joint	arthroscopic
cardio-	heart	cardiovascular
cranio-	skull	cranioplasty
derma-	skin	dermatitis
gastro-	stomach	gastrointestinal
hem-	blood	hemophilia
hepato-	liver	hepatitis
myo-	muscle	myocardial
nephro-	kidney	nephritis
osteo-	bone	osteoporosis
radio-	ray	radiology
sacro-	sacrum	sacroiliac
uro-	urinary organs	uropenia
vaso-	vessel	vasoconstrictor

Suffix	Definition	Example
-algia or -dynia	pain	neuralgia
-blast	early stage of a growth	cytotrophoblast
-ectomy	surgical removal	appendectomy
-itis	inflammation	bronchitis
-lysis	freeing of	dialysis
-oma	tumor	melanoma
-oscopy	viewing an organ	laparoscopy
-osis	process or condition	endometriosis
-otomy	cutting into	vasectomy
-pathy	abnormality	myopathy
-plasty	rebuilding or restoring	rhinoplasty
-pnea	breathing	apnea
-rrhea	flow	diarrhea
-scler(osis)	hardening	arteriosclerosis
-uria	pertaining to urine	glycosuria

Saving Money in the Hospital

Avoid unnecessary stays in the hospital. The daily hospital rate in some sections of the country is now as high as $1,000. And that doesn't include the costs for treatments, medicines or doctors' fees. The hospital should never be viewed as a place to get a good rest. Consider these tips:

- Choose outpatient services whenever you can. Many routine lab tests and diagnostic tests can be done for less money as an outpatient. You avoid the cost of an overnight stay in a hospital.
- As an inpatient, stay only the prescribed time that is necessary. Ask your doctor about home health care, which can provide a whole range of services at less cost than a hospital.
- Beware of duplication of tests. Be sure to ask the doctor what blood tests, X-rays and medical procedures you can expect.
- Be sure you know when checkout time is and make plans to observe it; otherwise, you're likely to be charged for an extra day's stay.
- If your health problem isn't an emergency, avoid being admitted to a hospital on a weekend. The hospital staff is reduced then, and testing will usually not begin until Monday.
- Use same day, or ambulatory, surgery for minor procedures (e.g., biopsy and cataract surgery). It is a big money-saver when compared to inpatient surgery.
- Keep a list of all services you receive in the hospital. Ask for an itemized bill so you can make sure you are billed correctly.

Types of Surgery

It's funny. People think of surgery as *major* when it happens to them and *minor* when it's being done to someone else. In reality, surgery is thought to be major when it involves any vital organs and/or requires a long time to perform. The following chart helps to classify various surgeries:

Curative - A procedure that rids the body of a problem or corrects a condition

Diagnostic - A procedure that helps in making a diagnosis about a suspected problem

Elective - A procedure that may or may not be done, depending upon the patient's wishes

Emergency - An immediate operation to save a life or maintain the use of a body part

Exploratory - A surgery that explores a body organ or body area for a suspected disorder

Palliative - A surgery that eases bodily pain, but doesn't cure the problem

Planned - A surgery set up well in advance of the actual operation date

Urgent - An operation that must be done within a matter of hours

Patient Rights

What rights and privileges can you expect from a hospital when you become a patient? According to the American Hospital Association (AHA), there are specific standards of care that all patients are entitled to. The AHA has developed a voluntary code, the Patient's Bill of Rights, which presents guidelines for both staff and patients:

- You have the right to considerate and respectful care.
- You have the right to obtain from your physician complete, current information concerning your diagnosis, treatment and prognosis in terms you can reasonably be expected to understand.
- You have the right to receive from your physician information necessary to give informed consent prior to the start of any procedure and/or treatment.
- You have the right to refuse treatment to the extent permitted by law, and to be informed of the medical consequences of your action.
- You have the right to privacy concerning your own medical care program, including all communications and records pertaining to your care.
- You have the right to expect that, within its capacity, a hospital must make a reasonable response to your request for services.
- You have the right to obtain information about any relationship of your hospital to other health care and educational institutions insofar as your care is concerned.
- You have the right to be advised if the hospital proposes to engage in or perform human experimentation affecting your care or treatment.
- You have the right to expect reasonable continuity of care.
- You have the right to examine and receive an explanation of your bill regardless of the source of payment.
- You have the right to know what hospital rules and regulations apply to your conduct as a patient.

Informed Consent

Every patient should be aware of the policy of informed consent, an ethical standard in medicine that implies that you have been given an explanation and fully understand your treatment. You should be able to explain in your own words what your treatment is about. You should know what the likelihood is that the medical procedure will accomplish what it's supposed to. The benefits and accompanying risks should always be identified clearly. You should also be notified if your treatment is experimental in nature.

The physician should review any alternatives available in lieu of surgery or other procedures. There are no guaranteed outcomes in medicine, but informed consent enables *you* to make a rational and educated decision about your treatment. It is also a tool that promotes greater understanding between you and your doctor and encourages joint decision-making.

Three principles of informed consent that involve your responsibility as a patient are:
- You cannot demand services that go beyond what are considered "acceptable" practices of medicine or that violate professional ethics.
- You must recognize that you may be faced with some uncertainties or unpleasantness.
- You should, if competent, be responsible for your choices and not pass them along to others.

Advance Directives

A federal law called the Patient Self-Determination Act requires hospitals to give you information about your rights as a patient under their care. Advance directives are a legal way for you to declare your wishes regarding the withholding or removal of life-sustaining care if you should suffer from a terminal illness, or if you should be in an incurable or irreversible mental or physical condition with no reasonable expectations of recovery.

There are two types of advance directives:
- **Living Will** - A document that spells out what medical treatment you would want or not want if you are unable to state it yourself. Most states have their own living will form or you can make up your own. You should discuss your living will with your family and physician.

- **Durable Power of Attorney (Health-Care Proxy)** - A document that names a person who would make treatment decisions for you if you are not able to make them yourself. Generally, it is a person who knows you and your values well and is in a good position to represent your wishes to your physician.

CHAPTER 5

HEALTH INSURANCE

Insurance Terms

Does it seem to you that health insurance policies are written in something other than simple English? Here are some terms that will help you understand a policy:

Assigned benefits - The doctor accepts payment directly from the insurance company.

Coinsurance - This means you pay a certain percentage (usually 20 percent) of the costs of a service. There may or may not be a set limit, after which the insurance coverage is 100 percent.

Copayment - This is a cost-sharing requirement in many health insurance policies in which the insured pays a percentage of or predetermined fee for the cost of the covered services.

Covered expenses - These are medical expenses that are paid for under the terms of a policy.

Deductible - This is the amount of money you must pay for medical expenses before the company pays anything.

Exclusion - This is a service that your health insurance company will not cover or pay for.

Preauthorization - This requirement calls for approval from the insurance company for certain services specified in the policy.

Preexisting condition - This is a health problem you had when the insurance took effect.

Stop-loss - This provision limits the amount you make in copayments to a maximum figure.

Usual and customary - This means the usual fees charged for medical services.

Waiting period - This period is one during which an insurance policy will not cover a problem.

Considering Your Needs

The right health insurance for you depends on your needs and the needs of your family. Policies vary—therefore, so do costs and what is covered. Be a wise shopper. Consider your needs before choosing health insurance. Ask these questions:

- Is my whole family covered?
- Are most services covered?
- Are routine checkups covered?
- Are well-care visits covered?
- Are immunizations covered?
- Is maternity care covered?
- Are there deductibles? What are they?
- Are there limits if my problem is chronic?
- How many days are covered in the hospital?
- Are psychological services covered?
- Can I choose my doctor? Can I be seen by the same doctor at each visit?
- Are specialist visits covered?

It's best to ask someone who knows a lot about health insurance for advice. Just because a friend, relative or co-worker chooses a certain health insurance policy doesn't mean it's right for you. Also, ask your employee benefits person or Employee Assistance Program (EAP) representative for information on the health insurance your company offers.

CHAPTER 6

MEDICAL DECISIONS

At some point in your life (maybe it's right now), you or a loved one may be faced with making a medical decision that could affect your quality of life. You can deal with this issue with greater ease when you have all the information you need. One way to get this information is to ask your doctor or health care professional all the right questions. This chapter will teach you what to ask.

Key Questions Checklist

The following is a summary of the key questions and recommendations that will assist you in making medical decisions. (Photocopy as needed.) Use them as a guide when visiting your doctor or health care professional. Check off the items you wish to discuss with your medical practitioner as the need arises:

1. **DESCRIPTION - What is my current complaint?**
   - ☐ What do I think the problem is?
   - ☐ When did it start?
   - ☐ What makes it better?
   - ☐ What makes it worse?
   - ☐ What are my signs and symptoms?
   - ☐ What daily habits are affected (e.g., eating, sleeping, activity, etc.)? Is it consistent or occurring only at certain times?

2. **DIAGNOSIS - What is my diagnosis?**
   - ☐ Can you explain the diagnosis to me in detail?
   - ☐ Is my condition chronic or acute?
   - ☐ If it is chronic, how will it affect my life?
   - ☐ Is my condition one that will be with me constantly or will it come and go?
   - ☐ If it will come and go, how often should I expect it?
   - ☐ Is there anything I can do to help prevent it?
   - ☐ Is my condition contagious? If yes, what should I do?
   - ☐ Is my condition genetic? If yes, what should I do?
   - ☐ How certain are you about this diagnosis?
   - ☐ Do you have any literature about my condition?
   - ☐ Is there a support group available?

3. **TREATMENT - What is the recommended treatment plan?**
   - ☐ Write down a description of the recommended treatment plan.
   - ☐ What results do you expect?
   - ☐ When can I expect to see results?

   If you are discussing surgery:
   - ☐ Give me a step-by-step account of the procedure, including anesthesia and recovery.
   - ☐ Also, consider getting a second opinion.

   If you are discussing a test:
   - ☐ What is the test called and how will it help identify what is wrong?
   - ☐ Will it give us specific or general information?
   - ☐ If the answer is general, where do we go from here?
   - ☐ How accurate and reliable is the test?
   - ☐ Is the test invasive or noninvasive?
   - ☐ What will I have to do to prepare for the test?

- [ ] Where do I go for the test?
- [ ] How and when will I get the test's results?
- [ ] Will more tests be necessary?

(Also see "Questions to Ask About Medications" on page 21.)

4. BENEFITS - What are the benefits of the treatment?

- [ ] What will be the specific benefits if I go ahead with the treatment?
- [ ] To what extent will the treatment improve my condition?
- [ ] Is there documented evidence that the recommended treatment will have a positive outcome?

5. RISKS - What are the potential risks of the treatment?

- [ ] List the possible risks and complications.
- [ ] Do the benefits outweigh the risks or vice versa?
- [ ] Make a list of the risks and benefits, rating each between one and five, to aid in your decision-making process. (One being not as important and five being very important.)

6. SUCCESS - What is the success rate for the treatment?

- [ ] What is the national success rate?
- [ ] What is the success rate at the hospital or medical facility where my treatment is planned?
- [ ] What is your success rate and experience with the surgery?
- [ ] How many procedures are the above success rates based on?
- [ ] Are there any personal factors that will affect my odds either way?
- [ ] How long will the results of my surgery or treatment last?

7. TIMING - When should I begin the treatment?

- [ ] When is the best time to get started with the treatment plan?

- [ ] Do I have to undergo treatment right away?
- [ ] If not, how long can I safely wait?
- [ ] Determine the best time for you to begin the treatment plan.

8. ALTERNATIVES - What are my options?

- [ ] What will happen if I decide to do nothing?
- [ ] What are my other options? (Include nonsurgical and outpatient alternatives if you are discussing surgery.)
- [ ] If you are not satisfied with your options, discuss this with your doctor. If you are still not satisfied, consider consulting another physician.
- [ ] Investigate every option that you are considering as thoroughly as the original treatment plan.

9. COST - How much will the treatment cost?

- [ ] What is the cost of the recommended treatment plan?
- [ ] Check with your insurance company to see what portion will be covered and whether you need to do anything to receive maximum coverage (e.g., seeking a second opinion and getting preauthorization).
- [ ] What related costs do I need to consider (e.g., time off work, child care, transportation, etc.)?

10. DECISION - What do I decide to do?

- [ ] You are now in a better position to make an intelligent, informed decision.
- [ ] Remember, you are ultimately responsible for your body and have the right to choose or refuse treatment.
- [ ] If you feel rushed or otherwise uncomfortable when discussing this information with your doctor, tell him or her how you feel.

Medical Decision Comparison Chart

Use this chart to help you compare different medical options that are available to you.
(Photocopy as needed.)

Diagnosis _____

	OPTION 1	OPTION 2	OPTION 3
Treatment			
Benefits			
Risks			
Success			
Timing			
Alternatives			
Cost			
Decision	Yes ☐ No ☐	Yes ☐ No ☐	Yes ☐ No ☐

WALLET-SIZE CHECKLIST

1. Diagnosis
- ☐ What is my diagnosis?
- ☐ Is my condition chronic or acute?
- ☐ Is my condition one that will be with me constantly?
- ☐ Is there anything I can do to help prevent it?
- ☐ Is my condition contagious or genetic?
- ☐ How certain are you about this diagnosis?

2. Treatment
- ☐ What is the recommended treatment?

If you are discussing medications:
- ☐ What will the medicine do for my particular problem?
- ☐ When, how often and for how long should I take the medicine?
- ☐ How long before the medicine starts working?
- ☐ Will there be side effects?
- ☐ Will there be interactions with other medications I am taking?

If you are discussing a test:
- ☐ What is the test called and how will it help identify the problem?
- ☐ Will it give us specific or general information?
- ☐ Will more tests be necessary?
- ☐ How accurate and reliable is the test?
- ☐ How should I prepare for the test?
- ☐ Where do I go for the test?
- ☐ How and when will I get the test's results?

If you are discussing surgery:
- ☐ Will you give me a step-by-step account of the procedure, including anesthesia and recovery?

3. Benefits vs. Risks
- ☐ What are the benefits if I go ahead with the treatment?
- ☐ What are the possible risks and complications?
- ☐ Do the benefits outweigh the risks or vice versa?

4. Success
- ☐ What is the success rate for the treatment?
- ☐ Are there any personal factors that will affect my odds either way?
- ☐ How long will the results of my treatment last?

5. Timing
- ☐ When is the best time to begin the treatment?
- ☐ When can I expect to see results?

6. Alternatives
- ☐ What will happen if I decide to do nothing?
- ☐ What are my other options?

7. Cost
- ☐ What is the cost of the recommended treatment?
- ☐ What related costs should I consider (e.g., time off work, child care, travel, etc.)?

8. Decision
- ☐ You can now make an informed decision.
- ☐ Remember, you have the right to choose or refuse treatment.
- ☐ If you feel rushed or uncomfortable when talking with your doctor, tell him or her how you feel.

© 1994, American Institute for Preventive Medicine

YOU AND YOUR DENTIST

An overall picture of a healthy person is incomplete if it doesn't include the vital role of proper dental care and good oral hygiene. A family dentist who is knowledgeable and prevention-oriented is a valued part of everyone's health care team.

The Dental Checkup

The following components ensure a proper examination of your mouth by a dentist:
- Visual check of the soft tissues (tongue, cheek, throat and gums) for redness and puffiness or white discoloration
- Check of the bite and jaw joints
- Measurement of any pockets that may have developed between the teeth and the gums. (This is a check for periodontal problems.)
- Full set of X-rays (if they haven't been taken recently)
- Questioning of the patient about any areas of concern

When to Visit Your Dentist

- Every six months for a cleaning and checkup
- If your gums bleed easily or are swollen, reddened or soft
- If you notice a change in your bite
- If you have an injury to a tooth or it is dislodged due to an accident. (It can often be replanted if seen by a dentist immediately.)
- If you have any discomfort from a tooth
- If you have a tendency to grind your teeth, experience pain near the jaw joint or have chronic headaches

Dental Specialties

The American Dental Association recognizes a number of different dental specialties:

Endodontics - Disease prevention and treatment of root pulp (the living tissue that conveys sensation to the tooth)

Oral surgeon (maxillofacial surgeon) - Surgical treatment of jaw and mouth injuries, diseases or tooth extraction

Orthodontics - Correction of mouth deformities or tooth irregularities, often through braces or functional appliances

Pedodontics - Care of children's teeth

Periodontics - Preventive care and treatment of structures that surround and support the teeth (e.g., gums)

Prosthodontics - Rehabilitation of oral problems with such devices as bridges, crowns or dentures

Public health dentistry - Control of dental disease through community dental programs

All of these specialties require at least two additional years of advanced training after dental school.

CHAPTER 8

MENTAL HEALTH

People who are mentally healthy feel good about themselves and comfortable with others. They are also able to deal with the demands, challenges and changes presented in everyday life.

Everyone, regardless of age, race, sex or economic status, is subject to emotional upsets. You can feel down, angry or anxious in response to a variety of things, and such feelings can come and go. When these feelings are disturbing, interfere with daily life and/or linger for weeks or months, they may signal a problem that requires professional assistance. According to the National Institute for Mental Health, at any given time, approximately 40 million Americans (about one in six) experience a mental disorder that interferes with employment and/or daily life.

Mental Health Facts

- About 25 percent of the people who seek medical help for physical problems actually have troubled emotions.
- The most common reasons people seek mental health treatment are for depression and anxiety.
- Between eight and 14 million Americans suffer from depression each year.
- Approximately 80 to 90 percent of all depressed people respond to treatment.
- Approximately 10 percent of Americans have phobias.
- Some 12.5 million Americans are drug abusers or chemically dependent, and 13 million are dependent on alcohol.

- Nearly 25 percent of the elderly who are thought to be senile actually suffer some form of mental illness that can be treated effectively.
- Therapy does not have to take a long time. Nearly half of the people who enter therapy will complete it in seven sessions or less.

It's Smart to Ask for Help

Many people are reluctant to seek mental health services because of the "stigma" of having an "emotional" problem. Society has a tendency to view mental health issues differently from medical ones. When someone breaks a leg, has chest pains or needs to get a prescription, that person will see a doctor. However, when people experience depression, excessive fears or a problem with alcohol, they may be embarrassed to seek help. Many people view these conditions as "weaknesses" that they should be able to handle themselves. Unfortunately, this view keeps them from getting the professional help that can help them deal with and/or solve these problems.

To recognize a problem and receive psychological help is not a sign of weakness at all. Rather, to do so is a sign of strength. Also, taking part in your company's Employee Assistance Program (EAP)—if it has one—or seeing a therapist is completely confidential. No information will be released to anyone without your permission.

Reasons to Seek Help

The following symptoms usually signal the need for professional help. Only a trained professional can diagnose and determine the treatment needed:

- Thinking or talking about suicide
- Seeing or hearing things that aren't actually present
- Suspiciousness or paranoia
- Strange or grandiose ideas
- Crippling or excessive anxieties (phobias or fears)
- Wide mood swings (extreme highs and lows)
- Prolonged depression and apathy (a sense of hopelessness, loss of pleasure in life, confusion or constant frustration)
- Marked personality change
- Compulsive behaviors (e.g., overspending, overeating, excessive exercising)
- Marked changes in eating or sleeping patterns
- Excessive anger or hostility; destructive, abusive or violent behavior
- Problems with the law
- Difficulty with authority
- Abuse of alcohol and/or other drugs
- Difficulty interacting with other people (spouse, parents, children, co-workers and friends)
- Denial of obvious problems; strong resistance to receiving help
- Social withdrawal and isolation
- Inability to cope with the loss of a loved one
- Extreme jealousy
- Preoccupation with physical illness
- Overall decline in job performance
- Problems on the job
- A feeling that you've lost control of your life
- Inability to cope with problems or daily activities such as school, job or personal needs
- Sexual problems

Common Mental Health Conditions

Anxiety disorder - Characterized by unrealistic or excessive worry about any real or imagined life circumstances (e.g., finances, social performance). Persons experiencing anxiety may have rapid pulse and/or breathing rate, racing or pounding heart, dry mouth, sweating, trembling, shaking, shortness of breath, faintness, tension or stomach problems.

Critical incident stress syndrome - Psychological symptoms and/or physical conditions caused by a specific traumatic event. Examples include workplace traumas such as threatened or actual acts of violence and injury or death. It is similar to post-traumatic stress syndrome where people who have experienced a critical event often suffer from acute anxiety, depression and feeling out of control. They may also have nightmares and/or flashbacks of the event.

Dependent personality - Characterized by dependent and submissive behavior. This person has difficulty making decisions without a tremendous amount of advice from others. Persons with dependent personalities will even allow others to make important decisions for them and are overly concerned with other people liking them.

Depression - A condition marked by sadness, hopelessness, helplessness, pessimism and a loss of interest in life. Symptoms of depression include long-lasting crying spells, fatigue, loss of interest or pleasure in ordinary activities (including sex), changes in eating and sleeping patterns, lack of concentration, and thoughts of suicide or death.

Hypochondria - A condition characterized by a preoccupation with one's health. People with hypochondria falsely believe they have some disease even though physical examinations show otherwise.

Hysterical personality - A common feature of this disorder is a consistent pattern of being excessively emotional as a means of obtaining attention. Hysterics constantly look for reassurance and approval from others and do not feel comfortable in situations where they are not the center of attention.

Jealousy - Normal jealousy is usually a harmless condition in which people feel someone or something they like or love might be taken away by another person. Excessive jealousy, however, is an intense, mentally painful condition that causes the sufferer to become suspicious and always be on the lookout for signs that he or she is losing a desired person or object. These people become obsessed with their fears and often cannot concentrate on anything else.

Manic-depression - A mental illness characterized by mood swings from elation and/or euphoria to severe depression. Extreme irritability is common during the euphoria phase of the disease. A phase can last anywhere from several days to several months before another mood swing. It usually occurs before the age of 35 and affects 1 percent of the population at some time in their lives.

Narcissistic personality - This disorder is characterized by an excessive sense of self-importance. Narcissists exaggerate their accomplishments and abilities and expect to be viewed as special even if their achievements do not warrant it.

Obsessive-compulsive disorder - An anxiety disorder where the sufferer has persistent, involuntary thoughts or images (obsessions) and engages in ritualistic acts (e.g., washing his or her hands) according to certain self-imposed rules (compulsions).

Panic attack - A brief period of acute anxiety that can occur without warning. Symptoms include shortness of breath, chest discomfort, heart palpitations, sweating and choking.

Paranoid personality - A pattern of thinking and behaving characterized by suspiciousness, mistrust of others and over-sensitivity. People experiencing this make an effort to find evidence that confirms their prejudices or attitudes.

Passive-aggressive personality - Describes people who are both passive and aggressive at the same time. They express their hostility in indirect and nonviolent ways such as procrastinating, forgetfulness, habitual tardiness and lying. They resent anyone making demands of them and, through their aggravating behavior, make sure they do not comply with these demands.

Phobia - An anxiety disorder in which the individual feels terror, dread or panic when faced with a feared object, situation or activity. Examples include simple phobias such as a fear of snakes; social phobias such as the fear of speaking in front of other people; and complex phobias such as agoraphobia, which is the fear of being in places or situations where escape might be difficult or embarrassing.

Post-traumatic stress disorder - A condition where a person reexperiences a traumatic past event like a wartime situation, hostage-taking or rape. Symptoms include nightmares, flashbacks of the event, excessive alertness and emotional numbness to people and activities.

Schizophrenia - A group of mental disorders in which there are severe disturbances in thinking, mood and behavior. The sufferer experiences delusions, hallucinations, disordered thinking and/or inappropriate emotions.

Substance abuse - Uncontrollable misuse of drugs (both legal and illegal) and/or alcohol on a regular basis even though doing so interferes with daily life.

CHAPTER 9

STAYING WELL

A new interest is taking hold today: the interest people have in making themselves healthy. In greater numbers than ever before, the American public wants to do those things that will promote health and increase longevity. Exercise salons are booming, health foods are readily accessible, cigarette smoking is the exception and not the rule, and joggers and walkers are all around. We have come a long way from Mark Twain's philosophy that "the only way to keep your health is to eat what you don't want, drink what you don't like and do what you'd rather not."

It's encouraging to see people's desire to make their lifestyles the best they can be. The emphasis is also shifting from traditional medicine, which is designed to treat illness, to doing those things that prevent sickness from occurring in the first place.

The public wants to become better health consumers as well. We recognize warning signs. We read labels. We know when a doctor is or is not needed. We are opening our eyes to the risk factors for conditions such as heart disease, diabetes and cancer.

This chapter deals with eight topics that are important to good health as well as to prevention of disease.

Cigarette Smoking: Packing It In

It is not easy to quit smoking cigarettes. This is because smoking involves both physical and psychological components. Nicotine is a physically addictive substance. After an initial rejec-

tion by the body, a tolerance level develops in the smoker and withdrawal symptoms occur when nicotine is withheld. Cigarettes also produce a psychological dependence. The desire to smoke is triggered by certain situations, emotions and a need to inhale and exhale something.

Smoking Facts

- Cigarette smoking is our nation's number one preventable cause of illness and premature death. Over 440,000 people in the U.S. die from the effects of smoking each year.
- After inhaling, 70 to 90 percent of the chemical compounds in a cigarette stay in the smoker's lungs.
- Cigarette smokers are 15 times more likely to get lung cancer, 16 times more likely to have emphysema, 10 times more likely to have bronchitis and twice as likely to have a heart attack than nonsmokers.
- Nonsmokers who inhale secondhand smoke from a burning cigarette have an increased risk of lung cancer and heart disease as well.
- Pregnant women who smoke are cutting off oxygen to their developing fetus as well as altering the blood pressure and heart rate of the baby. Low-birth-weight babies, spontaneous abortions and stillbirths are more prevalent in smokers.
- Medical research has found that each cigarette smoked takes 15 minutes off a person's life, on average.
- Children of smokers have twice the incidence of respiratory ailments as the children of nonsmokers.
- According to the American Cancer Society, eight out of 10 smokers would like to quit.

The "Warm Pheasant" Plan to Quit Smoking

You've heard of quitting cigarettes "cold turkey"—all at once, in an unflinching moment of resolution. Well, that works for some, but not all smokers. In fact, there are as many ways to quit smoking as there are brands of cigarettes for sale. If you're like Mark Twain who said, "Quitting smoking is easy. I've done it over 100 times," you might want to try the "warm pheasant" method. Unlike the cold-turkey approach, this three-phase plan allows you to continue to smoke while you prepare to quit, psychologically and physically.

Phase I: Preparing to Quit

This phase takes approximately one week:
- Mark a "quit" date on your calendar one week in advance.
- Keep track of each cigarette you smoke by making a slash mark on a piece of paper tucked in the wrapper of your cigarette pack.
- Every time you have an urge to light up, wait 10 minutes.
- Collect your cigarette butts in a "butt bottle." (The mere sight of so many spent cigarettes will graphically demonstrate just how much you really smoke in a week.)

Phase II: Quitting

This phase takes approximately one to two weeks:
- Throw away all your cigarettes and hide all smoking paraphernalia like matches, lighters and ashtrays.
- Whenever you have an urge to smoke, take a deep breath through your mouth and slowly exhale through pursed lips. Repeat five to 10 times.
- Change your routine to eliminate familiar smoking cues. If you always light up when driving to work, take a different route. Or substitute a walk for your usual coffee-and-cigarette break. Or sit in a chair you don't customarily use when relaxing or watching television at home.
- Take up activities you don't normally associate with smoking. Enroll in a cooking class, visit a nonsmoking friend or go swimming at your local YMCA or YWCA, for example.
- Keep your hands busy by holding something such as a pen, Nerf Ball or rubber band.
- In place of cigarettes, substitute other things that will provide oral gratification (e.g., sugarless gum or mints, toothpicks or coffee stirrers).
- Avoid drinking coffee and alcohol or eating foods high in sugar such as candy and pastries. They cause biochemical changes in the body that increase your desire for a cigarette.
- Create a piggy bank. Put the money you used to spend on cigarettes in a jar and watch it add up.
- Place a rubber band on your wrist and snap it every time you get an urge to smoke.

Phase III: Staying off Cigarettes

Allow three months for this final phase:
- Always remember that the craving to smoke will pass, whether you smoke or not.
- Renew your commitment to stay off cigarettes each day.
- Beware of saboteurs, usually other smokers, who may try to encourage you to light up. Assert your right to not smoke.
- Talk to a nonsmoking buddy for support.
- Make a list of good things you've noticed since you quit (e.g., food tastes better, you cough less and your clothes don't smell bad).
- Continue to practice the behavior modification techniques listed in the quitting phase.

Source: The Smokeless Program, developed by the American Institute for Preventive Medicine, Farmington Hills, Michigan, 1994.

Stress: Learning to Cope

Do you know what stress is?
- Stress is the body's nonspecific response to any increased demand placed upon it.
- Stressors are those events, objects or thoughts that will cause the stress response to occur.

Keeping Track of Stress Signals

Many of us have symptoms of stress every day without realizing it. To recognize the signals your body is sending you, read over this partial list of stress symptoms. Make a mental note or place a check next to those symptoms that you've experienced when under stress. Place two checks by symptoms you experience frequently. Write in any other symptoms you experience when feeling stressed. (Symptoms of stress could indicate a physical problem and should be checked out before assuming you are simply not coping well.)

Symptoms of Stress

- Nervous tic
- Clearing throat
- Clenching hands
- Gritting teeth
- Feeling lonely
- Queasy stomach
- Vomiting
- Diarrhea
- Headache
- Backache
- Neck ache
- Hives
- Constipation
- Depression
- Rash

- Jittery feelings
- Rapid heartbeat
- Sweating
- Sexual difficulties
- Dry mouth and throat
- Irritability
- Emotional instability
- Inability to concentrate
- Accident proneness
- Stuttering
- Insomnia
- Forgetfulness
- Frequent urination
- Nightmares
- Negative thoughts

- Pacing
- Foot tapping
- Overeating
- Smoking
- Drinking
- Feeling fearful
- Crying
- Fatigue

- Faintness or dizziness
- Lack of interest
- Low energy level
- Temper outbursts
- _____
- _____
- _____
- _____

Conditions Related to Stress

Research has revealed a clear link between physical illness and stress. In some cases, stress plays an important part in the nature and severity of illness. In fact, the American Academy of Family Physicians states that approximately two-thirds of all visits to the family doctor are for stress-related disorders. Read the following list. Make additions to the list if you feel that stress contributes to a condition not listed.

Conditions Associated With or Made Worse by Stress

- Acne
- Alcoholism
- Allergies
- Arthritis
- Asthma
- Backaches
- Cancer
- Colitis
- Common cold
- Coronary heart disease
- Eating disorders
- Eczema
- Gout
- Headaches
- High blood pressure
- Insomnia

- Intestinal disorders
- Low back pain
- Lowering of the body's immune system
- Nervous breakdown
- Neurosis
- Premenstrual syndrome (PMS)
- Stroke
- Temporomandibular joint syndrome (TMJ)
- Ulcers
- _____
- _____
- _____
- _____
- _____
- _____

Life Events Questionnaire

Is there a connection between the number of major life events a person experiences in a year and the likelihood of illness? Drs. Thomas Holmes and Richard Rahe think so. They reached this conclusion after questioning 7,000 people about the number of life events they went through in one year. The people who scored highest on this questionnaire experienced the highest amount of physical illness in the year following the test. Since major life changes can produce stress-induced illness, take a look at how the past year's life events add up for you.

Instructions: Place a check in the column labeled "Happened" for those events that occurred in the past 12 months. Then record your score with the event value for each. Total the score for each column, then add those numbers to get a grand total.

Event Rank	Event Value	Hap-pened	Your Score	Life Event	Event Rank	Event Value	Hap-pened	Your Score	Life Event
1	100	___	___	Death of a spouse	24	29	___	___	Trouble with in-laws
2	73	___	___	Divorce	25	28	___	___	Outstanding personal achievement
3	65	___	___	Marital separation					
4	63	___	___	Jail term	26	26	___	___	Spouse begins or stops work
5	63	___	___	Death of close family member	27	26	___	___	Begin or end of school
6	53	___	___	Personal injury or illness	28	25	___	___	Change in living conditions
7	50	___	___	Marriage	29	24	___	___	Revision of personal habits
8	47	___	___	Fired from job	30	23	___	___	Trouble with boss
9	45	___	___	Marital reconciliation	31	20	___	___	Change in work hours or conditions
10	45	___	___	Retirement					
11	44	___	___	Change in health of family member	32	20	___	___	Change in residence
					33	20	___	___	Change in schools
12	40	___	___	Pregnancy	34	19	___	___	Change in recreation
13	39	___	___	Sexual difficulties	35	19	___	___	Change in church activities
14	39	___	___	Gain of new family member	36	18	___	___	Change in social activities
15	39	___	___	Business readjustment	37	17	___	___	Mortgage or loan less than $50,000*
16	39	___	___	Change in financial state					
17	37	___	___	Death of close friend	38	16	___	___	Change in sleeping habits
18	36	___	___	Change in line of work	39	15	___	___	Change in number of family get-togethers
19	35	___	___	Change in number of arguments with spouse					
					40	15	___	___	Change in eating habits
20	31	___	___	Mortgage over $50,000*	41	13	___	___	Vacation
21	30	___	___	Foreclosure of mortgage/loan	42	12	___	___	Christmas
					43	11	___	___	Minor violations of the law
22	29	___	___	Change in duties at work				___	**TOTAL COLUMN 2**
23	29	___	___	Son or daughter leaving home				+ ___	**TOTAL COLUMN 1**
		___		**TOTAL COLUMN 1**				= ___	**GRAND TOTAL**

* The financial amount was increased by $40,000 from the original Life Events Questionnaire to reflect current economic conditions.

Scoring

- People who score less than 199 have a very mild risk.
- People who score 200 to 299 have a more moderate risk of developing physical illness in the next 12 months.
- People who score 300 or more have a strong risk of developing physical illness in the next 12 months.

(These scores represent only a likelihood of getting sick and not a definite prediction.)

Tips for Stress Management

- Maintain a regular program of healthy eating, good health habits and adequate sleep.
- Exercise regularly. This promotes physical fitness and emotional well-being.
- Don't let your emotions get "bottled up" inside. Share your feelings with others.
- Learn to manage your time efficiently.
- Avoid unnecessary arguments or quarrels.
- Do a "stress rehearsal." Prepare for stressful events by imagining yourself feeling calm and handling the situation well.
- Minimize your exposure to things that cause distress.
- Practice a relaxation technique daily.
- Several times a day do a "body check" for tensed muscles and let them relax.
- Do deep-breathing exercises.
- Be a Good Samaritan. Spend time helping others.
- Balance work and play.
- Plan some "me time" daily.
- Engage in activities you enjoy and look forward to.
- Discover the "elf" in yourself. Learn to have fun.
- He who laughs, lasts. Improve your laugh life.
- Participate in activities with people who share your interests.
- Reward yourself with little things that make you feel good.
- Challenge yourself to do something new.
- Surround yourself with cheery people. Avoid stress carriers.
- Shun the "superman" or "superwoman" syndrome. No one is perfect.
- Set realistic goals for yourself.
- Be flexible in dealing with people and events. Avoid "psychosclerosis," a hardening of the *attitudes*.
- Accept the things you cannot change in yourself or others.
- Forgive yourself for mistakes.
- Take satisfaction in your accomplishments. Don't dwell on your shortcomings.
- Develop and maintain a positive attitude. View changes as positive challenges, opportunities or blessings.
- Seek professional help if needed.

Fitness: Get Fit, Stay Fit

Physical fitness has many benefits:

- Stress, boredom and depression are minimized as exercise seems to take the edge off daily tension.
- Skin tone is improved through fitness.
- When our bodies demand more oxygen (e.g., in climbing stairs), it's no problem.
- Muscle tone is revitalized; strength, endurance and even posture can improve.
- Fitness allows your heart to function with less strain placed upon it.
- Our self-esteem tends to improve as we see good things in the mirror.
- Blood circulation gets better and better.
- We sleep better.
- Our appetite for food is more manageable and our digestive process works better.
- Greater flexibility and ease are experienced in the joints.
- Physical exercise increases the number of calories that are burned. In fact, calories are burned at a 15-percent-higher rate for up to six hours after activity.

Beginning an Exercise Program

There are some basic points to keep in mind when beginning an exercise program:

- Before beginning strenuous exercise, it is advisable that you consult your physician, particularly if you have been inactive for an extended period of time, are substantially overweight, are over 35 years of age and/or have a medical problem.
- Choose an activity plan that is right for you. Take into consideration where it will be done, what equipment is needed, whether it will be done with others, if it can be done in bad weather, what the cost is and, most important, whether you will enjoy it.
- Ease into your exercise program. Start off with activities of low intensity, frequency and duration, then build up your pace over the next several weeks. A good rule to follow is that if you can't talk while exercising, you're overdoing it.
- Do warm-up exercises before the activity. Loosen up your muscles by stretching and/or walking for five minutes. When the activity is done, cool down with five more minutes of walking and/or stretching.
- Select an appropriate time and place to do your exercise. Get into a routine in which the activity is done at the same time each day. Wait at least two hours after eating before doing a strenuous activity. If you exercise before a meal, wait about 25 minutes before you eat.
- For good results you should exercise at least three times a week for at least 20 minutes each session.
- Be in tune with your body while exercising. If muscles or joints start to hurt, ease up. It is usually not necessary to stop all activity for minor soreness. Be aware of the warning signs of serious health problems.
- Don't overdress. Not only is there no benefit to excessive sweating, but it can even be dangerous.
- Read about fitness and exercise.

- Talk to a person who practices good fitness habits.
- The first step is the hardest, but also the most important.

Four Popular Physical Activities to Consider

Bicycling - Bicycling is a good exercise to do with others and is a method of transportation as well. It provides wonderful conditioning for the legs and can improve cardiovascular fitness. Safety precautions are important when bicycling outdoors, so make sure you wear a bicycle helmet. To improve cardiovascular fitness, cycling should be done at least three times a week for 40 to 60 minutes each time. A stationary bicycle that has a resistance adjuster is good for regular exercise. It's certainly convenient since you can read or watch TV while you pedal away, and the weather doesn't interfere with your exercising.

Jogging - Jogging is an excellent fitness activity for improving your overall fitness level. With proper progression and little difficulty, people who are unaccustomed to exercise can advance from being walkers and walk-joggers ("woggers") to joggers. Correct posture, pace, number of times per week and proper attire are all factors in its effectiveness.

Swimming - Swimming has long been a popular exercise form with people who suffer from orthopedic problems or obesity because it reduces pressure on the musculoskeletal system. Swimming can produce relaxation and sound sleep patterns. Compared to jogging, 100 yards of swimming is roughly equivalent to 400 yards of jogging.

Walking - Walking is the most popular form of physical activity. If done on a regular basis, walking can not only help you to lose weight, but will relax you as well. There are some other advantages to walking: It can be done anywhere and anytime; it's free; you already know how to do it; and it can be done by almost anyone. Body posture is important to make your walking as efficient as possible. Keep these pointers in mind when walking:

- Hold your head erect.
- Keep your back straight.
- Point your toes straight ahead.
- Keep your abdomen flat.
- Swing your arms loosely at your sides.
- Land on your heel and roll forward off the ball of your foot.
- Wear shoes that are cushioned and provide support.
- If you become breathless, you're walking too fast.
- Don't compete with others—you're not in a race.
- Make your walk a pleasant experience.

Nutrition: Eating for Life

Eating right plays a pivotal role in good health and in disease prevention. The foods you choose can help lower your risk for heart disease, stroke, diabetes, osteoporosis and certain cancers. Do yourself a favor: Eat well to feel well and be well.

The Dietary Guidelines for Americans

The Dietary Guidelines for Americans, formulated by the Department of Agriculture and the Department of Health and Human Services, cover the most up-to-date advice from nutrition scientists and are the basis of federal nutrition policy. They suggest that you:

- Eat a variety of foods to get the energy, protein, vitamins, minerals and fiber you need for good health.
- Maintain healthy weight to reduce your chances of having high blood pressure, heart disease, stroke, certain cancers and the most common kind of diabetes.

- Choose a diet low in fat, saturated fat and cholesterol to reduce your risk of heart attack and certain types of cancer. Because fat contains over twice the calories of an equal amount of carbohydrates or protein, a diet low in fat can help you maintain a healthy weight.
- Choose a diet with plenty of vegetables, fruits and grain products, which provide needed vitamins, minerals, fiber and complex carbohydrates, and which can help you lower your intake of fat.
- Use sugars only in moderation. A diet with lots of sugars has too many calories and too few nutrients for most people and can contribute to tooth decay.
- Use salt and sodium only in moderation to help reduce your risk of high blood pressure.
- If you drink alcoholic beverages, do so in moderation. Alcoholic beverages supply calories, but little or no nutrients. Drinking alcohol is also the cause of many health problems and accidents and can lead to addiction.

What is the Food Guide Pyramid?

An easy way to follow the Dietary Guidelines for Americans is to choose foods daily using the Food Guide Pyramid. The pyramids of Egypt have withstood the passage of time. Likewise, the Food Guide Pyramid can be used throughout a lifetime as a good foundation of what Americans should eat every day. It is not a rigid prescription, but instead is a general guide that lets you choose a healthy diet right for you and members of your family.

The pyramid calls for eating a variety of foods from each group to get the nutrients you need. At the same time, you can adjust the number of servings you eat from each group to get the right amount of calories (and grams of fat) you need to lose or gain weight or maintain a healthy weight.

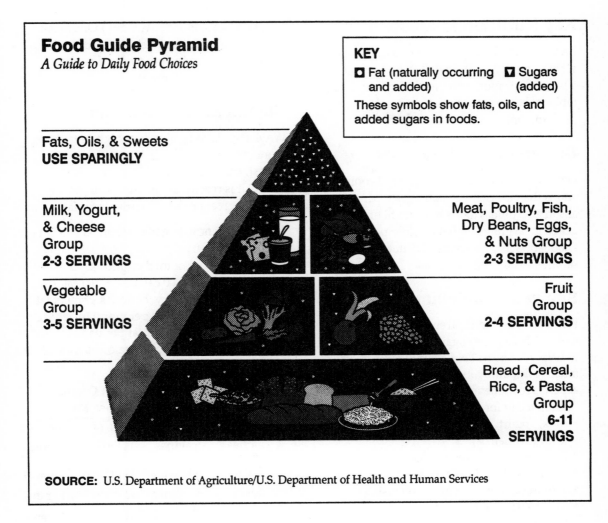

Food Guide Pyramid
A Guide to Daily Food Choices

KEY
◻ Fat (naturally occurring ▼ Sugars
and added) (added)
These symbols show fats, oils, and
added sugars in foods.

Fats, Oils, & Sweets
USE SPARINGLY

Milk, Yogurt,
& Cheese
Group
2-3 SERVINGS

Meat, Poultry, Fish,
Dry Beans, Eggs,
& Nuts Group
2-3 SERVINGS

Vegetable
Group
3-5 SERVINGS

Fruit
Group
2-4 SERVINGS

Bread, Cereal,
Rice, & Pasta
Group
**6-11
SERVINGS**

SOURCE: U.S. Department of Agriculture/U.S. Department of Health and Human Services

What Counts As a Serving?

- Bread, Cereal, Rice and Pasta
  - 1 slice of bread
  - 1 ounce of ready-to-eat cereal
  - ½ cup of cooked cereal, rice or pasta

- Vegetable
  - 1 cup of leafy, raw vegetables
  - ½ cup of other vegetables
  - ¾ cup of vegetable juice

- Fruit
  - 1 medium apple, banana or orange
  - ½ cup of chopped, cooked or canned fruit
  - ¾ cup of fruit juice

- Milk, Yogurt and Cheese
  - 1 cup of milk or yogurt
  - 1½ ounces of natural cheese
  - 2 ounces of processed cheese

- Meat, Poultry, Fish, Dry Beans,
  Eggs and Nuts
  - 2 to 3 ounces of cooked, lean meat,
    poultry or fish
  - ½ cup of cooked dry beans, 1 egg, or
    2 tablespoons of peanut butter
    (Each counts as 1 ounce of lean meat.)

Key Nutrition Issues

Balance is the key. Know what to say yes to, what to moderate and what to go easy on. Say yes to five or more servings of fruits and vegetables a day to get vitamins, minerals, dietary fiber and anticancer substances.

Say yes to dietary fiber

Dietary fiber comes from plant foods only and is the part that goes undigested and unabsorbed. Animal foods have no fiber. Aim to get 20 to 35 grams of dietary fiber per day. Food labels list the grams of dietary fiber per serving. Read them.

Say yes to calcium

Why? It is needed to strengthen bones and teeth, to help guard against osteoporosis and to help your heart beat, your blood clot, your muscles flex and your nerves react. Health experts recommend 800 to 1,500 milligrams of calcium a day for adults. Good food sources are:
- Milk, yogurt, cheese (Choose nonfat and low-fat varieties.)
- Broccoli, collard greens, kale, spinach
- Legumes, dried beans, peas
- Tofu (if calcium is used in processing)
- Salmon, sardines (with bones)
- Calcium-fortified juices, cereals, breads, etc.

Use sugar, salt, sodium and alcohol in moderation

- **Sugar** - Many foods that contain large amounts supply calories, are limited in nutrients and can contribute to tooth decay.
- **Salt and Sodium** - Most Americans eat more salt and sodium than they need. (Salt contains 40 percent sodium, 60 percent chloride.) The recommended amount of sodium is between 2,400 and 3,000 milligrams per day.
- **Alcohol** - Moderate use means no more than one to two drinks per day: one per day for women, two per day for men. (Women who are trying to conceive or are pregnant should not drink alcoholic beverages.) One drink equals 12 ounces regular beer, four to five ounces wine, one-and-one-half ounces distilled spirits (80 proof).

Say no to too much fat

Why? Populations with diets high in fat have more obesity and certain types of cancer (breast, colon, prostate). How much is too much? It is recommended that you get less than 30 percent of total calories from fat.

To figure out how to get less than 30 percent of calories from fat:
- Take 30 percent of total calories. Example: .30 x 1,200 calories = 360 calories.
- Divide the answer by 9 calories/gram of fat (fat contains 9 calories per gram) to get the upper limit of grams of fat per day. Example: 360 calories ÷ 9 calories/gram of fat = 40 grams of fat.

For this many calories	Maximum Grams of Fat per Day		
	30% of calories	25% of calories	20% of calories
1,200	40 grams	34 grams	28 grams
1,500	50 grams	42 grams	34 grams
1,800	60 grams	50 grams	40 grams
2,000	67 grams	56 grams	44 grams

Read food labels to find out how many grams of fat one serving of a food item contains.

Say no to saturated fat

Why? More than anything else in the diet, saturated fat raises blood cholesterol. Saturated fats are generally solid at room temperature. Examples of foods that are high in saturated fat:
- Coconut oil
- Palm oil
- Animal fats
- Dairy foods with fats
- Cocoa butter

About cholesterol

Cholesterol is an odorless, white, waxy substance manufactured only by animals. It is present in every cell in all parts of the body, including the brain and nervous system, muscle, skin, liver, intestines, heart and skeleton.

There are two sources of cholesterol: The cholesterol manufactured by the body, mainly in the liver, and dietary cholesterol found in the animal foods that we eat. Examples of foods with cholesterol are:
- Organ meats, such as liver and kidneys
- Eggs yolks
- Meats, poultry and fish
- Fats in dairy products

Plant foods have no cholesterol.

In excess, dietary cholesterol can contribute to hardening of the arteries. It is recommended that we do not eat more than 300 milligrams of dietary cholesterol per day.

Measuring Blood Cholesterol

Your blood cholesterol can be measured using a blood sample taken from your finger or your arm. The federal government has established the following guidelines for individuals:

Total cholesterol level
Less than 200 mg/dl . . . . Desirable
200-239 mg/dl . . . . Borderline High
More than 240 mg/dl . . . . High

A fasting blood test is not needed to measure total blood cholesterol. Your doctor will probably order a fasting blood test, however, if your total blood cholesterol is elevated. A fasting blood test will reveal a more complete "cholesterol profile." It will give measurements of types of lipoproteins—"packages" in which cholesterol travels in the blood. Two lipoproteins of interest are:

Low-density lipoproteins (LDL), which
carry most of the cholesterol in the blood. LDLs deposit cholesterol in the artery walls and are often referred to as "bad cholesterol."

High-density lipoproteins (HDL), which contain a small amount of cholesterol. HDLs help remove cholesterol from the blood and, therefore, are called "good cholesterol."

LDL and HDL cholesterol levels give a better picture of your risk for coronary heart disease than your total cholesterol level alone. A *high* LDL-cholesterol level and/or *low* HDL-cholesterol level increases your risk. The following guidelines are used today:

LDL cholesterol
Less than 130 mg/dl . . . . Desirable
130-159 mg/dl . . . . Borderline High
More than 160 mg/dl . . . . High

HDL cholesterol
Less than 35 mg/dl . . . . High Risk
More than 55 mg/dl . . . . Low Risk

Note: LDLs and HDLs are not found in foods.

Some health experts use a ratio of total cholesterol divided by HDL to determine risk for heart disease.

Total cholesterol/HDL (ratio)
More than 6.0 . . . . High Risk
Less than 4.0 . . . . Low Risk

About triglycerides

Triglycerides are fat-like substances carried through the bloodstream to the tissues. The bulk of the body's fat tissue is in the form of triglycerides, stored for later use as energy. We get triglycerides from the fat in our foods, both animal and plant sources. Normal fasting blood triglyceride levels range from 40 to 160 mg/dl. They are considered elevated if fasting levels are over 250 mg/dl. To lower elevated triglycerides, do the following:
- Lose weight if you are overweight.
- Eat a low-fat diet.
- Limit alcohol.
- Limit sugar and foods with sugar.
- Exercise regularly.

In addition to dietary measures, some people may need medicine to help lower cholesterol and/or triglycerides. Check with your health care professional.

Weight Control: "Chewsing" Well

Millions of Americans are caught up in the daily struggle to shed unwanted pounds. The link between obesity and such medical conditions as diabetes, high blood pressure and heart disease has been well-established. These threats to our health, however, don't always provide the incentives we need to change.

Only a small percentage of Americans who try to lose weight seem to keep it off—in part because it is not easy to change old habits. Liquid potions, diet pills, powders, crash or fad diets do not prove successful over the long run and can even be harmful.

The three key ingredients for successful weight loss are:
- Regular, physical activity
- Reduction of caloric intake, especially from fat
- Modification of eating and exercise behaviors

What should you do?

- Set up a regular exercise program.
- Follow the federal Dietary Guidelines for Americans (see page 42).
- Use the Food Guide Pyramid (see page 43), but opt for choices in each level that are low in fat.

- **FATS, OILS, SWEETS GROUP**
  - *LOW IN FAT*: Light mayonnaise and margarines, nonfat and low-fat salad dressing
  - *AVOID*: Butter, lard, stick margarine, coconut oil and palm oil. Use liquid vegetable oils in small amounts.

- **MILK, YOGURT, CHEESE GROUP**
  - *LOW IN FAT*: Skim, ½% milk, plain nonfat yogurt, part skim and nonfat cheeses (2 to 3 grams of fat or less per ounce)
  - *LIMIT*: Whole milk, 2% milk, regular cheese, (cheddar, Swiss, American), ice cream, whole-milk yogurt, cream cheese, sour cream, yogurt with fruit preserves

- **MEAT, POULTRY, FISH, DRY BEANS, NUTS, EGG GROUP**
  - *LOW IN FAT*: Lean meats, poultry (remove skin before eating), egg white (3 to 4 regular eggs/week), any fresh, frozen fish (not fried), tuna in water, dry beans, peas, legumes
  - *LIMIT*: Fatty meats and luncheon meats (like bologna), hot dogs (turkey or meat), sausage, nuts and peanut butter

- **VEGETABLE GROUP**
  - *LOW IN FAT*: Any fresh, frozen (plain) vegetables, raw vegetable salads
  - *LIMIT*: Vegetables prepared in cream, butter, or cheese sauce, creamy vegetable salads such as potato salad, cole slaw

- **FRUIT GROUP**
  - *LOW IN FAT*: Fresh, frozen or canned fruits (in their own juice or water)
  - *LIMIT*: Avocado (¼ of 1 avocado has around 9 grams of fat)

- **BREAD, CEREAL, RICE, PASTA GROUP**
  - *LOW IN FAT*: Bread, rolls, English muffins, whole grain breads preferred over white-enriched, unsweetened or low-sugar ready-to-eat cereals (Shredded wheat, Cheerios, Grape Nuts, Total, Wheaties, etc.), hot cereals (oatmeal, cream of wheat, rice, etc.), bulgur, plain pasta, rice, couscous, low-fat crackers, popcorn (no salt)
  - *LIMIT*: Croissants, doughnuts, coffee cakes, danish, pies, cookies, granola bars and cereal, cheese and high-fat crackers

---

- **COMBINATION FOODS**
  - *LOW IN FAT*: Stir-fried vegetables and rice or pasta, with small amounts of lean meats, sandwiches with lean meats (turkey, ham, chicken, tuna), small hamburgers, garden salads with nonfat or small amounts of low-fat dressing, de-fatted soups, stews with greater proportion of vegetables, beans, pasta or rice than meat, burritos, spaghetti, lasagna, etc., (use less meat and cheese), pizza with mostly vegetables, less cheese, no fatty meats
  - *LIMIT*: Fried meat and fish sandwiches, large double-decker hamburgers and cheeseburgers, taco salad, hot dogs, nachos with cheese, pizza with double cheese and high-fat meats like pepperoni and sausage

Follow Behavior Modification Techniques for Weight Control

Use these suggestions to change the way you eat:

- Eating pace
  - Eat slowly. Chances are you will eat less.
  - Chew and swallow each bite thoroughly before beginning another.
  - Take sips of water between bites.

- Eating mood
  - Make a point to eat only when relaxed. (Many people eat to reduce tension.)
  - Instead of thinking of "not eating," think of showing respect for your body by refusing to overeat.
  - Concentrate on feelings of being bloated or stuffed before you overeat. Be aware of these negative physical sensations. This will help you limit your food intake.

- Eating out
  - Choose restaurants where a variety of low-fat foods are available. Decide what you'll eat ahead of time.
  - Don't starve yourself all day prior to dining out.
  - Avoid "all-you-can-eat" restaurants.
  - Consider ordering "a la carte" or "half orders" to keep portions small.

- Eating with others
  - Beware of "saboteurs" who try to undermine your weight-loss efforts. They may feel threatened by your success.
  - Tell others about your long-term weight-loss goals.
  - Meet friends for a walk instead of lunch.

- Self rewards
  - Spend some time imagining yourself at your healthy body weight. Visualize in detail how you look, feel and think as the healthier you.
  - Give yourself positive reinforcement each day you follow your eating plan. Choose something that's a little special (e.g., a stroll in the park, a long-distance call, some "me time").

- Keep saying positive self-statements to yourself. Say "I am in control" or "I choose to respect myself." This will go a long way when you find yourself wanting to eat at inappropriate times.

- Miscellaneous techniques
  - Know the difference between appetite and hunger. Appetite is a psychological desire for food, while hunger is a true physical need for it.
  - Use smaller-sized plates for meals.
  - To avoid impulse buying at the grocery store, shop only from a well-planned list and never shop when hungry.
  - Help eliminate your desire for food by yelling "stop!"
  - Plan your snacks in advance.
  - Put on tight clothes if you feel a desire to binge.
  - Don't eat just because others do. Wait until you are really hungry.
  - Above all, maintain a positive attitude. Commit to being a positive thinker. Focus on what you can do and what rewards come from eating well and exercising. They will result in improved health, a better mental attitude, more energy, improved appearance and performance and more.

Alcohol: Use Without Abuse

The effects of alcohol vary from person to person. The following factors influence the intoxicating properties of alcohol:

- Amount of food already in the stomach
- Body weight
- Presence of other drugs already in the system
- Pace that drinks are consumed
- Mental and emotional condition
- Individual level of tolerance

The Effects of Alcohol

There is a relationship between the blood-alcohol concentration in your system and how you are affected by it. The chart that follows describes what you can expect as more and more alcohol is consumed.

Amount of Distilled Spirit Consumed in 2 hours (ounces)	Alcohol in Blood (percent)	Typical Effects (vary per individual)
3	0.05	Loosening of judgment, thought and restraint; release of tension; carefree sensation
4.5	0.08	Tensions and inhibitions of everyday life lessened
6	0.10	Voluntary motor action affected; awkward hand and arm movements; walk and speech clumsy
10	0.20	Severe impairment, staggering, loud, incoherent, emotionally unstable, very drunk; 100 times greater risk of traffic accident
14	0.30	Deeper areas of brain affected; parts affecting stimulus response and understanding confused, stuporous
18	0.40	Asleep, difficult to arouse, incapable of voluntary action, equivalent of surgical anesthesia
22	0.50	Coma, anesthesia of centers controlling breathing and heartbeat; death

Know Your Limit [1]

Body Weight (in lbs.)	# of Drinks [2] During a 2-Hour Period									
100	1	2	3	4	5	6	7	8	9	10
120	1	2	3	4	5	6	7	8	9	10
140	1	2	3	4	5	6	7	8	9	10
160	1	2	3	4	5	6	7	8	9	10
180	1	2	3	4	5	6	7	8	9	10
200	1	2	3	4	5	6	7	8	9	10
220	1	2	3	4	5	6	7	8	9	10
240	1	2	3	4	5	6	7	8	9	10

Be Careful Driving BAC* to .05	Driving May Be Impaired BAC .05-.09 [3]	Do Not Drive BAC .10 and up

[1] This chart provides averages only. Individual effects may vary and factors such as food in the stomach, medication and fatigue can affect your tolerance.

[2] One drink is 1¼ oz. of 80-proof liquor, 12 ounces of beer, or four ounces of wine.

[3] The BAC percentages for impairment and intoxication vary from state to state.

*BAC = Blood-Alcohol Content

Developed by Techniques for Alcohol Management. Used with permission.

If you're in doubt about your ability to drive, play it safe. Don't drive!

Preventing Alcohol Problems

Here are some guidelines to follow to prevent the onset of problems due to alcohol:

- Be aware of the blood-alcohol concentration danger levels.
- Don't develop a routine of social drinking or a pattern of drinking at a particular time of the day.
- Eat some food along with a drink and never start to drink on an empty stomach.
- Avoid social pressures to drink. Be assertive in your choice not to drink. Remember, parties are for socializing, not for getting intoxicated.
- Get help if you suspect an alcohol dependency problem. Don't wait until the problem worsens.
- Remember, an entire family suffers when one member has an untreated alcohol problem.
- Check with your doctor about drinking alcohol while taking prescription and over-the-counter medication.
- Don't drive if you've been drinking and don't be a passenger of someone who has been drinking.
- If you have a drink, drink it slowly. Never gulp it down due to thirst. If thirsty, drink water first.
- Avoid alcohol if you're pregnant.
- Skip that offer of "one for the road."
- Be wary of unfamiliar drinks and choose not to consume them.
- Be aware that nothing will sober you up but time. Your liver will only metabolize about one ounce of alcohol per hour.

Safety: Tips for Home

Most accidents happen at home. If you think your house is "home, safe home," take a look around. At first glance it may look orderly, but certain trouble spots can lead to cuts, falls, burns or other injuries. The following room-by-room checklist can alert you to accidents waiting to happen:

Kitchen

- Cleaners and dangerous chemicals should be stored out of children's reach.
- Scissors, knives, ice picks and other sharp tools should be stored separately from other utensils and out of the reach of children.
- Towels, curtains and other flammable materials should hang a safe distance from heat sources like the stove.
- Kitchen fans and stove ventilation exhausts should be clean and in good working order.
- Electrical cords should run a safe distance from the sink or range.
- Electrical outlets should not be overloaded.
- A sturdy step stool should be available to help reach high cabinets.
- Vinyl floors should be cleaned with non-skid wax.
- A nonskid floor mat should be in place in front of the sink.
- The kitchen should be well-lit.

Bedroom

- Electrical cords should be tucked away from foot traffic and in good working order.
- Electrical outlets should not be overloaded.
- Electric blankets should not be covered by bedspreads or other blankets when in use.
- Carpeting should be secured to the floor.
- A night-light should be put between the bed and the bathroom or hallway.
- The bedroom telephone should be easy to reach, even from the floor, if necessary.

- Ashtrays, irons, electric hair curlers and other potential fire hazards should be located away from bedding, curtains or other flammable material.
- Smoke detectors should be located near entrances to rooms, and their batteries should be checked often and replaced when needed.
- Emergency exit routes should be planned, discussed and practiced.

Bathroom

- Floor mats should have skid-proof backing.
- Rubber mats or adhesive-backed strips should be in place in the bathtub or shower stall.
- A support bar should be securely installed in the bathtub or shower stall.
- Hair dryers, electric shavers or other electric appliances should be kept away from water and unplugged when not in use.
- A light switch should be located near the bathroom entrance or entrances.

Halls and Stairs

- Halls and stairs should be well-lit, with a light switch at each end of a stairway.
- If a staircase is dimly lit, the top and bottom steps should be marked with reflective tape.
- Sturdy hand rails should be securely installed on both sides of each stairway.
- Floor covering on stairs and in halls should be skid-proof or carpeted and not creased or frayed.
- Stairways should be clear of shoes, books, toys, tools and other clutter.
- When young children are in the house, gates should block access to stairways.

Basement and Garage

- To avoid confusion and misuse, all chemicals and cleaners should be kept in their original containers and out of children's reach.
- Hazardous chemicals should be kept under lock and key and out of children's reach.
- Sharp or otherwise potentially hazardous tools should be in good working order and kept off-limits to children.

- Gasoline and other flammable materials should be stored away from heat sources and in airtight containers (outside the home, if possible).
- Buy a radon test kit from your state department of health or department of environmental protection, or contact the Environmental Control Agency (230 South Dearborn Street, Chicago, IL 60604) for information on radon testing. (Radon is an invisible gas that causes health problems if it builds up in homes and can't escape.) If your residence tests high for radon, hire a reliable radon expert to help you reduce levels of this gas.

Elsewhere Around the House

- Outdoor porches and walkways should be kept clear of ice in winter weather.
- Window screens should be securely fastened, especially if small children are around.
- Do not have poisonous plants in your yard or inside your house.
- Do not leave children unattended near swimming pools and playground equipment.
- Take steps to remedy unsafe situations as soon as possible.

Pregnancy: Planning a Healthy Baby

The general rule is that healthy moms have healthy babies. If you plan to become pregnant, take the following steps to be sure your baby gets off to a good start:
- Consider genetic tests or counseling if you or your partner has a family history of genetic disorders, if you are 35 or older or if your partner is 60 or older.
- Have a complete medical exam, including a gynecological exam. A number of medical conditions, including obesity, high blood pressure, diabetes, sexually transmitted diseases, having AIDS or the AIDS virus (HIV), smoking, alcohol use, nutritional deficiencies

and Rh negative blood factor (after the first pregnancy, if the father is Rh positive) can jeopardize the health of mother and child.

- Take measures to control and/or treat all medical conditions and take care of your health before you get pregnant. If you have a chronic medical condition, ask your doctor how it may affect your pregnancy and whether or not you should change or adjust any medication you are taking.
- Check with your doctor about the effects of any prescription or over-the-counter medication you take.
- If you're taking birth control pills, use an alternative form of birth control for three months before trying to become pregnant.
- If you're markedly overweight, plan to lose excess pounds before becoming pregnant.
- Exercise regularly.
- Start prenatal vitamins while trying to get pregnant. This may help prevent certain birth defects such as neural tube defects (e.g., spina bifida). Continue to take vitamin- and mineral supplements throughout your pregnancy, as prescribed by your doctor.

You and your baby will do best if you follow these guidelines:
- Contact your doctor as soon as you think you are pregnant.
- See your doctor at least once a month during your pregnancy.
- Ask your doctor or a dietitian to outline a meal plan that meets the special nutritional needs created by pregnancy.
- Drink at least eight glasses of water every day.
- Avoid caffeine, alcohol, nicotine and illicit drugs, as they can harm you and your unborn baby.
- Consult your doctor before taking any medication.
- Follow your doctor's advice about weight gain. The amount of weight you gain should depend on your weight and health status before you became pregnant, as well as your ethnic background.
- Continue to exercise in moderation with your practitioner's permission.

- Practice relaxation and other stress-control techniques. (Doctors think emotional stress may constrict the blood supply to the uterus and placenta, the baby's sole source of oxygen and nutrients.)
- Enroll in childbirth preparation classes even if you have attended these for other pregnancies.
- If you own a cat, arrange for someone else to empty the litter box. Cat excrement can transmit a disease called toxoplasmosis. If you're infected while pregnant, your baby may be stillborn, born prematurely or suffer serious damage to the brain, eyes or other parts of the body.
- Be informed. Know the warning signs of pregnancy complications. These include increasing blood pressure and early labor. Getting treatment early is important.

Preventing Premature Labor

A pregnant woman who starts to have her baby too soon is in premature labor. A full-term pregnancy is about 40 weeks. Babies born before 37 weeks are considered premature and may have health problems because they were born early.

The cause of premature labor is not completely understood. Any pregnant woman can have premature labor. The following conditions are associated with an increased risk of having a premature baby:
- Pregnant with twins, triplets, etc.
- Previous premature birth
- Smoking, drinking alcohol, misusing drugs
- Abnormally shaped uterus
- Daughter of a mother who took DES (diethylstilbestrol—a drug used in the 1940s-1970s by pregnant women for morning sickness and other reasons)
- Infection of the female organ(s)
- Younger than 18 or older than 35
- Unusual life pressure or stress
- Bleeding
- Two or more second-trimester abortions or miscarriages

This is not an all-inclusive list. If you have questions about these conditions, discuss them with your practitioner.

Being at an increased risk does not mean a woman will have a premature baby. Whether you are at risk or not, learn the warning signs and how to feel your uterus (womb) to tell if you are in labor. It is possible to prevent a baby from being born too early in some cases if early warning signs are recognized and steps are taken to stop labor. The following are warning signs of preterm labor:
• Contractions of the uterus
• Menstrual-like cramps that come and go or don't go away
• Pelvic pressure, which feels like the baby is pushing down, that comes and goes
• Low, dull backache that comes and goes or doesn't go away
• Abdominal cramping with or without diarrhea
• Fluid leaking from the vagina
• Fever of 100.4°F or higher and/or chills

Remember that premature labor is usually not painful. If you have any of the signs of premature labor, do the following:
• Lie down, tilted toward your left side for one hour. Do not lie flat on your back.
• Drink two to three glasses of water or juice during this hour.
• Keep feeling your stomach for uterine contractions.

If the signs do not go away in one hour or if you have fluid leaking from your vagina, do not wait. Call your doctor!

When you call, tell your nurse or doctor:
• Your name
• When your baby is due
• What signs you are having
• How often you are having contractions

SECTION II

COMMON HEALTH PROBLEMS

About This Section

Getting sick costs more than ever before. All these health care costs are going up:
- Insurance Rates
- Copayments
- Deductibles
- Tests
- Prescriptions
- Doctor office and health clinic visits

You have to make a lot of decisions when you get sick, such as:
- Should I go to the emergency room?
- Should I call my doctor?
- Can I wait and see if it gets better?
- Can I take care of it myself?
- What self-treatments should I perform?

This section of *Self-Care* can help answer these and other important questions. Detailed in this section are 92 common health problems and what you can do when you have one of them.

Sometimes you can treat these problems with self-care. Sometimes you need medical help. *Self-Care* can help you ask the right questions and find the answers to take care of your health. Each health problem discussed in this section is divided into three parts:

- Facts about the problem: What it is, what causes it, symptoms and treatments
- Yes and no questions to help you decide if you should get help fast, call your doctor, see your doctor or provide self-care
- A list of Self-Care Procedures for the problem

How to Use This Section

- Find the problem in the table of contents in the beginning of the book and go to that page. The problems are listed in alphabetical order.
- Read about the problem, what causes it (if known), its symptoms and treatments.
- Ask yourself the "Questions to Ask." Start at the top of the flowchart and answer yes or no to each question. Follow the arrows until you get to one of these answers:
  - Seek Emergency Care
  - See Doctor
  - Call Doctor
  - Provide Self-Care

What the Instructions Mean

Seek Emergency Care

 You should get help fast. Go to the hospital emergency room or call for emergency medical service (EMS) from your city EMS department or local ambulance service.

Make sure you know a phone number for emergency medical help. Write it down near your phone and in the "Emergency Phone Numbers" list in the front of this book.

See Doctor

 The term doctor can be used for a number of health care providers. They include:

- Your physician
- Your health maintenance organization (HMO) clinic, primary doctor or other designated health professional
- Walk-in clinic or urgent care center
- Physician's assistants (P.A.'s), Certified Nurses (C.N.'s), who work with your doctor
- Home health care provider
- Your dentist

When you see the "See Doctor" symbol, you should do so as soon as you can. You may need medicine or treatment to keep the problem from getting worse.

Call first and ask for an appointment or for immediate care. Tell the nurse or receptionist what's wrong if you can't talk to your doctor directly. If you can't be seen soon, ask for a referral. A referral from your doctor can help you get to see someone else who can help you.

Call Doctor

 Call your doctor and state the problem. He or she can decide what you should do. He or she may:

- Tell you to make an appointment to be seen
- Send you to a laboratory for tests
- Prescribe medicine or treatment over the phone
- Give you specific instructions to treat the problem

Provide Self-Care

 You can probably take care of the problem yourself if you answered no to all the questions. Use the Self-Care Procedures that are listed. But call your doctor if you don't feel better in a reasonable amount of time. You may have some other problem.

CHAPTER 10

EYE, EAR, NOSE AND THROAT PROBLEMS

Earache

Earaches can be slight or very painful. They are a sign that something is wrong. The most common cause of earaches is plugged eustachian tubes. These tubes go from the back of the throat to your middle ear. When eustachian tubes get blocked, fluid gathers, causing pain. Things that make this happen include infections of the middle ear, colds, sinus infections and allergies. Other things that can cause ear pain include changes in air pressure in a plane, something stuck in the ear, too much ear wax, tooth problems and ear injuries.

Very bad ear pain should be treated by a doctor. Treatment will depend on its cause. Most often this includes pain relievers, antibiotics (if infection is involved), methods to dry up or clear the blocked ear canal and whatever else is necessary to treat the source of the pain. You can, however, use Self-Care Procedures if ear pain is slight and produces no other symptoms. One example is with a mild case of "swimmer's ear," which affects the outer ear (see Self-Care Procedures).

Prevention

Much can be done to prevent earaches. Heed the old saying "Never put anything smaller than your elbow into your ear." This includes cotton-tipped swabs, bobby pins, your fingers, etc. Doing so could damage your eardrum. When you blow your nose, do so gently, one nostril at a time. Don't smoke. Smoking and secondhand smoke can increase the risk of infection for you and persons around you, especially if they are prone to ear infections.

Questions to Ask

With the earache do you also have these symptoms:
- Stiff neck
- Fever
- Drowsiness
- Nausea, vomiting

 YES → **SEEK EMERGENCY CARE**

 NO

Did the pain start after a blow to the ear or recent head trauma? **YES** → **SEEK EMERGENCY CARE**

 NO

Are any of these things present in an infant or small child especially following an upper respiratory infection, a cold, air travel or in a child with a history of ear problems:
- Constant pulling, touching or tugging at one or both ears
- Fever
- Constant crying despite being comforted
- Ear or ears that are hot and sensitive to the touch
- Unresponsiveness to loud noises, a bell or to the sound of your voice
- Irritability and sleeplessness especially at night or when lying down

 YES → **SEE DOCTOR**

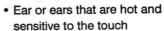 **NO**

With the earache, do you also have hearing loss, ringing in the ears, dizziness or nausea? **YES** → **SEE DOCTOR**

 NO

flowchart continued on next page

Self-Care Procedures

To reduce pain:

- Place a warm washcloth or heating pad (set on low, adults only) next to the ear. Some health professionals recommend putting an ice bag or ice in a wet washcloth over the painful ear for 20 minutes.
- Take acetaminophen, aspirin, ibuprofen or naproxen sodium. *Note: Do not give aspirin or any medication containing salicylates to anyone 19 years of age or younger, unless directed by a physician, due to its association with Reye's syndrome, a potentially fatal condition.*

Are there signs of infection such as:

- Fever (especially 102°F or higher)
- Sticky, green or bloody discharge
- *Severe* ear pain and/or increased pain when wiggling the earlobe

 YES →

SEE DOCTOR

NO

To open up the eustachian tubes and help them drain:

- Sit up.
- Prop your head up when you sleep.
- Yawn. (This helps move the muscles that open the eustachian tubes.)
- Chew gum or suck on hard candy. This is especially helpful during pressure changes that take place during air travel, but can also be useful during the middle of the night if you wake up with ear pain. (Do not give to children under age five.)
- Stay awake during takeoffs and landings when traveling by air.
- Take an oral decongestant such as Sudafed, which can dry up the fluid in the ear that causes the pain. Decongestant nasal sprays can be used, but only for up to three days or as directed by your doctor. Take a decongestant:
  - At the first sign of a cold if you have gotten ear infections often after previous colds
  - One hour before you land when you travel by air if you have a cold or know your sinuses are going to block up
- Take a steamy shower.
- Use a cool-mist vaporizer, especially at night.
- Drink plenty of cool water.
- Gently, but firmly, blow through your nose while holding both nostrils closed until you hear a pop. This will help promote ear drainage and can be done several times a day.
- Feed a baby his or her bottle in an upright position, not with the child lying down.

Is the earache persistent, more than mild, and does it occur after:

- A mild ear injury
- Hard or repeated nose blowings
- Sticking an object of any kind in the ear
- A cold, or sinus or upper respiratory infection
- Swimming, and is *extremely painful* when the earlobe is wiggled or touched
- Exposure to extremely loud noises (e.g., rock concerts, heavy machinery)

YES →

SEE DOCTOR

NO

Has a small object or insect entered the ear that cannot be easily or safely removed?

YES →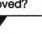

SEE DOCTOR

NO

Does the earache occur with jaw pain, headache or a clicking sound when opening and closing the mouth?

YES →

CALL DOCTOR

NO

PROVIDE SELF-CARE

In treating a mild case of swimmer's ear, the goal is to clean and dry the ear's outer canal without doing further damage to the top layer of skin. What you can do:

- Shake your head to expel trapped water after swimming or showering.
- Dry the ear canal. Using a clean facial tissue, twist each corner into a tip and gently place each tip into the ear canal for 10 seconds. Repeat with the other ear using a new tissue.
- Use an over-the-counter product such as Swim-Ear. Apply drops into the ears to fight infection. Follow package directions.
- Do not remove earwax. This coats the ear canal and protects it from moisture.

To avoid getting swimmer's ear:

- Wear wax or silicone earplugs that can be softened and shaped to fit your ears. They are available at most drugstores.
- Wear a bathing cap to help keep water from getting into your ears.
- Don't swim in dirty water.
- Swim on the surface of the water instead of underneath it.

Eyestrain From Computer

Office workers have their share of work-related hazards. People who use video display terminals (VDTs) may often complain of eyestrain, pain, stiffness in their backs and shoulders, and stress. These complaints can be a result of:

- Using a VDT for long time periods
- Improper positioning of the VDT
- Poor lighting
- Poor posture
- Tight deadlines

VDT users can protect themselves from the physical problems that go with using them with the Self-Care Procedures listed.

Questions to Ask

Do you still have eyestrain, pain and stiffness in back and shoulders despite using Self-Care Procedures listed?

YES

CALL DOCTOR

NO

PROVIDE SELF-CARE

Self-Care Procedures

To prevent eyestrain:

- Reduce glare. Keep the VDT away from windows. Turn off or shield overhead lights. Use a glare-reducing filter over the screen. Wear clothes that won't make you a source of glare.
- Place your paperwork close enough that you don't have to keep refocusing when switching from the screen to the paper. Use a paper holder.
- Place the screen so that your line of sight is 10 to 15 degrees (about one-third of a 45-degree angle) below horizontal.
- Dust off the screen often.
- Blink often to keep your eyes from getting dry. Use "artificial tear" eyedrops if needed.
- Tell your eye specialist that you use a VDT. Glasses and contacts worn for other activities may not be good for work on a VDT. (With bifocals, the near vision part of the lens is good for looking down, as when you read, but not straight ahead, as you do when looking at a video display screen. So you may need single-vision lenses for VDT work.)
- If the image on the VDT screen is blurred, dull or flickering, have the screen serviced right away.
- Try to keep the VDT screen two feet away from your eyes.

To prevent muscle tension when you work on a VDT:

- Use a chair that supports your back and can be easily adjusted to a height that feels right for you.
- Take a 15-minute break, if you can, for every two hours you use a VDT. Get up and go for a short walk, for example.
- Do stretching exercises of the neck, shoulder and lower back every one to two hours.
  - Rotate your head in a circular motion, first clockwise, then counterclockwise.
  - Shrug your shoulders up, down, backward and forward.
  - While standing or sitting, bend at the waist, leaning first to the left, then to the right.

Hay Fever

Despite its name, hay fever has nothing to do with hay or fever. A nineteenth-century physician called it this because he began to sneeze every time he entered a hay barn. But hay fever is, in fact, a reaction of the upper respiratory tract to anything to which you may be allergic. The medical term for hay fever is allergic rhinitis. Symptoms include itchy, watery eyes; runny, itchy nose; congestion and sneezing. Hay fever is most common in spring and fall, but some people have it all year. You can try to avoid things that give you hay fever. Talk to your doctor if that doesn't help. He or she may prescribe antihistamines, decongestants or nasal sprays. Here are a few tips on these medications:

- Antihistamines stop your body from making histamine, a substance your body makes when you are exposed to an allergen. Histamine causes many allergic symptoms. For best results, take the antihistamine 30 minutes before going outside. *Note: Some over-the-counter antihistamines may cause more drowsiness than prescription ones. Also, care should be taken when driving and operating machinery since antihistamines can make you drowsy.*

- Decongestants shrink the blood vessels in your nose and do not usually cause drowsiness.
- Don't use a nasal spray for more than three days at a time unless directed by your doctor. You may become dependent on it.

It is best to take what your doctor prescribes instead of experimenting with over-the-counter products on your own.

Your doctor may prescribe other things, such as cromolyn sodium or steroids. He or she may suggest allergy shots if your hay fever is very bad. First, you take a skin test. Then you get shots that have a tiny bit of the allergen. The shots help your body get used to the allergen so that your system is not so sensitive.

Questions to Ask

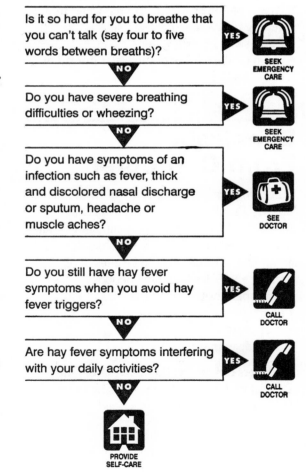

Is it so hard for you to breathe that you can't talk (say four to five words between breaths)? **YES** → SEEK EMERGENCY CARE

NO

Do you have severe breathing difficulties or wheezing? **YES** → SEEK EMERGENCY CARE

NO

Do you have symptoms of an infection such as fever, thick and discolored nasal discharge or sputum, headache or muscle aches? **YES** → SEE DOCTOR

NO

Do you still have hay fever symptoms when you avoid hay fever triggers? **YES** → CALL DOCTOR

NO

Are hay fever symptoms interfering with your daily activities? **YES** → CALL DOCTOR

NO

PROVIDE SELF-CARE

Self-Care Procedures

- Try to stay away from things that give you hay fever: Let someone else do outside chores. Mowing the lawn or raking leaves can make you very sick if you are allergic to pollen from grains, trees or weeds. It's a problem if you are allergic to molds, too.
- Keep windows and doors shut and stay inside when the pollen count or humidity is high. Early morning is sometimes the worst. Put an air conditioner or air cleaner in your house, especially in your bedroom. Be sure to clean the filter often.
- Try to keep dust, mold and pollen away from you at home and work:
  - Dust and vacuum your home often. Wear a dust-and-pollen mask if necessary.
  - Wash rugs.
  - Take carpets and drapes out of your bedroom.
  - Cover your mattress with a plastic cover.
  - Do not use a feather pillow.
  - Stay away from stuffed animals. They collect dust.
  - Don't have pets. If you must, keep them outside the house.
  - Don't hang sheets and blankets outside to dry. Pollen can get on them.
  - Shower, bathe and wash your hair following heavy exposure to pollens, dust, etc.
- Avoid tobacco smoke and other air pollutants.

Hearing Loss

Do people seem to mumble a lot lately? Do you have trouble hearing in church or theaters? Is it hard to pick up what others say at the dinner table or at family gatherings? Does your family ask you to turn down the volume on the TV or radio?

These are signs of gradual, age-related hearing loss called presbycusis. High-pitched sounds are the ones to go first. Hearing loss from presbycusis cannot be restored, but hearing aids,

along with the Self-Care Procedures listed, can be helpful.

Hearing loss can also result from other things:
- Acoustic trauma, which may be caused by a blow to the ear or exposure to excessive noise. Excessive noise includes that generated by low-flying airplanes and types of heavy, loud machinery.
- Blood vessel disorders including high blood pressure
- A blood clot that travels to nerves in the ear
- Ear wax that blocks the ear canal
- Chronic middle-ear infections or an infection of the inner ear
- Ménière's disease (a disease marked by excess fluid in canals of the inner ear)
- Multiple sclerosis
- Syphilis
- Brain tumor

Babies and young children should have their hearing checked during routine office visits. You may suspect a hearing problem in your child if he or she isn't properly responding to sounds. You may also notice that he or she is not learning to speak as quickly as expected. Children can be born with hearing loss or develop it from an ear or upper respiratory infection.

Questions to Ask

In a child: Does the child not respond to any sound, even a whistle or loud clap? Did the child's mother have German measles when pregnant with the child? Does the child not respond to sounds after:
- Recent earache or upper respiratory infection
- Airplane travel

YES

SEE DOCTOR

NO

flowchart continued on next page

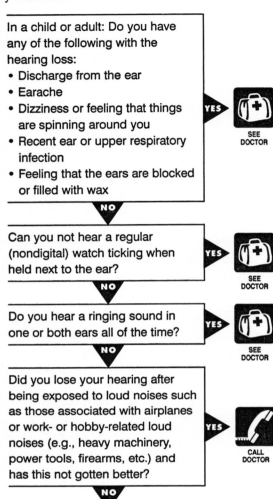

In a child or adult: Do you have any of the following with the hearing loss:
- Discharge from the ear
- Earache
- Dizziness or feeling that things are spinning around you
- Recent ear or upper respiratory infection
- Feeling that the ears are blocked or filled with wax

YES → SEE DOCTOR

NO ↓

Can you not hear a regular (nondigital) watch ticking when held next to the ear?

YES → SEE DOCTOR

NO ↓

Do you hear a ringing sound in one or both ears all of the time?

YES → SEE DOCTOR

NO ↓

Did you lose your hearing after being exposed to loud noises such as those associated with airplanes or work- or hobby-related loud noises (e.g., heavy machinery, power tools, firearms, etc.) and has this not gotten better?

YES → CALL DOCTOR

NO ↓

PROVIDE SELF-CARE

Self-Care Procedures

For gradual, age-related hearing loss (presbycusis):
- Ask people to speak clearly, distinctly and in a normal tone.
- Look at people when they are talking to you. Watch their expressions to help you understand what they are saying. Ask them to face you.
- Try to limit background noise when having a conversation.

- In a church or theater, sit up front.
- To rely on sight instead of sound, install a buzzer, flasher or amplifier on your telephone, door chime and alarm clock. Also, an audiologist (hearing therapist) may be able to show you other techniques for "training" yourself to hear better.

To clear earwax: (Use only if you know that the eardrum is not perforated. Check with your doctor if you are in doubt.)
- Lie on your side. Using a syringe or medicine dropper, carefully squeeze a few drops of lukewarm water into your ear (or have someone else do this). Let the water remain there for 10 to 15 minutes and then shake it out.
- Do this again but use a few drops of hydrogen peroxide, mineral oil or an over-the-counter cleaner such as Murine Ear Drops or Debrox. Let the excess fluid flow out of the ear.
- After several minutes, follow the same procedure using warm water again, letting it remain there for 10 to 15 minutes. Tilt the head to allow it to drain out of the ear.

You can repeat this entire procedure again in three hours if the earwax has not cleared.

To prevent hearing loss:
- Don't put cotton-tipped swabs, fingers, bobby pins and such in your ear.
- Don't blow your nose with too much force. It is better to gently blow one nostril at a time with a tissue or handkerchief held loosely over the nostril.
- Avoid places that have loud noises (airports, construction sites, etc.). Protect your ears with earplugs.
- Keep the volume low on such items as personal stereos and car stereos. If someone else can hear the music when the earphones are on your head, the volume is too loud.
- Follow your doctor's advice for disorders that can cause hearing loss (e.g., high blood pressure, Ménière's disease, etc.).
- Avoid prolonged use of or overdosing on drugs that cause hearing loss (e.g., heavy use of aspirin, streptomycin, quinine).

Also be aware of things that can help you hear sounds if your hearing is impaired:
- Hearing aids. (See your health care provider.)
- Devices made to assist in hearing sounds from the TV and radio
- Special equipment that can be installed in your telephone by the telephone company
- Portable devices made especially to amplify sounds. (These can be used for movies, classes, meetings, etc.)

Hiccups

Hiccups are simple enough to explain. Your diaphragm (the major muscle involved in breathing that sits like a cap over the stomach) goes into spasm. Things that promote hiccups are:
- Eating too fast, which causes you to swallow air along with food
- Eating fatty foods to the point where they make the stomach full enough to irritate the diaphragm

According to a doctor who studies hiccups, there is a hiccup center in the brain that triggers a spasm of the esophagus setting in motion the cycle leading to hiccups. This, he thinks, is a protective mechanism to keep a person from choking on food or drink. Luckily, hiccups are generally harmless and don't last very long.

Questions to Ask

Do the hiccups occur with:
- Severe abdominal pain and
- Spitting up blood or blood in the stools

YES → **SEEK EMERGENCY CARE**

NO ↓

Have the hiccups lasted longer than eight hours in an adult or three hours in a child?

YES → **CALL DOCTOR**

NO ↓

flowchart continued in next column

flowchart continued

Have the hiccups started only after taking prescription medicine?

YES → **CALL DOCTOR**

NO ↓

PROVIDE SELF-CARE

Self-Care Procedures

Luckily, there's no shortage of hiccup cures, and better still, most of them work (although some baffle medical science). A study reported in the *New England Journal of Medicine* found that one teaspoon of ordinary table sugar, swallowed dry, cured hiccups immediately in 19 out of 20 people (some of whom had been hiccuping for as long as six weeks). If this doesn't stop the hiccups right away, repeat it three times at two-minute intervals. (For young children, use a teaspoon of corn syrup.) Other popular folk remedies worth trying include:
- Hold your tongue with your thumb and index finger and gently pull it forward.
- With your neck bent backward, hold your breath for a count of 10. Exhale immediately and drink a glass of water.
- Breathe into and out of a paper (not plastic) bag.
- Swallow a small amount of finely cracked ice.
- Massage the back of the roof of your mouth with a cotton swab. A finger works equally well.
- Eat dry bread slowly.
- Drink a glass of water rapidly.

Laryngitis

Disc jockeys get laryngitis. So do actors, politicians and others who talk for hours. But ordinary people who overuse their voices get laryngitis, too. Perhaps you cheer too loudly and too often at a basketball game. Or perhaps you lose your voice for no apparent reason.

Air pollution or spending an evening in a smoky room can irritate the larynx (voice box) and cause laryngitis. Infections, too, can inflame the larynx. When your larynx is irritated or inflamed, your voice becomes hoarse, husky and weak. Sometimes laryngitis is painless, but you may get a sore throat, fever or dry cough, a tickling sensation in the back of the throat, or have trouble swallowing. Smoking, drinking alcohol, breathing cold air and continuing to use already-distressed vocal cords can make the situation worse.

Questions to Ask

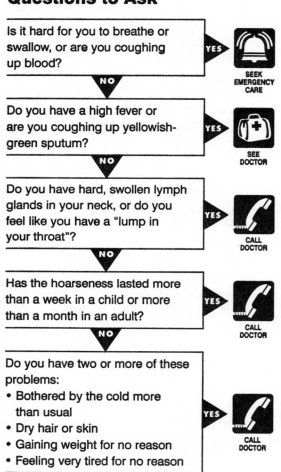

Is it hard for you to breathe or swallow, or are you coughing up blood?

YES → **SEEK EMERGENCY CARE**

NO ↓

Do you have a high fever or are you coughing up yellowish-green sputum?

YES → **SEE DOCTOR**

NO ↓

Do you have hard, swollen lymph glands in your neck, or do you feel like you have a "lump in your throat"?

YES → **CALL DOCTOR**

NO ↓

Has the hoarseness lasted more than a week in a child or more than a month in an adult?

YES → **CALL DOCTOR**

NO ↓

Do you have two or more of these problems:
• Bothered by the cold more than usual
• Dry hair or skin
• Gaining weight for no reason
• Feeling very tired for no reason

YES → **CALL DOCTOR**

NO ↓

PROVIDE SELF-CARE

Self-Care Procedures

• Don't talk if you don't need to. Use a notepad and pencil to write notes instead. If you must speak, do so softly, but don't whisper.
• Use a cool-mist humidifier in your home, especially in your bedroom.
• Drink lots of warm drinks. Tea with honey is good.
• Gargle with warm salt water (¼ teaspoon of salt in ½ cup of water).
• Take a hot shower or steam bath.
• Don't smoke. Stay away from places with smoky air.
• Suck on cough drops, throat lozenges or hard candy. (Do not give to children under age five.)
• Take aspirin, acetaminophen, ibuprofen or naproxen sodium. *Note: Do not give aspirin or any medication containing salicylates to anyone 19 years of age or younger, unless directed by a physician, due to its association with Reye's syndrome, a potentially fatal condition.*

Nosebleeds

Nosebleeds are usually a childhood problem, a scary but minor bout with broken blood vessels just inside the nose. They're caused by a cold, frequent nose blowing and picking, allergies, a dry environment, using too much nasal spray or a punch or other blow to the nose.

Not all nosebleeds are minor. Some are serious, such as heavy bleeding from deep within the nose (called a posterior nosebleed) that's hard to stop. This type usually strikes the elderly and is most commonly caused by hardening of nasal blood vessels, high blood pressure, drugs to treat blood clots, primary bleeding disorders like hemophilia or by a tumor in the nose.

Questions to Ask

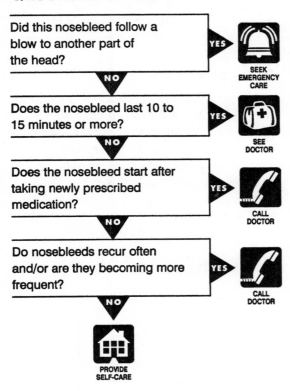

Did this nosebleed follow a blow to another part of the head? **YES** → SEEK EMERGENCY CARE

NO ↓

Does the nosebleed last 10 to 15 minutes or more? **YES** → SEE DOCTOR

NO ↓

Does the nosebleed start after taking newly prescribed medication? **YES** → CALL DOCTOR

NO ↓

Do nosebleeds recur often and/or are they becoming more frequent? **YES** → CALL DOCTOR

NO ↓

PROVIDE SELF-CARE

Self-Care Procedures

Although there are lots of ideas about how to treat minor nosebleeds, the following procedure is recommended by the American Academy of Otolaryngology-Head and Neck Surgery.

- Sit with your head leaning forward.
- Pinch the nostrils shut, using your thumb and forefinger in such a way that the nasal septum (the nose's midsection) is being gently squeezed.
- Hold for 15 uninterrupted minutes, breathing through your mouth.
- At the same time, apply cold compresses (such as ice in a soft cloth) to the area around the nose.
- For the next 24 hours, make sure your head is elevated above the level of your heart.
- Also, wait 24 hours before blowing your nose, lifting heavy objects or exercising strenuously.

Note: If you are unable to stop a nosebleed by using the Self-Care Procedures, call your doctor.

Pinkeye

Pinkeye is an inflammation of the conjunctiva, the underside of both the upper and lower eyelids and the covering of the white portion of the eye. The medical term for this is conjunctivitis. Some causes of pinkeye along with possible solutions are:

- Allergic reaction to airborne pollens, dust, mold spores and animal dander or direct contact with chlorinated water or cosmetics. If you can't avoid the allergens, antihistamines can help. So can certain eye drops. Ask your doctor which one(s) to use.
- Bacterial conjunctivitis (noted by a puslike discharge). Warm compresses, along with an antibiotic ointment or prescription drops, can help. When treated correctly, bacterial conjunctivitis will clear up in two to three days, but you should continue to use the medicine as prescribed by your doctor.
- Viral conjunctivitis is a complication of a cold or flu. This type has less discharge but more tearing than the bacterial form. Antibiotics don't work. Viral conjunctivitis can take 14 to 21 days to clear up.

Questions to Ask

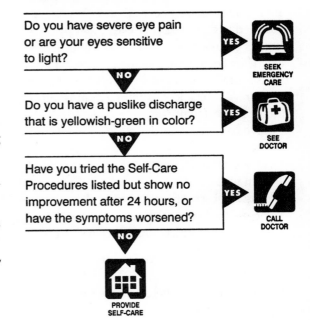

Do you have severe eye pain or are your eyes sensitive to light? **YES** → SEEK EMERGENCY CARE

NO ↓

Do you have a puslike discharge that is yellowish-green in color? **YES** → SEE DOCTOR

NO ↓

Have you tried the Self-Care Procedures listed but show no improvement after 24 hours, or have the symptoms worsened? **YES** → CALL DOCTOR

NO ↓

PROVIDE SELF-CARE

Self-Care Procedures

Here are some ways to relieve the symptoms of pinkeye:

- Don't touch the eye area with your fingers. If you must wipe your eyes, use tissues.
- With your eyes closed, apply a washcloth soaked in warm (not hot) water to the affected eye three to four times a day for at least five minutes at a time. (These soaks also help to dissolve the crusty residue of pinkeye.)
- Use over-the-counter eye drops. They may soothe irritation and help relieve itching.
- Avoid wearing eye makeup until the infection has completely cleared up. (And never share makeup with others.)
- Don't cover or patch the eye. This can make the infection grow.
- Don't wear contact lenses while your eyes are infected.
- Wash your hands often and use your own towels. Pinkeye is very contagious and can be spread from one person to another by contaminated fingers, washcloths or towels.

Sinus Problems

Your sinuses are behind your cheekbones and forehead and around your eyes. Healthy sinuses drain almost a quart of water every day. They keep the air you breathe wet. Your sinuses can't drain right if they are infected and swollen. Your chances of getting a sinus infection increase if you:

- Have hay fever
- Smoke
- Have a nasal deformity or sinuses that don't drain well
- Have an abscess in an upper tooth
- Sneeze hard with your mouth closed or blow your nose too much when you have a cold

Symptoms of a sinus infection are:
- Head congestion
- Nasal congestion and discharge (usually yellowish-green)

- Pain and tenderness over the facial sinuses
- Pain in the upper jaw
- Recurrent headache that changes with head position and disappears shortly after getting out of bed
- Fever

Sinus complications can be serious. Your doctor can tell if you have a sinus infection with a physical exam, a laboratory study of a sample of your nasal discharge and X-rays of the sinuses. You may need prescriptions for an antibiotic, a decongestant as well as a nasal spray and/or nose drops. These work to clear the infection and reduce congestion. (Severe cases may require surgery to drain the sinuses.)

Questions to Ask

Do you have two or more of the following:
- A fever over 101°F
- Greenish-yellow or bloody-colored nasal discharge
- A severe headache that doesn't get better when you take aspirin or acetaminophen or that is worse in the morning or when you bend forward
- Pain between the nose and lower eyelid
- A feeling of pressure inside the head
- Eye pain, blurred vision or changes in vision
- Pain in the cheek or upper jaw
- Swelling around the eyes, nose, cheeks and forehead
- Trouble sleeping or thinking clearly

YES

SEE DOCTOR

NO

PROVIDE SELF-CARE

Self-Care Procedures

A cool-mist humidifier can help. Wet air helps make mucus thin. You can put a warm wash-cloth or compress on your face, too. This can help with the pain. Here are some more tips:

- Drink plenty of water and other liquids.
- Take aspirin or acetaminophen, ibuprofen or naproxen sodium for pain. *Note: Do not give aspirin or any medication containing salicylates to anyone 19 years of age or younger, unless directed by a physician, due to its association with Reye's syndrome, a potentially fatal condition.*
- Take an over-the-counter (OTC) decongestant pill, or an OTC pill for pain such as Tylenol Sinus that also includes a decongestant. (Older men should check with their doctors before taking decongestants. Decongestants that have ephedrine can give older men urinary problems.)
- Use nose drops only for the number of days prescribed. Repeated use of them creates a dependency. Your nasal passages "forget" how to work on their own and you have to continue using drops to keep nasal passages clear. To avoid picking up germs, never borrow nose drops from others, and don't let anyone else use yours. Throw the drops away after treatment.

Sore Throats

Sore throats range from a mere scratch to pain so severe that even swallowing saliva hurts. Often the cause of all this misery can be either a virus or bacteria. Viral sore throats are the more common of the two and don't respond to antibiotics; bacterial ones do. So it's important to know what kind of bug is roughing up your throat. A sore throat can result from a fungal infection, too. In this case, an antifungal drug is used to treat it.

Bacterial sore throats are most often caused by streptococcus (strep throat) and usually bring a high fever, headaches and swollen, enlarged

neck glands with them. Viral sore throats generally don't. But even doctors have trouble diagnosing a sore throat based on symptoms alone. (A child with a bacterial sore throat may have no other symptoms, for example.) And if left untreated, serious complications, including abscesses, kidney inflammation or rheumatic heart disease, could arise from a strep throat. So your doctor may take a throat culture. If strep or other bacteria are the culprit, he or she will prescribe an antibiotic. Be sure you take all of the antibiotic.

Questions to Ask

Is it very hard for you to breathe, are you unable to swallow your own saliva, or are you unable to say more than three or four words between breaths?

SEEK EMERGENCY CARE

NO

Do you have any of the following problems with the sore throat:
- Fever
- Swollen, enlarged neck glands
- Headache
- General achy feeling
- Ear pain
- Bad breath
- Skin rash
- Loss of appetite
- Vomiting
- Abdominal pain
- Chest pain
- Dark urine

YES

SEE DOCTOR

NO

Do your tonsils or back of the throat look bright red or have visible pus deposits?

YES

SEE DOCTOR

NO

flowchart continued on next page

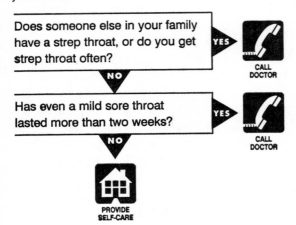

Does someone else in your family have a strep throat, or do you get strep throat often? **YES** — CALL DOCTOR

NO

Has even a mild sore throat lasted more than two weeks? **YES** — CALL DOCTOR

NO

PROVIDE SELF-CARE

Self-Care Procedures

You can take some steps to relieve sore throat discomfort:

- Gargle every few hours with a solution of ¼ teaspoon of salt dissolved in ½ cup of warm water.
- Drink plenty of warm beverages, such as tea (with or without honey), and eat soup.
- For strep throat, eat and drink cold foods and liquids such as frozen yogurt, popsicles and ice water.
- Use a cool-mist vaporizer or humidifier in the room where you spend most of your time.
- Don't smoke. Smoke can aggravate sore throats and make you more susceptible to them.
- Don't eat spicy foods.
- Suck on a piece of hard candy or a medicated lozenge every so often. (Do not give to children under age five.)
- Take aspirin or acetaminophen for the pain or fever (or both). *Note: Do not give aspirin or any medication containing salicylates to anyone 19 years of age or younger, unless directed by a physician, due to its association with Reye's syndrome, a potentially fatal condition.*
- Do not get in close contact with anyone you know who has a sore throat.

Sty

A sty is a small boil or bacterial infection in a tiny gland of the eyelid. If the oil-producing glands on the upper or lower rim of the eyelid become infected, they become swollen and painful. A sty is tiny at first, but it can blossom into a bright red, painful sore.

Eventually, a "baby" sty will come to a head and appear yellow, because it accumulates pus. Generally, the tip will face outward, and the sty will break open and drain on its own.

Questions to Ask

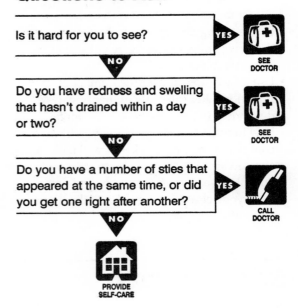

Is it hard for you to see? **YES** — SEE DOCTOR

NO

Do you have redness and swelling that hasn't drained within a day or two? **YES** — SEE DOCTOR

NO

Do you have a number of sties that appeared at the same time, or did you get one right after another? **YES** — CALL DOCTOR

NO

PROVIDE SELF-CARE

Self-Care Procedures

You can relieve the discomfort of a sty by following these steps:

- Apply warm (not hot) wet compresses to the affected area three or four times a day for five to 10 minutes at a time.
- Avoid situations that expose your eyes to excessive dust or dirt.
- Don't poke or squeeze the infected area, no matter how tempted you may be to pop the sty. Most sties respond well to home care and don't require further treatment.

Tinnitus (Ringing in the Ears)

Imagine hearing a ringing noise in your head that doesn't go away. This maddening noise, called tinnitus, can range in volume from a ring to a roar. It affects nearly 36 million Americans, most of them older adults. Seven million people are so seriously bothered by tinnitus that living a normal life is not possible. In fact, tinnitus can interfere with work, sleep and normal communication with others.

Like a toothache, tinnitus isn't a disease in itself, but a symptom of another problem. Examples are:
- Earwax blocking the ear canals
- Food allergies
- Reactions to medications
- Middle-ear trauma or infections
- Blood vessel abnormalities in the brain
- Ear nerve damage (due to exposure to loud noise)
- Anemia
- Ménière's disease
- Diabetes
- Brain tumors (rarely)

And sometimes, tinnitus is due simply to advancing age. It often accompanies loss of hearing. Occasionally, tinnitus is temporary and will not lead to deafness. Treatment is aimed at finding and treating the problem that causes the tinnitus.

Questions to Ask

Do you have severe pain in the ears, forehead or over the cheekbones, a severe headache, dizziness and/or sudden loss of hearing?

YES →
SEEK EMERGENCY CARE

NO ↓

flowchart continued in next column

flowchart continued

Have you been taking aspirin or other medications containing salicylates such as Trilisate or Disalcid (which are sometimes used to treat arthritis), and do you have these problems with ringing in the ears?
- Nausea
- Vomiting
- Dizziness
- Rapid breathing
- Hallucinations

YES →
SEEK EMERGENCY CARE

 NO ↓

Along with ringing in the ears, do you have one or more of the following?
- Dizziness
- Vertigo
- Unsteadiness in walking
- Loss of balance
- Vomiting
- Difficulty hearing sounds or speech of others

YES →
SEE DOCTOR

NO ↓

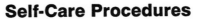

PROVIDE SELF-CARE

Self-Care Procedures

- For mild cases of tinnitus, play the radio or a "white noise" tape (white noise is a low, constant sound) in the background to help mask the tinnitus.
- Biofeedback or other relaxation techniques can help you reduce stress, calm down and concentrate, shifting your attention away from the tinnitus.
- Exercise regularly to promote good blood circulation.
- Ask your doctor about a recently developed tinnitus masker, which looks like a hearing aid. Worn on the ear, it makes a subtle noise that masks the tinnitus without interfering with hearing and speech.

- If the noises started during or after traveling in an airplane, try pinching your nostrils and blowing through your nose. Chewing gum or sucking on hard candy may help prevent the ear popping and ringing sounds in the ear from happening when you do fly. (Do not give to children under age five.) Also, it is prudent to avoid flying when you have an upper respiratory tract infection.
- Limit your intake of caffeine, alcohol, nicotine and aspirin.
- To prevent damage to the ear, wear earplugs when exposed to loud noises such as heavy machinery.

CHAPTER 11

RESPIRATORY PROBLEMS

Asthma

About 10 million Americans suffer the wheezing, chest tightness and breathing difficulty that typify asthma. Doctors call it an episodic disease because acute attacks alternate with symptom-free periods. Asthma is a physical problem, not an emotional one (although stress, anxiety or frustration can worsen asthma), and it can be severe enough to disrupt people's lives. It is a complex disorder that needs to be treated by a doctor who can monitor its condition.

Asthma cuts down the air flow in the lungs. This makes it hard to breathe and can cause wheezing. (Other things can cause wheezing, too. Something may be stuck in the throat, or there may be an infection. Always tell your doctor about wheezing, especially if your child has it.)

A variety of triggers can set off asthma attacks:
- Having an upper respiratory tract infection or bronchitis
- Breathing an allergen like pollen, mold, animal dander or particles of dust, smoke or other irritants
- Eating certain foods or taking certain drugs
- Exercising too hard
- Breathing cold air
- Experiencing emotional distress

Asthma attacks range from mild to severe, so treatment varies. Generally, asthma is too complex to treat with over-the-counter preparations. A doctor should monitor your condition.

He or she may prescribe one or more of these for your asthma:
- Bronchodilators, either in oral, inhaled or aerosol form, which open airways to make breathing easier
- Steroids, either in oral or aerosol form, to counteract an allergic reaction, and when other drugs are not successful for your asthma
- Cromolyn sodium to be inhaled before an attack that is triggered by allergies or exercise. This won't work once the attack starts. When used with steroids, though, it may help prevent asthma attacks.

Questions to Ask

Is it so hard for you to breathe that you can't say four or five words between breaths? Or does your chest feel tight? Or do you have wheezing that doesn't go away? **YES** →

SEEK EMERGENCY CARE

NO ↓

Does your asthma attack not respond to home treatment or prescribed medicine? **YES** →

SEE DOCTOR

NO ↓

Do you have signs of an infection (e.g., fever), or are you coughing up anything that is green, yellow or blood-colored? **YES** →

SEE DOCTOR

NO ↓

Are your asthma attacks coming more often or getting worse? **YES** →

SEE DOCTOR

NO ↓

PROVIDE SELF-CARE

Self-Care Procedures

Asthmatics can do a number of things to help themselves:
- Drink plenty of liquids (2 to 3 quarts a day) to keep secretions loose.
- Find out what triggers your asthma, and get rid of things that bother you at home and at work.
- Make a special effort to keep your bedroom allergen-free.
  - Sleep with a foam or cotton pillow, not a feather one.
  - Wash mattress pads in hot water every week.
  - Use throw rugs, not carpeting.
  - Don't use drapes.
  - Vacuum and dust often. Wear a dust-filter mask when you do.
- Avoid using perfumes.
- Don't smoke. Try to avoid air pollution.
- Wear a scarf around your mouth and nose when you are outside in cold weather. Doing so will warm the air as you breathe it in and will prevent cold air from reaching sensitive airways.
- Stop exercising if you start to wheeze.
- Don't take foods or medicines that have sulfites. Sulfites are in wine and many shellfish. They bother many people with asthma.
- Sit up during an asthma attack. Don't lie down.
- Install an electronic air filter in your central heat or air conditioning, or use portable air cleaners to keep the air clean. Change and/or wash furnace and air-conditioner filters regularly.
- If you have a portable humidifier or vaporizer, use distilled instead of tap water. Clean and dry the appliance after each use.
- Keep your asthma medicine handy. Take it as soon as you start to feel an attack.
- Some people with asthma are allergic to aspirin. Use acetaminophen instead.

Bronchitis

If you've ever had a cough that felt as though it started down in your toes, or if you've ever started coughing and couldn't stop, you may have had bronchitis. Bronchitis can be either acute or chronic, depending on how long it lasts and how serious the damage.

Acute bronchitis is generally caused by an infectious agent (like a virus or bacterium) or an environmental pollutant (like tobacco smoke) that attacks the mucous membranes within the windpipe or air passages in your respiratory tract, leaving them red and inflamed. This type often develops in the wake of a sinus infection, cold or other respiratory infection and can last anywhere from three days to three weeks.

Signs of acute bronchitis are:
- Cough that has little or no sputum
- Chills, low-grade fever (usually less than 101°F)
- Sore throat and muscle aches
- Feeling of pressure behind the breastbone or a burning feeling in the chest

Treatment may include a doctor's prescription for:
- Bronchodilators (drugs that open up the bronchial passages)
- Antibiotics

In chronic bronchitis, the airways produce too much mucus. It's enough to cause a daily cough that brings up the mucus, continuing for as long as three months or more, for more than two years in a row. Many people, most of them smokers, develop emphysema (destruction of the air sacs) along with chronic bronchitis. Because chronic bronchitis results in abnormal air exchange in the lung and causes permanent damage to the respiratory tract, it's much more serious than acute bronchitis.

Signs of chronic bronchitis are:
- A cough that is productive (i.e., one that produces mucus or phlegm)
- Shortness of breath upon exertion (in early stages)
- Shortness of breath at rest (in later stages)

People living in heavily industrialized areas exposed to air pollution, workers exposed to metallic dust or fibers and people who smoke are most susceptible to chronic bronchitis. In fact, cigarette smoking is the most common cause of chronic bronchitis. So quitting is essential and may bring complete relief.

Treatment includes:
- Stopping smoking and avoiding second-hand smoke
- Avoiding or reducing exposure to air pollution and chemical irritants
- Avoiding exposure to cold, wet weather
- Using cough medicines with an expectorant

Questions to Ask

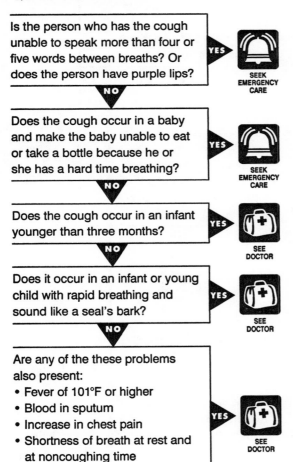

Is the person who has the cough unable to speak more than four or five words between breaths? Or does the person have purple lips?
YES → SEEK EMERGENCY CARE
NO ↓

Does the cough occur in a baby and make the baby unable to eat or take a bottle because he or she has a hard time breathing?
YES → SEEK EMERGENCY CARE
NO ↓

Does the cough occur in an infant younger than three months?
YES → SEE DOCTOR
NO ↓

Does it occur in an infant or young child with rapid breathing and sound like a seal's bark?
YES → SEE DOCTOR
NO ↓

Are any of the these problems also present:
- Fever of 101°F or higher
- Blood in sputum
- Increase in chest pain
- Shortness of breath at rest and at noncoughing time
- Vomiting
YES → SEE DOCTOR
NO ↓

flowchart continued in next column

---

flowchart continued

Have you been exposed to chemicals at work or at home such as those in new carpet or tobacco smoke?
YES → CALL DOCTOR
NO ↓

PROVIDE SELF-CARE

Self-Care Procedures

- Use a cool-mist humidifier or vaporizer.
- Take aspirin or acetaminophen for fever and aches. *Note: Do not give aspirin or any medication containing salicylates to anyone 19 years of age or younger, unless directed by a physician, due to its association with Reye's syndrome, a potentially fatal condition.*
- Rest.
- Drink plenty of liquids like water, clear soup and tea.
- Don't smoke.
- Stay away from air pollution as much as you can. Use air conditioning, air filters, and a filter mask for your nose and mouth if you need to. Stay inside when air pollution is heavy, if you get bronchitis easily.
- Instead of using cough suppressants, use expectorants. Take bronchodilators and/or antibiotics as prescribed by your doctor.

Common Cold

About 30 million Americans are coughing, sneezing and blowing their noses while you read this. What's wrong with them? They have the most common illness we know, the common cold. The common cold usually lasts three to seven days and the average person gets three or four a year. The things that come with a cold are:
- Sneezing
- Runny nose

- Fever of 101°F or less
- Sore throat
- Dry cough

How do you get colds? Colds are caused by viruses. You can get a cold virus from mucus on other people's hands—such as from a hand-shake—when they have colds. You can also pick up the virus on towels, telephones or money. Then someone else gets the virus from you. It goes on and on. Cold viruses also travel through coughs and sneezes.

Prevention

- Wash your hands often. Keep them away from your nose, eyes and mouth.
- Try not to touch people or their things when they have a cold.
- Get lots of exercise. Eat and sleep well.
- Use a handkerchief or tissues when you sneeze, cough or blow your nose. This helps to keep you from passing your germs to others.
- Use a cool-mist vaporizer or humidifier in your bedroom in the winter.

Questions to Ask

Do you have any of these problems with the cold:
- Quick breathing or trouble breathing
- Wheezing
- Feeling weak or low on energy
- Feeling jumpy or easily angered
- Delirium. (Delirium can make you restless or confused. Sometimes you see things that aren't there. Watch out for this especially in children.)

 YES

SEE DOCTOR

NO

flowchart continued in next column

flowchart continued

Do you have any of these problems with the cold:
- Earache
- Bright red sore throat or sore throat with white spots
- Coughing that lasts more than 10 days
- Coughing up something yellowish-green or gray
- Fever over 103°F in an adult under 50
- Fever of 102°F or higher in a person 50 to 60 years old
- Fever of 101°F or higher in a person over 60
- Fever over 104°F in a child under 12
- A bad smell from the throat, nose or ears

YES

SEE DOCTOR

NO

Do you have pain or swelling over your sinuses that gets worse when you bend over or move your head? (Your sinuses are behind your cheekbones, eyes and forehead.) Watch out for this especially when you also have a fever of 101°F or higher.

YES

SEE DOCTOR

NO

PROVIDE SELF-CARE

Self-Care Procedures

Time is the only cure for a cold. Some things can make you feel better, though. Here are some hints for fighting a cold:
- Rest in bed if you have a fever.
- Drink lots of hot or cold drinks. They help clear out your respiratory tract. This can help prevent other problems, like bronchitis.
- Take aspirin, acetaminophen, ibuprofen or naproxen sodium for muscle aches and pains.

Note: Do not give aspirin or any medication containing salicylates to anyone 19 years of age or younger, unless directed by a physician, due to its association with Reye's syndrome, a potentially fatal condition.

- Gargle with warm salt water, drink tea with honey and lemon or suck on throat lozenges for a sore throat. (Do not give lozenges to children under age five.)
- Breathe from a cool-mist vaporizer or humidifier to help quiet a cough.
- Eat chicken soup. It helps clear out mucus.
- Check with your doctor about taking vitamin C. This seems to make some people feel better when they have a cold and may help keep them from getting a cold, even though this has never been medically proven.

Coughs

A lot of things can make you cough:
- An infection
- An allergy
- Cigarette smoke
- Something stuck in your windpipe
- Dry air

Coughing can be a sign of many ailments. Your body uses coughing to clear your lungs and airways. Coughing itself is not the problem. What causes the cough is the problem. There are three kinds of coughs:

Productive - A productive cough brings up mucus or phlegm.

Nonproductive - A nonproductive cough is dry and doesn't bring up any mucus.

Reflex - A reflex cough comes from a problem somewhere else, like the ear or stomach.

How to treat your cough depends on what kind it is, what caused it and what your other symptoms are. Treat the cause and soothe the irritation. Stay away from smoking and second-hand smoke, especially when you have a cough. Smoke hurts your lungs and makes it harder for your body to fight infection.

Questions to Ask

Do you have these problems:
- Trouble breathing and inability to say more than four or five words between breaths. (A baby or small child may be unable to cry, eat, or drink a bottle.)
- Chest pain
- Fainting
- Coughing up blood

 YES **SEEK EMERGENCY CARE**

NO

Is the person who has the cough a baby or small child? If so, does he or she have these problems, too:
- The cough sounds like a seal's bark (high and whistling)
- A fever of 102° to 103°F

YES **SEE DOCTOR**

NO

Did the cough start suddenly and last an hour or more without stopping?

YES **SEE DOCTOR**

NO

Are wheezing, shortness of breath, rapid breathing or swelling of the abdomen, legs and ankles present with the cough?

YES **SEE DOCTOR**

NO

If the person with the cough is an adult, is there a fever of 102°F or higher?

YES **SEE DOCTOR**

NO

Do you have any of these problems with the cough?
- Weight loss for no reason
- Tiredness
- A lot of sweating at night

YES **SEE DOCTOR**

NO

Does your chest hurt only when you cough, and does the pain go away when you sit up or lean forward?

YES **SEE DOCTOR**

NO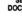

flowchart continued on next page

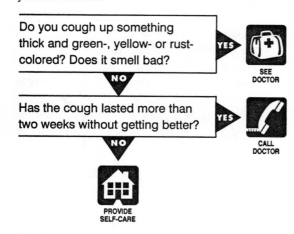

Do you cough up something thick and green-, yellow- or rust-colored? Does it smell bad? **YES** → SEE DOCTOR

NO

Has the cough lasted more than two weeks without getting better? **YES** → CALL DOCTOR

NO

PROVIDE SELF-CARE

Self-Care Procedures

For productive coughs (coughs that bring up mucus):

- Drink plenty of liquids. Water helps loosen mucus and soothe a sore throat. Fruit juices are good, too.
- Use a cool-mist vaporizer, especially in the bedroom. Put a humidifier on the furnace.
- Take a shower. The steam can help thin the mucus.
- Ask your pharmacist for an over-the-counter expectorant. Robitussin is one kind.
- Stop smoking cigarettes, cigars and/or pipes. Stay away from places where people smoke.

For nonproductive coughs (coughs that are dry):
- Drink plenty of liquids.
- Drink hot drinks like tea with lemon and honey to soothe the throat.
- Suck on cough drops or hard candy. (Do not give these to children under age five.)
- Take an over-the-counter cough medicine that has dextromethorphan. Robitussin-DM is one of these.
- Try a decongestant if you have postnasal drip. You feel postnasal drip at the back of your throat. Decongestants help dry it out.
- Make your own cough medicine. Mix one part lemon juice and two parts honey. (Don't give this to children younger than one year.)

Other tips include:
- Don't give children under age five small objects like paper clips and buttons or foods like peanuts and popcorn. A small child can easily get something caught in the throat or windpipe. Even adults should be careful to chew and swallow foods slowly.
- Don't smoke. Stay away from secondhand smoke.
- Stay away from chemical gases that can hurt your lungs.
- Exercise. Start easy and work up slowly. You will make your breathing muscles stronger. You will fight infection better, too.

Flu

"Oh, it's just a touch of the flu," some say, as if they had nothing more than a cold. Yet each year 50,000 people in the U.S. die from pneumonia and other complications of the influenza virus, or flu.

Cold and flu symptoms resemble each other, but they differ in intensity. A cold generally starts out with some minor sniffling and sneezing, but the flu hits you all at once: You're fine one hour and in bed the next. A cold rarely moves into the lungs; the flu can cause pneumonia. You may be able to drag yourself to work with a cold, but with a flu you may be too ill to leave your bed.

You probably have the flu if you get these symptoms suddenly and severely:
- Dry cough
- Sore throat
- Severe headache
- General muscle aches or backache
- Extreme fatigue
- Chills
- Fever up to 104°F
- Pain when you move your eyes, or burning eyes

Muscle aches and fatigue are the biggest signs of the flu. These are normally absent with a cold.

Prevention

To avoid getting the flu in the first place:

- Get plenty of rest, eat well, and exercise regularly. These will help you resist picking up the flu.
- Get a flu shot before each flu season if you are over age 65 or have a chronic medical illness that makes it hard for you to fight infection.

Questions to Ask

Do you have any of these problems with the flu:
- Inability to speak more than four or five words between breaths
- Purple lips
- Chest pain
- Spitting up blood
- Fever, stiff neck and lethargy

YES → SEEK EMERGENCY CARE

NO ↓

Do you have any of these problems with the flu:
- Earache
- Sinus pain
- Something thick coming from the nose, ears or chest

YES → SEE DOCTOR

NO ↓

Is your fever and/or other symptoms like coughing getting worse?

YES → CALL DOCTOR

NO ↓

Did a deer tick bite you 10 days to three weeks before you got sick? Were you in the woods or somewhere else where ticks live?

YES → CALL DOCTOR

NO ↓

Have you had the flu more than a week and not felt better after trying any of the Self-Care Procedures listed? Or have new symptoms developed?

YES → CALL DOCTOR

NO ↓

flowchart continued in next column

---

flowchart continued

Have you had any side effects from taking any prescribed or over-the-counter medicine?

YES → CALL DOCTOR

NO ↓

PROVIDE SELF-CARE

Self-Care Procedures

There's no cure for the flu. It has to run its course. Generally, if you are in good health, you can treat the flu on your own. The best way to do that is to get plenty of rest so your body can fight off the virus. Try these tips, too:

- Drink lots of hot (but not scalding) drinks. They soothe your throat, help unplug your nose and replace water you lose by sweating.
- Gargle with warm strong tea or warm salt water.
- Suck on cough drops or hard candy. (Do not give these to children under age five.)
- Let yourself cough if you are bringing up mucus. Your body needs to get rid of it. Ask you pharmacist for an over-the-counter expectorant.
- Don't drink milk or eat dairy foods for a couple of days. They make mucus thick and hard to cough up.
- Wash your hands often. Be sure to wash after blowing your nose and before cooking. This also helps stop you from giving the flu to others.
- Take aspirin, acetaminophen, ibuprofen or naproxen sodium. *Note: Do not give aspirin or any medication containing salicylates to anyone 19 years of age or younger, unless directed by a physician, due to its association with Reye's syndrome, a potentially fatal condition.*
- Use a cool-mist vaporizer or humidifier, especially in the bedroom. This will increase the moisture in the air. (Clean after each use.)

CHAPTER 12

SKIN PROBLEMS

Acne

Acne is a skin condition marked by pimples such as whiteheads, blackheads or even raised, red ones that hurt. These pimples show up on the face, neck, shoulders and/or back. Acne mostly strikes teenagers and young adults. For some, acne or the scars it can leave persist into adulthood. Acne results when oil ducts below the skin get clogged with secretions and bacteria. Factors that help cause acne include:

- Normal increase in the levels of the hormone androgen during adolescence
- Changes in hormone levels before a woman's menstrual period or during pregnancy
- Rich moisturizing lotions or heavy or greasy makeup
- Emotional stress
- Nutritional supplements that have iodine
- Cooking oils, tar or creosote in the air. Creosote is often used as a wood preservative.
- Putting pressure on the face by sleeping on one side of the face or resting your head in your hands
- Birth control pills, steroids, anticonvulsive medications and lithium (the latter used to treat some forms of depression)

Most cases of acne can be treated with the Self-Care Procedures listed. When this is not enough, a doctor can prescribe topical ointments, Retin A cream or gel and/or antibiotics.

Questions to Ask

Is your acne very bad and do you have signs of an infection with it (e.g., fever and swelling)?	**YES**	SEE DOCTOR

NO

flowchart continued in next column

flowchart continued

Are the pimples big and painful?	**YES**	CALL DOCTOR

NO

Have you tried the Self-Care Procedures and they haven't helped, or have the Self-Care Procedures made your skin worse?	**YES**	CALL DOCTOR

NO

PROVIDE SELF-CARE

Self-Care Procedures

Time is the only cure for acne, but these tips may help:

- Keep your skin clean. Wash often with plain soap and water.
- Use a washcloth. Work the soap into your skin gently for a minute or two. Rinse well.
- Use a clean washcloth every day. Bacteria, which can give you more pimples, love a wet washcloth.
- Try an astringent lotion, degreasing pads or a face scrub.
- Ask your doctor for the name of a good acne soap.
- Leave your skin alone! Don't squeeze, scratch or poke at pimples. They can get infected and leave scars.
- Use an over-the-counter lotion or cream that has benzoyl peroxide. (Some people are allergic to benzoyl peroxide. Try a little on your arm first to make sure it doesn't hurt your skin.) Follow the directions as listed.
- Wash after you exercise or sweat.

- Wash your hair at least twice a week.
- Keep your hair off your face.
- For men: Wrap a warm towel around your face before you shave. This will make your beard softer. Always shave the way the hair grows.
- Don't spend too much time in the sun.
- Don't use a sunlamp.
- Use only water-based makeup. Don't use greasy or oily creams, lotion or makeup.

Athlete's Foot

It smells bad. It's itchy. It's persistent. It's contagious. And it attacks the skin between the toes (usually the third and fourth). What is it? Fungus of the foot, better known as athlete's foot.

People usually get athlete's foot from walking barefoot over wet floors around swimming pools, locker rooms and public showers that are contaminated with the fungus, which feasts on moisture. Athlete's foot has these signs and symptoms:
- Moist, soft red or gray-white scales on the feet, especially between the toes
- Cracked, peeling, dead skin areas
- Itching
- Sometimes small blisters on the feet

Questions to Ask

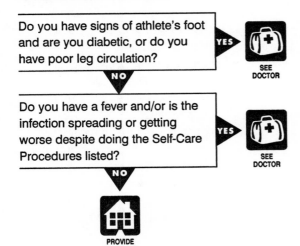

Do you have signs of athlete's foot and are you diabetic, or do you have poor leg circulation? **YES** → SEE DOCTOR

NO ↓

Do you have a fever and/or is the infection spreading or getting worse despite doing the Self-Care Procedures listed? **YES** → SEE DOCTOR

NO ↓

PROVIDE SELF-CARE

Self-Care Procedures

If you get athlete's foot:
- Wash your feet twice a day, especially between your toes, and dry the area thoroughly. Do not, however, use deodorant soaps.
- Apply an over-the-counter antifungal powder, cream or spray between your toes and inside of your socks and shoes.
- Wear clean socks made of cotton or wool. (Natural fibers absorb moisture.) Change your socks during the day to help your feet stay dry.
- Wear shoes that provide some ventilation, such as sandals or canvas loafers, whenever you can.
- Alternate shoes daily to let each pair air out between wearings.

Burns

Burns can result from dry heat (fire), moist heat (steam, hot liquids), electricity, chemicals or radiation (including sunlight). Treatment for burns depends on:
- The depth of the burn (whether it is first-, second- or third-degree)
- How much area of the body is affected
- The location of the burn

First-degree burns affect only the outer layer of skin. The skin area appears dry, red and mildly swollen. A first-degree burn is painful and sensitive to the touch. Mild sunburn and brief contact with a heat source (e.g., a hot iron) are examples of first-degree burns. First-degree burns should feel better within a day or two. They should heal in about a week if there are no complications. (See Self-Care Procedures.)

Second-degree burns affect the lower layers of the skin as well as the outer skin. They are painful and swollen and show redness and blisters. The skin also develops a weepy, watery surface. Examples of second-degree burns are severe sunburn, burns caused by hot liquids and a flash from gasoline. Self-Care Procedures can be used to treat many second-degree burns, depending on where the burns are and how much area is affected.

Third-degree burns affect the outer and deeper skin layers as well as any underlying tissue and organs. They appear black and white and charred. The skin is swollen and underlying tissue is often exposed. The pain felt with third-degree burns may be less than with first- or second-degree burns or none at all because nerve endings may be destroyed. Pain may be felt around the margin of the affected area, however. Third-degree burns usually result from electric shocks, burning clothes, severe gasoline fires, etc. They always require emergency treatment. They may result in hospitalization and sometimes require skin grafts.

Questions to Ask

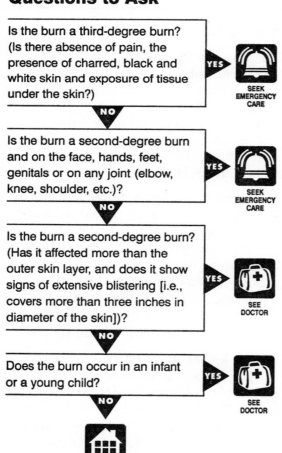

Is the burn a third-degree burn? (Is there absence of pain, the presence of charred, black and white skin and exposure of tissue under the skin?) **YES** → SEEK EMERGENCY CARE

NO

Is the burn a second-degree burn and on the face, hands, feet, genitals or on any joint (elbow, knee, shoulder, etc.)? **YES** → SEEK EMERGENCY CARE

NO

Is the burn a second-degree burn? (Has it affected more than the outer skin layer, and does it show signs of extensive blistering [i.e., covers more than three inches in diameter of the skin])? **YES** → SEE DOCTOR

NO

Does the burn occur in an infant or a young child? **YES** → SEE DOCTOR

NO

PROVIDE SELF-CARE

Self-Care Procedures

For first-degree burns:
- Cool the area right away. Place the affected area in a container of cold water or under cold running water. Do this for at least five to 10 minutes or until the pain is relieved. This will also reduce the amount of skin damage. (If the affected area is dirty, gently wash it with soapy water first.)
- Do not apply ice or cold water for too long a time. This may result in complete numbness leading to frostbite.
- Keep the area uncovered and elevated, if possible. Apply a dry dressing if necessary.
- Do not use butter or other ointments (e.g., Vaseline).
- Avoid using local anesthetic sprays and creams. They can slow healing and may lead to allergic reactions in some people.
- Call your doctor if after two days you show signs of infection (fever of 101°F or higher, chills and increased redness, swelling or pus in the infected area) or if the affected area is still painful.
- Take aspirin, acetaminophen, ibuprofen or naproxen sodium to relieve pain. *Note: Do not give aspirin or any medication containing salicylates to anyone 19 years of age or younger, unless directed by a physician, due to its association with Reye's syndrome, a potentially fatal condition.*

For second-degree burns (that are not extensive and are less than three inches in diameter):
- Immerse the affected area in cold (not ice) water until the pain subsides.
- Dip clean cloths in cold water, wring them out and apply them over and over again to the burned area for as long as an hour. Blot the area dry. Do not rub.
- Do not break any blisters that have formed.
- Avoid applying antiseptic sprays, ointments, creams. Once dried, dress the area with a single layer of loose gauze that does not stick to the skin. Hold in place with bandage tape that is placed well away from the burned area.

- Change the dressing the next day and every two days after that.
- Prop the burn area higher than the rest of the body, if possible.
- Call your doctor if there are signs of infection (e.g., fever of 101°F or higher, chills and increased redness and swelling or pus in the affected area) or if the burn shows no sign of improvement after two days.

Cold Hands and Feet

Some people wear mittens and heavy socks year-round, even in warm weather, indoors and out, because their hands and feet are always cold. A number of factors may be responsible, including:
- Poor circulation due to coronary heart disease
- Raynaud's disease (disorder that affects the flow of blood to the fingers and sometimes to the toes)
- Frostbite
- Working with vibrating equipment (like a jackhammer)
- A side effect of taking certain medications
- An underlying disease affecting blood flow in the tiny blood vessels of the skin. (Women smokers may be prone to this condition.)
- Stress

Symptoms to look for are:
- Fingers or toes turning pale white or blue, then red, in response to cold
- Tingling or numbness
- Pain during the white phase of discoloration

Questions to Ask

Have your hands or feet had prolonged exposure to subfreezing temperatures which may have resulted in frostbite? (Frostbite symptoms are tingling and redness followed by paleness [white or bluish appearance] and numbness of affected areas.)

YES

SEEK EMERGENCY CARE

NO

Do your hands or feet turn pale, then blue then red, and get painful and numb when exposed to the cold or stress?

YES

CALL DOCTOR

NO

PROVIDE SELF-CARE

Self-Care Procedures

If wearing gloves and wool socks and staying indoors where it's warm are nuisances and don't help, try these other warm-up tips:
- Don't smoke. It impairs circulation.
- Avoid caffeine. It constricts blood vessels.
- Avoid handling cold objects. Use ice tongs to pick up ice cubes, for instance.
- With fingers outstretched, swing your arms in large circles, like a baseball pitcher warming up for a game. This may increase blood flow to the fingers. (Skip this tip if you have bursitis or back problems.)
- Do not wear footwear that is tight-fitting.
- Wiggle your toes. It may help keep them warm as a result of increased blood flow.
- Practice a relaxation technique such as biofeedback.

Corns and Calluses

All too often, corns and calluses are the price we pay for neglecting our feet. Corns and calluses are very much alike; they just differ in where they occur.

Corns show up on the bony area on top of the toes and the skin between the toes. Corns feel hard to the touch, are tender and have a roundish appearance. A small, clear spot called a hen's eye may form in the center.

Calluses can occur on any part of the body that goes through repeated pressure or irritation. Common places are on the heels or balls of the feet, on the hands and on the knees. Calluses are flat, painless thickenings of the skin.

Corns and calluses form as a protective response. They are extra cells made in a skin area that gets repeated rubbing or squeezing from such things as:
- Footwear that fits poorly
- Activities that put pressure on the hands, knees and feet

If Self-Care Procedures do not get rid of corns and calluses, a family doctor or foot doctor (podiatrist) may need to be consulted. He or she can scrape away the hardened tissue and peel away the corn with stronger solutions. (Sometimes warts lie underneath corns and need to be treated, too.)

Questions to Ask

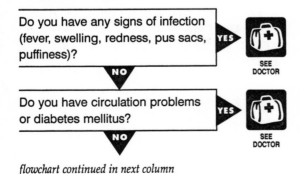

flowchart continued in next column

flowchart continued

Do you have one or both of these problems even after following the Self-Care Procedures:
- Continued or worse pain
- No improvement after two to three weeks

YES — CALL DOCTOR

NO — PROVIDE SELF-CARE

Self-Care Procedures

For corns:
Never pick at corns or use toenail scissors or clippers, a razor blade or any other sharp tool to cut off corns. You may injure your skin or trigger an infection. Instead:
- Get rid of shoes that fit poorly, especially if they squeeze your toes together.
- Soak your feet in warm water to soften the corn.
- Cover the corn with a protective, nonmedicated pad, usually available in drugstores. (A piece of foam rubber or moleskin will do in a pinch.)
- If the outer layers of a corn have peeled away, apply a nonprescription liquid of five to 10 percent salicylic acid and cover the area with a small bandage.
- Take your shoe to a shoe-repair person and ask that he or she sew a metatarsal bar onto your shoe to use when a corn is healing.

For calluses:
Never try to get rid of a callus by cutting it with a sharp tool. Instead:
- Soak your feet in warm water to soften the callus, then pat dry.
- Rub the callus gently with a pumice stone.
- Cover calluses with protective pads, available in drugstores.
- Check for poorly fitting shoes or other sources of pressure that may lead to calluses.

- Wear gloves if doing a hobby or work that puts pressure on the hands.
- Wear knee pads for activities that put pressure on your knees.

Cuts, Scrapes and Punctures

Cuts, scrapes and punctures all make you bleed, but there are differences among them:

- Cuts slice the skin open. Close cuts so they won't get infected.
- Scrapes hurt only the top part of your skin. They can hurt more than cuts, but they heal quicker.
- Punctures stab deep. Leave punctures open so they won't get infected.

You can treat most cuts, scrapes and punctures yourself. But you should go to the emergency room if you are bleeding a lot, or if you are hurt very badly. Blood gets thicker after bleeding for a few minutes. This is called clotting, which slows down bleeding. Press on the cut to help slow down the bleeding. You may have to apply pressure for 10 minutes for a bad cut. Sometimes a cut needs stitches. Stitches help the cut heal.

Questions to Ask

Is the bleeding from a cut, scrape or puncture severe:
- Is the person in shock?
- Does blood spurt from the wound?
- Has the person lost a lot of blood? (½ cup for an adult, less for a child)?
- Is the cut still bleeding a lot after 10 minutes of applied pressure?

 YES

SEEK EMERGENCY CARE

NO

flowchart continued in next column

---

flowchart continued

Does the cut need stitches?
- Is it deep? (Does it go down to the muscle or bone?)
- Is it on the head or face?
- Is it longer than an inch on a body part that bends such as an elbow, knee or finger?
- Do the edges of the cut skin hang open?

 YES

SEEK EMERGENCY CARE

NO

Is the cut still bleeding after 20 minutes of applied pressure, even if it is a small cut?

 YES

SEE DOCTOR

NO

Are there signs of infection a day or two after the injury:
- Fever of 101°F or higher
- Redness, swelling, tenderness at or around the wound
- Pain that gets worse instead of better
- Sick feeling

YES

SEE DOCTOR

NO

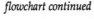
PROVIDE SELF-CARE

Self-Care Procedures

For cuts and scrapes:
- Clean around the wound with soap and water. (It's okay if some gets into the cut, but it may hurt.)
- Press on the cut to stop the bleeding. Do this for up to 10 minutes if you need to. Use a sterile bandage or a clean cloth. Use a clean hand if you don't have a bandage or cloth. (Dry gauze can stick to the wound, so try not to use it.) Don't use a Band-Aid.
- Press on the cut again if it keeps bleeding. Get help if it is still bleeding after 20 or more minutes. Keep pressing on it while you wait for help.

- Lift the part of the body with the cut higher than the person's heart. This slows down blood flow to that spot.
- Put first-aid cream on the cut when it is clean and dry. Use a sterile cloth or cotton swab. Try Polysporin, Neosporin or Johnson & Johnson First-Aid Cream.
- Put one or more Band-Aids on the cut. Do it this way:
  - Put the Band-Aid across the cut so it can help hold the cut together.
  - The sides of the cut should touch, but not too tightly. Don't let them overlap.
  - Don't touch the cut with your hand.
  - You can use a butterfly bandage if you have one.
  - Use more than one bandage for a long cut.
  - For scrapes, make a bandage from gauze and first-aid tape.
- Leave the bandage on for 24 hours. Change the bandage every day or two. Change it more often if you need to. Be careful when you take the bandage off. You don't want to make the cut bleed again. Wet gauze before you pull it off.
- Take aspirin, acetaminophen, ibuprofen or naproxen sodium for pain. Don't take aspirin every day unless your doctor tells you to. Aspirin can keep blood from clotting if you take it for a long time. *Note: Do not give aspirin or any medication containing salicylates to anyone 19 years of age or younger, unless directed by a physician, due to its association with Reye's syndrome, a potentially fatal condition.*
- Call your doctor right away if you have not had a tetanus shot in the last 10 years. Ask if you need a shot. If you don't have a doctor, call your local health department.

For punctures that cause minor bleeding:
- Let the wound bleed to clean itself out.
- Take out anything that caused the puncture. Use clean tweezers. (Dip the tweezers in alcohol for five minutes to clean them. Or you can hold a lit match to the ends.) *Don't pull anything out of a puncture wound if blood gushes from it or if it has been bleeding a lot. Get emergency care.*

- Wash the wound with warm water and soap, or take a bath or shower to clean it.
- Leave the wound open. You can cover it with a bandage if it is big or still bleeds a little.
- Soak the wound in warm, soapy water two to three times a day.

Eczema

Eczema is a chronic skin problem. A chronic problem lasts a long time and can come and go. Most people get eczema on the head, face, neck or the insides of their elbows, wrists and knees. It looks like small blisters and crusty scales. Both children and adults get eczema. It runs in families. People who have asthma often have eczema, too. Eczema is usually worse when you are a child. Then it gets better and may even go away. But some people have eczema all their lives. The following can worsen eczema:
- Wool clothes
- Sweating
- Stress
- Hard weather, especially very hot, humid weather
- Foods like eggs, milk, seafood and wheat
- Cosmetics, dyes, medicines, deodorants, skin lotions, permanent press clothes and other things you may be allergic to

Questions to Ask

Are there any signs of infection with the eczema? Do you have a fever? Or is the eczema very crusty and runny?

YES → SEE DOCTOR

NO ↓

Has the rash lasted for a long time?

YES → CALL DOCTOR

NO ↓

PROVIDE SELF-CARE

Self-Care Procedures

Your doctor should treat eczema. But you can do a lot to make it better:

- Don't take baths too often. Add bath oil to the water. Or take quick showers.
- Use warm water instead of hot when you take a bath or shower.
- Use a mild soap or no soap on the eczema.
- Stay away from wool clothes and blankets.
- Use a light, nongreasy lotion on your skin after you wash. Pick one that's unscented.
- Try to keep from sweating. For example, don't wear too many clothes for the weather.
- Wear rubber gloves when you do housework. Put a little cornstarch inside the gloves. Or try latex gloves lined with cotton.
- Stay away from food, chemicals, cosmetics and other things that make your eczema worse.
- Don't scratch! Scratching eczema only makes it worse. It can get infected. Keep your fingernails short.

Frostbite

Each year, 9,000 to 10,000 Americans suffer the painful effects of frostbite. Yet preventing frostbite is remarkably simple.

Frostbite looks like a serious heat burn, but it's actually body tissue that's frozen and, in severe cases, dead. Most often, frostbite affects the toes, fingers, earlobes, chin and tip of the nose (i.e., unprotected extremities that freeze quickly). Danger signs are pain (initially), swelling, white skin, then numbness and eventually loss of function and absence of pain. Blisters may also develop.

Sheer cold causes frostbite, but wind chill speeds up heat loss and increases the risk. Depending on how long you're exposed and how cold or windy it is, frostbite can set in very slowly, or very quickly, before you know what's happening.

Prevention

Needless to say, frostbite is something you should try to prevent. Here are some "keep warm" precautions to take if you expect to spend any length of time in the cold:

- Layer your clothing. Many layers of thin clothing are warmer than one bulky layer. The air spaces trap body warmth close to the skin, insulating the body against cold. For example, wear two or three pairs of light- or regular-weight socks instead of one heavy pair.
- Avoid drinking alcohol or smoking cigarettes. Alcohol causes blood to lose heat rapidly, and smoking slows down blood circulation to the extremities.
- Stay indoors as much as possible during periods of extremely low temperature and high wind.

Questions to Ask

After exposure to cold temperature, do you experience:
- Pain, swelling, tingling or burning of the skin
- Skin color changing from white to red to purple
- Blisters
- Shivering
- Slurred speech
- Memory loss

YES

SEEK EMERGENCY CARE

NO

PROVIDE SELF-CARE

Self-Care Procedures

The old advice that says you should treat frostbite by rubbing the area with snow or soaking it in cold water is wrong. This treatment is ineffective and dangerous. Instead:

- Warm the affected area by soaking in a tub of warm water (101° to 104°F) and an antiseptic solution.

- Stop when the affected area becomes red, not when sensation returns. (This should take about 45 minutes. If done too rapidly, thawing can be painful and blisters may develop.)
- Keep exposed area elevated.
- Never massage a frostbitten area.
- Protect exposed area from the cold. It is more sensitive to reinjury.

Hair Loss

Most men and women experience hair loss as they get older; indeed, most men have some degree of baldness by age 60. This is quite normal and affects some persons more than others, especially if baldness runs in the family. Sudden or abnormal hair loss could, however, result from:

- Taking certain medications (like some used in treating cancer, circulatory disorders, ulcers or arthritis)
- Following a crash diet
- Hormonal changes such as with menopause
- A prolonged or serious illness

Some medical conditions lead to hair loss. These need treatment. They include:

- Hypothyroidism and ringworm (the latter a fungal infection that affects the scalp and/or hairs themselves)
- Areata, which causes areas of patchy hair loss, but does not affect the scalp. This condition improves rapidly when treated, but can even disappear within 18 months without treatment. Doctors may prescribe a topical steroid to be used once or twice a day.

For cosmetic reasons, some older persons wear wigs or toupees. Surgical hair transplant operations and the prescription drug Rogaine are treatment options for both men and women, in very select cases. (Wear a hat or use a sunscreen with a sun protection factor [SPF] of 15 or more on the bald parts of your head when your head is exposed to the sun. The risk of sunburn and skin cancer on the scalp increases with baldness.)

Questions to Ask

Do you experience one or more of the following:
- Unexplained fatigue and weight gain
- Feeling cold
- Numbness and tingling of hands and feet
- Slow heartbeat
- Coarse skin and hair
- Deepened or hoarse voice
- Depression
- Decreased sex drive

SEE DOCTOR

 NO

Has the hair loss occurred suddenly and in patches on the head? Is the scalp affected in any way such as with red or gray-green scales?

SEE DOCTOR

NO

Are there signs of infection (e.g., redness, tenderness, swelling and/or pain) at the site of hair loss?

SEE DOCTOR

NO

Does the hair loss occur from uncontrollably pulling out patches of hair?

CALL DOCTOR

NO

Have you begun losing your hair only after taking prescribed medicine for high blood pressure, high cholesterol, ulcers or arthritis?

CALL DOCTOR

NO

Do you want to find out about hair implants or the prescription drug (Rogaine) to treat naturally occurring hair thinning or baldness?

CALL DOCTOR

NO

PROVIDE SELF-CARE

Self-Care Procedures

To protect your hair from damage and loss:
- Avoid damaging hair care practices or use them infrequently. These include braiding, corn rolling; bleaching, dyeing, perming, straightening; hot curling irons and rollers, hair dryers, especially on a high setting.
- Use gentle shampoos and conditioners.
- Let your hair dry by patting it with a towel or by air drying.
- If you hair is damaged, cut it short or change your hairstyle to one that requires less damaging hair care practices.
- Take measures (e.g., yoga and other relaxation techniques) to reduce anxiety if this results in pulling out patches of hair.
- Don't be taken in by fraudulent claims for vitamin formulas, massage oils, lotions or ointments that promise to cure baldness. No existing potion or ointment will produce a full head of hair. The only remedy that comes close is the prescription drug Rogaine, originally developed as a blood pressure medication. Rogaine has shown promising results for some (but not all) cases of baldness. This applies to both men and women.
- Ask your doctor for a substitution medication if you are taking one that has caused hair loss. (Obviously, this may not be feasible with anticancer drugs.)

Hives

Hives, or urticaria, are red, raised, itchy welts. They appear, sometimes in clusters, on the face, trunk of the body, and, less often, on the scalp, hands or feet. Like the Cheshire cat in *Alice's Adventures in Wonderland*, hives can change shape, fade, then rapidly reappear. A single hive lasts less than 24 hours, but after an attack new ones may crop up for up to six weeks. According to estimates, nearly 20 percent of Americans will get hives at some time in their lives.

Hives can be (but aren't always) an allergic response to something you touched, inhaled or swallowed. Some common causes of hives include:
- Reactions to medications such as aspirin, sulfa and penicillin
- Animal dander (especially from cats)
- Cold temperatures
- Emotional or physical stress (including exercise)
- Foods (especially chocolate, nuts, shellfish or tomatoes)
- Infections
- Inhalants (especially pollen, mold spores or airborne chemicals)
- Insect bites
- Rubbing or putting pressure on the skin
- Exposure to chemicals
- Malignant or connective tissue disease

The cause of hives is not always known. But if you can identify the triggers (try keeping a diary), you may be able to prevent future outbreaks.

Questions to Ask

Do you have any of these problems:
- Shortness of breath and breathing difficulties
- Wheezing, dizziness
- Swollen lips, tongue and/or throat

YES

SEEK EMERGENCY CARE

NO

Did hives start after recently taking a medication? **YES**

CALL DOCTOR

NO

Do you have itching that is constant and/or severe, or do you have a fever? **YES**

CALL DOCTOR

NO

PROVIDE SELF-CARE

Self-Care Procedures

Here are some tips for a case of ordinary, nonthreatening hives:

- Don't take hot baths or showers. Heat worsens most rashes and makes them itch more.
- Apply cold compresses or take a warm bath.
- Wear loose-fitting clothing.
- Relax as much as possible. Studies have shown that relaxation therapy and even hypnosis help ease the itching and discomfort of hives.
- Ask your doctor whether or not you should take an antihistamine and have him or her recommend one. Antihistamines can help relieve itching and suppress hives. (Keep in mind that antihistamines can cause drowsiness and may make it dangerous for you to drive or perform other tasks requiring alertness.)
- Avoid taking aspirin, ibuprofen or naproxen sodium. They may aggravate hives.

Insect Stings

Warm-weather months often include run-ins with bees, wasps, mosquitos, fleas, spiders, etc.

As you'd expect, most people who have been stung know it. The most common symptoms are limited areas of pain and swelling with redness and itching. Beyond that, the symptoms of bee and wasp stings vary, depending on where you're stung and how sensitive you are to the sting.

People who are allergic to insect stings may have a severe reaction known as anaphylaxis (even if they've never had an allergic reaction to a sting before). The symptoms of a severe anaphylactic reaction include generalized swelling, wheezing, difficult breathing, a severe drop in blood pressure and sometimes coma and death. Needless to day, this is a medical emergency, so if you start to have a serious reaction to a sting, get medical help immediately.

If you've ever experienced an allergic reaction to an insect sting in the past, you should carry an emergency medical kit containing epinephrine (a drug to stop the body-wide reaction) and a hypodermic needle to inject it, an antihistamine, and an identification bracelet that lets others know you're allergic to insect stings. Also, people who have had severe reactions to bee or wasp stings should consider allergy shots as a protective measure.

Prevention

How can you avoid getting stung?

- Keep foods and drinks tightly covered. (Bees love sweet foods and soft drinks.)
- Avoid sweet-smelling colognes. Wear an insect repellent instead.
- Avoid looking like a flower. Choose white or neutral colors that won't attract bees.
- Wear snug clothing that covers your arms and legs, and don't go barefoot.
- Be careful when making home improvements such as removing shutters from the house. Bees often build hives behind shutters.
- Treat animals for fleas.

Questions to Ask

If you are stung by an insect, do you have these problems:
- Generalized swelling
- Throat feels closed up
- Wheezing
- Difficulty in breathing and/or swallowing
- Slurred speech
- Confusion
- Hives all over the body

YES — SEEK EMERGENCY CARE

Use "Bee Sting Kit" if you have one

NO

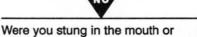

Were you stung in the mouth or on the tongue?

YES — SEEK EMERGENCY CARE

NO

flowchart continued on next page

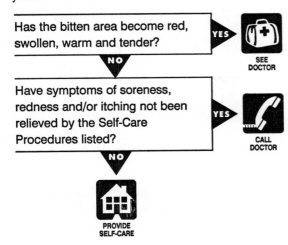

Has the bitten area become red, swollen, warm and tender? **YES** → SEE DOCTOR

NO

Have symptoms of soreness, redness and/or itching not been relieved by the Self-Care Procedures listed? **YES** → CALL DOCTOR

NO

PROVIDE SELF-CARE

Self-Care Procedures

- Gently scrape out the stinger, if there is one, as soon as possible.
- Don't pull or squeeze the stinger. It contains venom, and you'll end up re-stinging yourself. (This applies to bees only; yellow jackets, wasps and hornets don't lose their stingers.)
- Clean the sting area with soapy water.
- Apply ice to the sting immediately; it will minimize discomfort and prevent swelling and itching.
- Apply a paste made of meat tenderizer (like Accent) to the sting area. It seems to break down the protein in the venom.
- Take aspirin or acetaminophen, ibuprofen or naproxen sodium for the pain, and/or an antihistamine for the itching and swelling (provided you don't have to avoid these drugs for medical reasons). *Note: Do not give aspirin or any medication containing salicylates to anyone 19 years of age or younger, unless directed by a physician, due to its association with Reye's syndrome, a potentially fatal condition.*

Poison Ivy

During a walk through the woods—or even around your own garden—you can see birds, small animals and beautiful plants. But if you come in contact with poison ivy along the way, you may leave with an itchy rash as a souvenir of your trek.

The rash is caused by urushiol, a resin given off by poison ivy, poison oak and other related plants. Urushiol is an allergen, not a poison. Not everyone reacts to it. If you're allergic to the resin, however, and either touch the plant directly or come in contact with clothing or pets that have been exposed to it, you'll develop a rash of itchy, oozing blisters, sometimes with swelling.

Prevention

Knowing what poison ivy looks like is the key to prevent getting a rash. The old adage "Leaflets three, let it be" holds true.

Questions to Ask

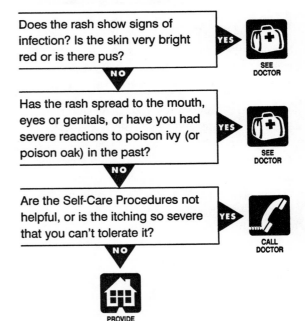

Does the rash show signs of infection? Is the skin very bright red or is there pus? **YES** → SEE DOCTOR

NO

Has the rash spread to the mouth, eyes or genitals, or have you had severe reactions to poison ivy (or poison oak) in the past? **YES** → SEE DOCTOR

NO

Are the Self-Care Procedures not helpful, or is the itching so severe that you can't tolerate it? **YES** → CALL DOCTOR

NO

PROVIDE SELF-CARE

Self-Care Procedures

If you have poison ivy, here's what to do:
- Remove and wash all clothes and shoes that have been contaminated. If an article isn't washable, isolate it in a ventilated area for three weeks.
- Bathe with soap and water, then apply rubbing alcohol to the exposed skin with cotton balls. Rinse with water afterward. Doing this within six hours of being exposed to the poison ivy may prevent a reaction.
- A rash may still develop two or three days after contact with the resin. If that happens, apply calamine lotion or 1 percent hydro-cortisone cream (available over-the-counter).
- Take an oral antihistamine such as diphen-hydramine (brand name Benadryl) to relieve itching.
- If weeping blisters develop, cover them with gauze and keep them wet with a solution of one tablespoon baking soda in one quart of water. (The fluid in blisters will not cause the rash to spread.)

Shingles

Shingles (herpes zoster) is a skin disorder triggered by the chicken pox virus (varicella zoster) that you first encountered as a child.

This virus is thought to lie dormant in the spinal cord until later in life. Shingles most often occurs between the ages of 50 and 70 in both men and women. Even though shingles is not as contagious as chicken pox, infants and people whose immunity is low should not be exposed to it. Besides aging, the risks for getting shingles increases with:
- Hodgkin's disease or other cancer
- Any illness in which infection-fighting systems are below par
- The use of anticancer drugs or any medica-tions that suppress the immune system (e.g., corticosteroids)
- Stress or trauma, either emotional or physical

Symptoms of shingles include:
- Pain, itching or tingling sensation before the rash appears.
- A rash of painful red blisters, which later crust over. Most often, the rash appears on the torso or side of the face and sometimes affects the eye. Only one side of the face or body is affected. Shingles is rarely present on both sides of the body.
- Though rare, fever and general weakness sometimes occur.

After the crusts fall off (usually within three weeks), pain can persist in the area of the rash. This usually goes away on its own after one to six months. Chronic pain can, however, last for months or years. The older you are, the greater the chances are that this is the case and the recovery time may also take longer.

Most cases of shingles are mild but can result in chronic, severe pain, blindness or deafness. So, to be on the safe side, if you get shingles let your doctor know.

Treatment for shingles includes:
- Pain relief with analgesics (codeine may sometimes be prescribed)
- Prescription medicines: Famvir and acyclovir (brand name Zovirax) oral and/or topical ointment. The sooner these medicines are started, the better the results.
- An antibiotic if the blisters become infected
- Antihistamines
- Corticosteroids
- Tranquilizers for a short time

Questions to Ask

With shingles, are you over 60 years of age, taking anticancer or other immunosuppressive drugs, or do you have a chronic illness? **YES** → **SEE DOCTOR**

NO ↓

Has the shingles affected your eyes? **YES** → **SEE DOCTOR**

NO ↓

flowchart continued on next page

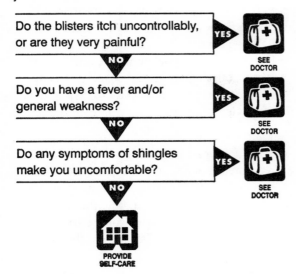

Do the blisters itch uncontrollably, or are they very painful? **YES** → SEE DOCTOR

NO ↓

Do you have a fever and/or general weakness? **YES** → SEE DOCTOR

NO ↓

Do any symptoms of shingles make you uncomfortable? **YES** → SEE DOCTOR

NO ↓

PROVIDE SELF-CARE

Self-Care Procedures

Following are things you can do (along with your doctor's treatment plan) to help relieve an active outbreak of shingles:

- Take an over-the-counter pain reliever such as acetaminophen, aspirin, ibuprofen or naproxen sodium, unless your doctor has given you prescription pain medicine. Ask your doctor which over-the-counter pain medicine is best for you. *Note: Do not give aspirin or any medication containing salicylates to anyone 19 years of age or younger, unless directed by a physician, due to its association with Reye's syndrome, a potentially fatal condition.*

- If possible, keep sores open to the air. Don't bandage them unless you live with or are around children or adults who have not yet had the chicken pox. They could pick up chicken pox from exposure to shingles.

- Don't wear restrictive clothing that irritates the area of the body where sores are present.

- Wash blisters, but never scrub them.

- Apply cool compresses, calamine lotion or baking soda to help alleviate the symptoms.

- Avoid drafty areas where you can get chilled.

Skin Rashes

Skin rashes come in all forms and sizes. Some are raised bumps; others are flat red blotches. Some are itchy blisters; others are patches of rough skin. Most rashes are harmless and clear up on their own within a few days. A few may need medical attention. The skin is one of the first areas of the body to react when exposed to something you or your child is allergic to.

The chart on page 92 lists information on some common skin rashes.

Questions to Ask

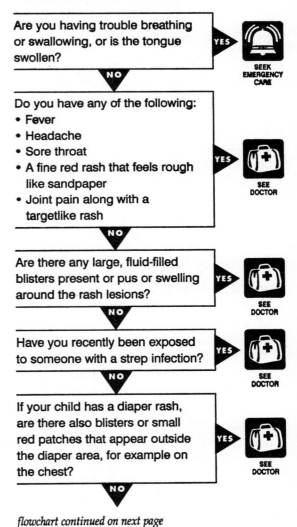

Are you having trouble breathing or swallowing, or is the tongue swollen? **YES** → SEEK EMERGENCY CARE

NO ↓

Do you have any of the following:
- **Fever**
- **Headache**
- **Sore throat**
- **A fine red rash that feels rough like sandpaper**
- **Joint pain along with a targetlike rash**

YES → SEE DOCTOR

NO ↓

Are there any large, fluid-filled blisters present or pus or swelling around the rash lesions? **YES** → SEE DOCTOR

NO ↓

Have you recently been exposed to someone with a strep infection? **YES** → SEE DOCTOR

NO ↓

If your child has a diaper rash, are there also blisters or small red patches that appear outside the diaper area, for example on the chest? **YES** → SEE DOCTOR

NO ↓

flowchart continued on next page

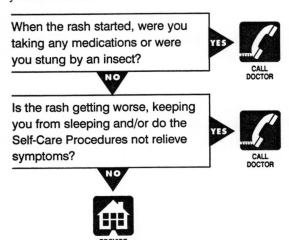

When the rash started, were you taking any medications or were you stung by an insect? **YES** → CALL DOCTOR

NO ↓

Is the rash getting worse, keeping you from sleeping and/or do the Self-Care Procedures not relieve symptoms? **YES** → CALL DOCTOR

NO ↓

PROVIDE SELF-CARE

Self-Care Procedures

Heat rash is best treated by staying in a cool, dry area. It will usually disappear within two to three days if you keep the skin cool. Things you can do:

- Take a bath in cool water, without soap, every couple of hours.
- Let your skin air dry.
- Apply calamine (not Caladryl) lotion to the very itchy spots.
- Put cornstarch in body creases such as inside elbows.
- Don't use ointments and creams that can block the sweat gland pores.

To treat diaper rash in a child:

- Change diapers as soon as they become wet or soiled (even at night if the rash is extensive).
- Wash your baby with plenty of warm water, not disposable wipes, to prevent irritating the skin. If the skin appears irritated, apply a light coat of zinc oxide ointment after the skin is completely dry.
- Keep the skin dry and exposed to air.
- Before putting on a fresh diaper, keep your baby's bottom naked on a soft, fluffy towel for 10 to 15 minutes.

- Put diapers on loosely so air can circulate under them. If disposable diapers are used, punch a few holes in them. Avoid ones with tight leg bands.
- Don't use plastic pants until the rash is gone.
- Wash cloth diapers in mild soap. Add ½ cup of vinegar to your rinse water to help remove what's left of the soap.

For temporary relief from the itchy rash typical of poison ivy, oak and sumac:

- As soon as possible, remove your clothes and shoes. Wash with soap and water to remove the plant oil from the skin. Rub the affected skin area with alcohol or alcohol wipes and then rinse with water. Wash all clothes and shoes you have on.
- Trim your nails. Try not to scratch. Keep busy with other activities.
- Soak the rash area in cool water or take baths with Aveeno (an over-the-counter colloidal oatmeal product) or put one cup of oatmeal in a tub full of water.
- Take a hot shower if tolerated. At first, the itching will get worse, but after a while it will stop, and the relief may last for hours. Repeat as soon as the itching starts again. Use calamine lotion every three to four hours.
- Apply a hydrocortisone cream. Put a very small dab of cream on the rash. Be careful not to rub and spread the poison. If you can see the cream on the skin, you've used too much. Repeat as needed every two to four hours. Do not use these creams near the eyes.
- Know how to recognize poison ivy, oak and sumac. Stay away from them.

Hives can be eased if you:

- Take an antihistamine such as Benadryl. Check the labels of cold medications that contain an antihistamine. Those that have diphenhydramine or chlorpheniramine are good choices. Know, though, that most antihistamines are likely to cause drowsiness.
- Cool off. Rub an ice cube over the hives, drape a washcloth dipped in cool water over the affected areas or take a cool-water bath.

- Rub your body with calamine lotion, witch hazel or zinc oxide.
- Find and eliminate the cause of the allergic reaction.

For cradle cap in babies:
- Use an antidandruff shampoo once a day, massaging your baby's scalp with a soft brush or washcloth for five minutes.
- Soften the hard crusts by applying mineral oil on the scalp before washing your child's hair. Be sure to thoroughly wash the oil out completely. Otherwise, the cradle cap condition may worsen.

To protect yourself from Lyme disease:
- Wear long pants tucked into socks and long-sleeve shirts when you walk through fields and forests. Light-colored, tightly woven clothing is best.
- Inspect yourself for ticks after outdoor activities.
- Remove any ticks found on the skin as follows:
  - Use tweezers to grasp the tick as close to the skin as possible.
  - Pull in a steady upward motion.
  - Try not to crush the tick because the secretions released may spread disease.
  - Wash the wound area and your hands with soap and water after removing ticks.
  - Save any removed ticks in a jar and take them to the doctor to aid in the diagnosis of Lyme disease.

The goals in treating chicken pox are to reduce and relieve the itching for comfort and to prevent scratching off the scabs which could start a secondary infection and/or leave scars.

For chicken pox in children:
- Encourage your child not to scratch the scabs. Keep him or her busy with other activities.
- Give your child a cool bath without soap, every three to four hours for the first couple of days at 15 to 20 minutes at a time. Add ½ cup of baking soda or colloidal oatmeal bath packet (e.g., Aveeno) to the bath water. Pat, do not rub, your child dry. Or dip a washcloth in cool water and place it on the itchy areas.
- Apply calamine (not Caladryl) lotion for temporary relief.
- Trim your child's fingernails to prevent infection caused by opened blisters. Scratching off the crusty scabs may leave permanent scars.
- Cover the hands of infants with cotton socks if they are scratching their sores.
- Wash your child's hands three times a day with an antibacterial soap, such as Safeguard or Dial, to avoid infecting the open blisters.
- Keep your child cool and calm. Heat and sweating make the itching worse. Also, keep your child out of the sun. Extra chicken pox will occur on parts of the skin exposed to the sun.
- Give your child Benadryl, an over-the-counter antihistamine, if the itching is severe or stops your child from sleeping. (See label for proper dosage.)
- Give your child acetaminophen (children's versions of the following: Tylenol, Tempra, Liquiprin, Datril, Anacin 3 or Panadol) for the fever. *Note: Do not give aspirin or any medication containing salicylates to anyone 19 years of age or younger, unless directed by a physician, due to its association with Reye's syndrome, a potentially fatal condition.*
- Give your child soft foods and cold fluids if he or she has sores in the mouth. Do not offer salty foods or citrus fruits that may irritate the sores.
- If necessary, have your child gargle with salt water (½ teaspoon to eight ounces of water) to help ease itching in the mouth.
- Reassure your child that the "bumps" are not serious and will go away in a week or so.

For adults with chicken pox:
- Follow any measures listed above that will bring relief. (Adults may take longer to recover from chicken pox and are more likely to develop complications. See your doctor if this is the case.)

For eczema, see Self-Care Procedures listed on page 83.

Common Skin Rashes

CONDITION OR ILLNESS	CAUSES	WHAT RASH LOOKS LIKE	SKIN AREAS AFFECTED	OTHER SYMPTOMS
Diaper Rash	Dampness and the interaction of urine and the skin	Small patches or rough skin, tiny pimples	Buttocks, thighs, genitals	Soreness, no itching
Cradle Cap	Hormones that pass through the placenta before birth	Scaly, crusty rash (in newborns)	Starts behind the ears and spreads to the scalp	Fine, oily scales
Heat Rash (Prickly Heat)	Blocked off sweat glands	Small red pimples, pink blotchy skin	Chest, waist, back, armpits, groin	Itching (may be a result of fever)
[1]Roseola	Herpes virus type-6	Flat, rosy red rash	Chest, abdomen	High fever 2 to 4 days before rash—child feels only mildly ill during fever
[1]Fifth Disease	Human parvovirus B19	Red rash of varying shades that fades to a flat, lacy pattern (rash comes and goes)	Red rash on facial cheeks; lacy rash can also appear on arms and legs	Mild disease with no other symptoms or a slight runny nose and sore throat
Eczema	Allergens	Dry, red, cracked skin, blisters that ooze and crust over. Sufficient scratching leads to a thickened rough skin.	On cheeks in infants; on neck, wrists, inside elbows and backs of knees in older children	Moderate to intense itching (may only itch first, then rash appears hours to days later)
[1]Chicken Pox[2]	Varicella/herpes zoster virus	Flat red spots that become raised resembling small pimples. These develop into small blisters that break and crust over.	Back, chest and abdomen first, then rest of body	Fatigue and mild fever 24 hours before rash appears—intense itching
[1]Scarlet Fever	Bacterial infection (streptococcal)	Rough, bright red rash (feels like sandpaper)	Face, neck, elbows, armpits, groin (spreads rapidly to entire body)	High fever, weakness before rash, sore throat, peeling of the skin afterward (especially palms)
[1]Impetigo	Bacterial infection of the skin	In infants, pus-filled blisters and red skin. In older children, golden crusts on red sores.	Arms, legs, face and around nose first, then most of body	Sometimes fever—occasional itching
Hives	Allergic reaction to food, insect bites, viral infection, drug or other substance	Raised red bumps with pale centers (resemble mosquito bites), shape, size and location of spots can change rapidly	Any area	Itching—in extreme cases, swelling of throat, difficulty breathing (may need emergency care)
Poison Ivy, Oak, Sumac	Interaction of oily resins of plant leaves with the skin	Red, swollen skin rash and lines of tiny blisters	Exposed areas	Intense itching and burning
Lyme Disease	Bacterial infection spread by deer tick bite(s)	Red rash that looks like a bull's-eye: raised edges surround the tick bites with pale centers in the middle. Rash starts to fade after a couple of days.	Exposed skin areas where ticks bite, often includes scalp, neck, armpit, groin	No pain, no itching at time of bite. Fever-rash occurs in the week following the bite(s).

[1] These conditions are contagious

[2] See pages 91 and 143-145 for more information on chicken pox

Sunburn

You should never get sunburned. It is not healthy, and it leads to premature aging, wrinkling of the skin and skin cancer.

Sunburn is caused by overexposure to ultraviolet (UV) light. This can be from the sun, sunlamps or even from some workplace light sources (e.g., welding arcs). Sunburn results in red, swollen, painful and sometimes blistered skin. Chills, fever, nausea and vomiting can occur if the sunburn is extensive and severe.

The risk for sunburn is increased for:
- Persons with fair skin, blue eyes and red or blond hair
- Persons taking some medications including sulfa drugs, tetracyclines, some diuretics and even Benadryl (an over-the-counter antihistamine)
- Persons exposed to industrial UV light sources
- Persons exposed to excessive outdoor sunlight

Sunburn can be prevented by using the following measures:
- Avoid the sun's rays between the hours of 10:00 a.m. and 4:00 p.m.
- Use sunblock with a sun protection factor (SPF) of 15 or more when exposed to the sun. The lighter your skin, the higher the SPF number should be. To be effective, sunscreen should be reapplied every hour and after swimming. Makeup is now available with sunscreening protection.
- Wear muted colors such as tan. Brilliant colors and white reflect the sun onto the face. Clothing is now available with sunscreening protection.
- Wear a hat when in the sun.

Questions to Ask

Are there any signs, even temporary ones, of dehydration, such as:
- Confusion
- Very little or no urine output
- Sunken eyes
- Wrinkled or saggy skin
- Extreme dryness in the mouth

YES

SEEK EMERGENCY CARE

NO

Do you have a fever of 102°F or higher or have severe pain or blistering with the sunburn?

YES

SEE DOCTOR

NO

PROVIDE SELF-CARE

Self-Care Procedures

- Cool the affected area with clean towels, cloths or gauze dipped in cool water or take a cool bath or shower.
- Take aspirin, acetaminophen, ibuprofen or naproxen sodium to relieve pain and headache and to reduce fever. *Note: Do not give aspirin or any medication containing salicylates to anyone 19 years of age or younger, unless directed by a physician, due to its association with Reye's syndrome, a potentially fatal condition.*
- Use an over-the-counter topical steroid cream such as Cortaid if the pain persists.
- Rest in a comfortable position, in a cool, quiet room.
- Drink plenty of water to replace fluid loss.
- Avoid using local anesthetic creams or sprays (e.g., Benzocaine or Lidocaine) or use sparingly because they cause allergic reactions in some people.

Varicose Veins

Varicose veins are swollen and twisted veins that look blue and are close to the surface of the skin. They are unsightly and uncomfortable. Veins bulge, throb and feel heavy. The legs and feet can swell. The skin can itch. Varicose veins may occur in almost any part of your body. They are most often seen in the back of the calf or on the inside of the leg between the groin and the ankle. Hemorrhoids (veins around the anus) can also become varicose. Causes and risk factors for varicose veins include:
- Obesity
- Pregnancy
- Hormonal changes at menopause
- Activities or hobbies that require standing for a long time
- A family history of varicose veins
- Past vein diseases such as thrombophlebitis (inflammation of a vein before a blood clot forms)

Medical treatment is not required for most varicose veins unless problems result, such as a deep-vein blood clot or severe bleeding which can be caused by injury to the vein.

Your doctor can take a venogram, a special X-ray of the vein, to tell if there are any problems. Surgery can be done to remove enlarged veins. Sclerotherapy can also be done on smaller veins. This procedure uses a chemical injection into the vein that causes it to close up. Other veins then take over its work. Both of these treatments, however, may bring only temporary success; following either, more varicose veins may develop.

Questions to Ask

Has the varicose vein become swollen, red, very tender or warm to the touch? **YES**
SEE DOCTOR

NO

flowchart continued in next column

flowchart continued

Are varicose veins accompanied by a rash or sores on the leg or near the ankle or have they caused circulation problems in your feet? **YES**
SEE DOCTOR

NO

PROVIDE SELF-CARE

Self-Care Procedures

To relieve and prevent varicose veins:
- Don't cross your legs when sitting.
- Exercise regularly. Walking is a good choice. It improves leg and vein strength.
- Keep your weight down.
- Avoid standing for prolonged periods of time. If your job or hobby requires you to stand, shift your weight from one leg to the other every few minutes.
- Wear elastic support stockings.
- Don't wear clothing or undergarments that are tight or constrict your waist, groin or legs.
- Eat high-fiber foods like bran cereals, whole grain breads, beans, fruits and vegetables to promote regularity. (Constipation contributes to varicose veins.)
- To prevent swelling, cut your salt intake.
- Exercise your legs. (From a sitting position, rotate your feet at the ankles, turning them first clockwise, then counterclockwise, using a circular motion. Next, extend your legs forward and point your toes to the ceiling, then to the floor. Then, lift your feet off the floor and gently bend your legs back and forth at the knees.)
- Elevate your legs when resting.
- Get up and move about every 35 to 45 minutes when traveling by air or even when sitting in an all-day conference. (Opt for an aisle seat in such situations.)

CHAPTER 13

DIGESTIVE PROBLEMS

Constipation

Constipation is when you have trouble having bowel movements. Abdominal swelling, straining during bowel movements, hard stools and the feeling of continued fullness even after a bowel movement are also signs of constipation. It can be very uncomfortable, but it usually doesn't signal disease or a serious problem. What factors cause or lead to constipation? A number of things do. These include:

- Not drinking enough fluids
- Not eating enough dietary fiber
- Not being active enough
- Using laxatives over a long period of time
- Taking certain medicines (e.g., some heart, pain and antidepressant medicines)
- Not going to the bathroom when you have the urge to have a bowel movement
- Medical problems such as hemorrhoids or an underactive thyroid gland

It is important to know that it is not necessary to have a bowel movement daily. What is more important is what is normal for you.

The "cure" for constipation generally consists of correcting the sort of habits that make bowel habits irregular. (See Self-Care Procedures.) You may also need to discuss measures with your doctor about medications and health conditions that could be causing you to be constipated.

Questions to Ask

Do you have any of these problems with the constipation:
- Fever
- Severe abdominal pain (especially located in the lower left section)
- Abdominal bloating
- Weight loss
- Very thin, pencil-like stools or blood seen in the stools

  YES → SEE DOCTOR

NO

Did you get constipated after taking prescribed or over-the-counter medicines and/or vitamins? **YES** → CALL DOCTOR

NO

Do you have persistent constipation despite using the Self-Care Procedures listed? **YES** → CALL DOCTOR

NO

 PROVIDE SELF-CARE

Self-Care Procedures

- Eat foods high in dietary fiber such as bran, whole-grain breads and cereals, fresh fruits and vegetables daily. They serve as natural stool softeners, thanks in part to their fiber content. One type of fiber absorbs water like a sponge, turning hard stools into large, soft easy-to-pass masses.
- Drink plenty of water and other liquids (at least eight glasses a day) to give the fiber plenty of water to absorb.

- Drink hot water, tea or coffee. These may help stimulate the bowel.
- Get plenty of exercise, to help your bowels move things along.
- Don't resist the urge to eliminate or don't put off a trip to the bathroom.
- Keep in mind that drugs such as antacids and iron supplements can be binding, and stay away from them if you get constipated easily. (Discuss this with your doctor first.)
- If necessary, for occasional constipation, you may need an over-the-counter stool softener, mild laxative or enema. (Check with your doctor ahead of time so you'll know what is best for you to take if and when you do get constipated.)

Ask your doctor about the use of "bulk-forming" laxatives such as Metamucil, Perdiem or Fiber Con. You may be able to use these daily, if necessary. Start out slowly and gradually increase how much you take. Also drink plenty of liquids with them. Bloating, cramping or gas may be noticed at first, but these symptoms should go away in a few weeks or less.

Do not use "stimulant" laxatives such as Ex-Lax, Dulcolax, Senokot or enemas, except occasionally, without your doctor's permission. In the long run, they can make you even more constipated, because your intestines can become lazy and won't work as well on their own. Long-term use of these laxatives can also lead to a mineral imbalance, cause problems with your body's use of other medicines and lower the amount of nutrients you absorb.

Diarrhea

Diarrhea is the frequent passing of watery, loose bowel movements. Almost everyone gets diarrhea once in a while. Usually, it lasts only a day or two and isn't serious. Many things can cause diarrhea:
- Infection by virus, bacteria or parasites
- Ingestion of bad water or spoiled food

- Food poisoning
- Allergies
- Emotional turmoil
- Too many laxatives
- Certain drugs (Antibiotics like tetracycline, Clindamycin and ampicillin can give you diarrhea.)
- Diverticulitis (a disease of the bowel)
- Inflammatory bowel disease, usually ulcerative colitis or Crohn's disease

Questions to Ask

If the person with diarrhea is a baby or child: Does the baby and/or child have any of these problems with the diarrhea:
- Sunken eyes
- Dry skin and dry mouth
- Dry diaper for more than 3 hours in a baby
- Passing no urine for more than 6 hours in a child
- Feeling weak and tired
- Very upset or cranky
- Weak cry

 YES

SEEK EMERGENCY CARE

NO

Does an adult have any of these problems with the diarrhea:
- Black stools
- Feeling very thirsty and not passing much urine
- Blood in the stool
- Severe pain in the stomach or buttocks
- Extremely dry mouth
- Wrinkled skin

YES

SEE DOCTOR

NO

Has the diarrhea lasted 48 hours or more? And/or does the person have a fever of 101°F or higher?

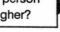 YES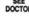

SEE DOCTOR

NO

flowchart continued on next page

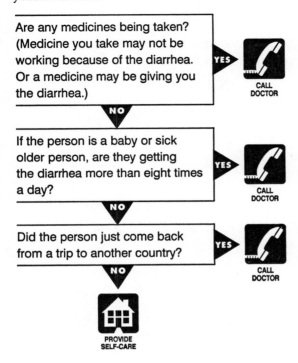

Are any medicines being taken? (Medicine you take may not be working because of the diarrhea. Or a medicine may be giving you the diarrhea.) **YES** → CALL DOCTOR

NO ↓

If the person is a baby or sick older person, are they getting the diarrhea more than eight times a day? **YES** → CALL DOCTOR

NO ↓

Did the person just come back from a trip to another country? **YES** → CALL DOCTOR

NO ↓

PROVIDE SELF-CARE

Self-Care Procedures

- Watch out for dehydration.
- Drink plenty of clear liquids. Sucking ice chips helps, too.
  - Adults should drink about two cups an hour unless they are vomiting.
  - Children over two years of age can drink up to two quarts a day. Ask your doctor for help if the child is thirsty, has cramps or seems weak or confused.
  - Ask your doctor what to give a child under two years of age. You can buy Pedialyte or Lytren (both are liquid and contain minerals) at most drugstores. While doctors recommend Pedialyte and Lytren for children, adults can take them, too.
- Here are some other clear liquids:
  - Water
  - Jell-O (liquid or solid)
  - Clear broth
  - Sodas like ginger ale, flat cola, 7-Up or Sprite
  - Weak tea with sugar

- Sport drinks like Gatorade
- A mixture of four teaspoons of sugar and one teaspoon of salt with four cups of water
- Don't drink very hot or very cold liquids.
- Don't drink apple juice, as it can worsen diarrhea, especially in children. Don't drink milk at this time either, as it too can worsen diarrhea.
- Eat little or no solids the first few days. Jell-O is okay. It counts as a clear liquid.

When the diarrhea starts to get better, follow these tips:
- Eat a B.R.A.T. diet. B.R.A.T. stands for ripe **b**ananas, **r**ice, **a**pplesauce and **t**oast. You should eat these foods before you try any others.
- Eat small amounts of soft foods like cooked potatoes. Stay away from meat, nuts, beans and dairy foods.
- Don't eat high-fiber foods like whole-grain bread or bran cereal.
- Don't eat foods that are hard to digest:
  - Raw fruits and vegetables
  - Fried foods
  - Sweets
- Don't drink coffee. (It's hard on your stomach.)
- Don't exercise too hard until the diarrhea is gone.
- Try an over-the-counter drug, such as Immodium A-D, Kaopectate or Pepto-Bismol. Wait at least 12 hours before taking these medicines, though. Let the diarrhea "run its course" to get rid of what caused it. *Note: Do not give aspirin or any medication containing salicylates, such as Pepto-Bismol, to anyone 19 years of age or younger, unless directed by a physician, due to its association with Reye's syndrome, a potentially fatal condition.*
- Follow these tips if the diarrhea was caused by an infection:
  - Wash your hands after you use the toilet.
  - Wash your hands before you cook.
  - Don't share towels with others.
  - Dry your hands with paper towels and throw the towels away.

Flatulence

Flatulence may be perfectly natural and something that everyone has at one time or another, but if you have more than your share, it's a major annoyance.

Where does all that gas come from? Often, it comes from swallowing air. It's also generated by intestinal bacteria that produce carbon dioxide and hydrogen (both odorless, by the way) in the course of breaking down carbohydrates and proteins in the food you eat. The minute quantities of other, more pungent gases gives flatus its characteristic odor. Eating certain foods, such as peas, beans and certain grains, produces noticeably more gas than eating other foods. All roughage in the diet will produce flatulence. A high-roughage diet, especially, will do this. When increasing dietary fiber in your diet, do so gradually. This will lessen the increase of flatus. Gas may signal a variety of other problems worth looking into:

- Lactose intolerance (inability to properly digest milk, cheese and other dairy products)
- Bacterial overgrowth in the intestines (often caused by certain antibiotics)
- Abnormal muscle contraction in the colon

Questions to Ask

Is the flatulence accompanied by severe steady pain in the upper abdomen, nausea and vomiting, or yellowing of the skin or eyes?

YES → SEE DOCTOR

NO ↓

Has the flatulence occurred only after taking a prescribed antibiotic?

YES → CALL DOCTOR

NO ↓

PROVIDE SELF-CARE

Self-Care Procedures

Common sense says eliminating food items that often cause gas (or eating them in small quantities) can go a long way toward reducing excess flatulence. Well-known offenders include:

- Apples
- Apricots
- Beans (dried, cooked)
- Bran
- Broccoli
- Brussels sprouts
- Cabbage
- Carrots
- Cauliflower
- Dairy products (for persons allergic to lactose)
- Eggplant
- Nuts
- Onions
- Peaches
- Pears
- Popcorn
- Prunes
- Raisins
- Sorbitol
- Soybean

(Eliminate or go easy on only the foods that affect you personally. With the exception of sorbitol, these foods listed are good sources of nutrients, so they should not be cut out altogether.)

- Keep a list of all the foods you eat for a few days and note when and the number of times you have gas. If you notice that you have excess gas after drinking milk, for example, try cutting down on it or eliminate it from your diet. See if the flatulence persists. Do the same for other suspecting foods.
- If you are lactose-intolerant use lactose-reduced dairy foods or add an over-the-counter (OTC) lactose-enzyme product such as Lactaid. These can be drops or tablets that you add to or consume with dairy products to help you digest the lactose they contain.
- Avoid swallowing air at mealtimes.
- The medication simethicone may help reduce flatulence by dispersing gas pockets (and preventing more from forming). It has no known side effects. Simethicone is available by prescription as well as over-the-counter under the brand name Mylicon.
- An OTC product called BEAN-O may curb flatulence caused by eating some foods.

Heartburn

Heartburn has nothing to do with your heart. The pain comes from stomach acid that backs up into your esophagus (the tube that connects your throat to your stomach). The esophagus passes behind the breastbone alongside the heart, so the irritation that takes place there feels like a burning feeling in the heart. All these things can cause heartburn:

- Taking aspirin, ibuprofen, naproxen sodium, arthritis medicine or cortisone
- Eating heavy meals
- Eating too fast
- Eating foods like chocolate, garlic, onions, peppermint, tomatoes or citrus fruits
- Lying down after a meal
- Smoking after eating
- Drinking coffee, even decaffeinated coffee
- Drinking alcohol
- Pregnancy
- Wearing tight clothing
- Being extremely overweight
- Swallowing too much air
- Stress
- Hiatal hernia (a bulging of the upper part of the stomach through the diaphragm)

Questions to Ask

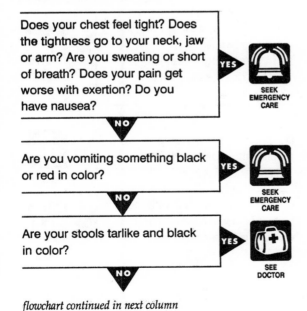

flowchart continued in next column

flowchart continued

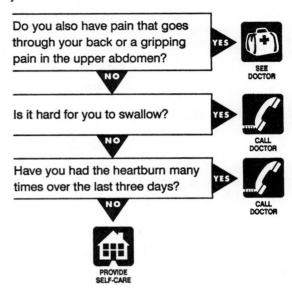

Self-Care Procedures

Stay away from foods you know give you heartburn. Try these tips, too:
- Sit straight. Stand up or walk around often. Don't bend over or lie down after you eat.
- Raise the head of your bed a little if you get heartburn at night. Try putting six-inch blocks under the head of your bed. Put them between the mattress and box springs or buy a wedge especially made for this.
- Keep your weight down. The top of your stomach can push up through your diaphragm if you're overweight. This can happen to pregnant women, too.
- Don't wear clothes that are tight around your stomach, like girdles.
- Eat small meals.
- Don't eat anything for three hours or less before going to bed.
- Take an over-the-counter (OTC) medicine, such as Pepcid AC Acid Controller or an antacid, if other treatments fail. Pepcid AC Acid Controller both relieves heartburn and can prevent it if taken one hour before eating meals which could result in heartburn. Antacids coat your stomach and fight stomach acid. Antacids come in liquid and tablet form. Talk to your doctor before taking antacids if you have heart disease, kidney disease or high blood pressure. Follow

package directions for Pepcid AC Acid Controller or antacids.

- Don't take baking soda. (Another name for baking soda is bicarbonate of soda or "bicarb" for short.) It seems to help at first, but the acid comes back worse later.
- Limit foods and drinks that contain air (e.g., baked goods, souffles, whipped cream and carbonated beverages)
- Don't drink through straws or bottles with narrow mouths.
- Don't smoke. It promotes heartburn.
- If you take aspirin, ibuprofen, naproxen sodium, arthritis medicines or cortisone, take them with food or milk.

Call your doctor if you have no relief after using Self-Care Procedures.

Hemorrhoids

Hemorrhoids are veins under the rectum or around the anus that are dilated or swollen. They are caused by repeated pressure in the rectal or anal veins. This pressure usually results from repeated straining to pass bowel movements. Rarely they result from benign or malignant tumors of the abdomen or rectum. The risk for getting hemorrhoids increases with:

- Constipation
- Low dietary fiber intake
- Pregnancy and delivery
- Obesity

Symptoms of hemorrhoids include:

- Rectal bleeding
- Rectal tenderness and/or itching
- Uncomfortable, painful bowel movements, especially with straining
- A lump that can be felt in the anus
- A mucous discharge after a bowel movement

Hemorrhoids are common and most people have some bleeding from them once in a while. Though annoying and uncomfortable, hemorrhoids are seldom a serious health problem. Reasons to seek medical treatment for hemorrhoids include:

- The presence of a painful blood clot in the hemorrhoid
- Excessive blood loss
- Infection
- The need to rule out cancer of the rectum or colon

If symptoms of hemorrhoids are not relieved with Self-Care Procedures listed or with time, medical treatment may be necessary. This includes:

- Cryosurgery which freezes the affected tissue
- Injecting a chemical into an internal hemorrhoid to shrink it
- Electrical or laser heat or infrared light to destroy the hemorrhoids
- Surgery called hemorrhoidectomy. One type, which requires general anesthesia, cuts out the hemorrhoids. Another, called ligation, uses rubber bands that are placed tightly over the base of each hemorrhoid causing them to wither away.

Questions to Ask

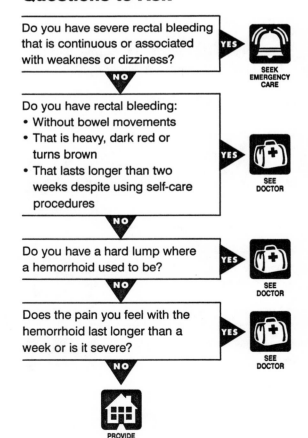

Do you have severe rectal bleeding that is continuous or associated with weakness or dizziness? **YES** → SEEK EMERGENCY CARE

NO

Do you have rectal bleeding:
- Without bowel movements
- That is heavy, dark red or turns brown
- That lasts longer than two weeks despite using self-care procedures

YES → SEE DOCTOR

NO

Do you have a hard lump where a hemorrhoid used to be? **YES** → SEE DOCTOR

NO

Does the pain you feel with the hemorrhoid last longer than a week or is it severe? **YES** → SEE DOCTOR

NO

PROVIDE SELF-CARE

Self-Care Procedures

- Take daily measures to produce soft, easily passed bowel movements such as:
  - Drink plenty of water and other fluids: at least 1½ to 2 quarts a day.
  - Eat foods with good sources of dietary fiber such as whole grain or bran cereals and breads, fresh vegetables and fruits.
  - Eat prunes and/or drink prune juice.
  - Add bran to your foods, if necessary (about three to four tablespoons per day).
  - Exercise regularly.
  - Pass a bowel movement as soon as you feel the urge. If you wait and the urge goes away, your stool could become dry and be harder to pass.
- Lose weight if you are overweight.
- Don't strain to have a bowel movement.
- Don't hold your breath when trying to pass a stool.
- Keep the anal area clean.
- Take warm baths.
- Use a sitz bath with hot water. A sitz bath device fits over the toilet. You can get one at a medical supply store or some pharmacies.
- Use moist towelettes or wet toilet paper after a bowel movement instead of dry toilet paper.
- Check with your doctor about using over-the-counter products such as:
  - Stool softeners
  - Zinc oxide preparations. Examples are Preparation H and Hemorid.
  - Medicated wipes such as Tucks
  - Medicated suppositories
- Don't sit too much because it can restrict blood flow around the anal area.
- Don't sit too long on the toilet.
- Don't read while on the toilet.
- For itching or pain, put cold compresses on the anus for 10 minutes up to four times a day.

Vomiting and Nausea

Vomiting is when you throw up what is in your stomach. Nausea is when you feel like you're going to vomit. Here are some common causes of nausea and vomiting:

- Viruses in the intestines (You can get diarrhea, too.)
- Morning sickness in pregnant women
- Some medications
- Spoiled food
- Eating or drinking too much

Some serious problems cause vomiting, too. Here are some of them:

- Appendicitis
- Brain tumors
- Acute glaucoma
- Stomach ulcers
- Hepatitis (inflammation of the liver)
- Meningitis (inflammation of membranes that cover the brain and spinal cord)

Questions to Ask

Do you have any of these problems along with the vomiting:
- Stiff neck, fever and headache
- Black or bloody vomit
- Severe pain in and around one eye
- Blurry eyesight
- A head injury that happened a short time ago

 YES

 SEEK EMERGENCY CARE

NO

Dehydration is when your body loses too much water. Do you have any of these signs of dehydration:
- Feeling confused
- Very little or no urine
- Sunken eyes
- Wrinkled or saggy skin

YES

 SEEK EMERGENCY CARE

 NO

flowchart continued on next page

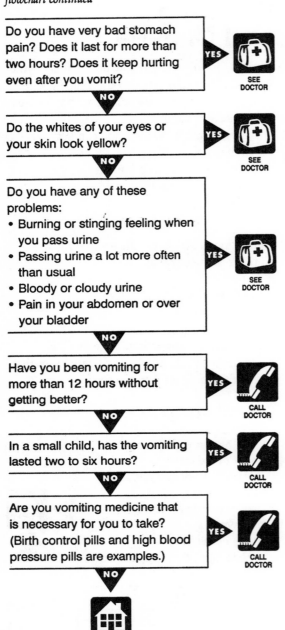

Do you have very bad stomach pain? Does it last for more than two hours? Does it keep hurting even after you vomit? — **YES** — SEE DOCTOR

NO

Do the whites of your eyes or your skin look yellow? — **YES** — SEE DOCTOR

NO

Do you have any of these problems:
• Burning or stinging feeling when you pass urine
• Passing urine a lot more often than usual
• Bloody or cloudy urine
• Pain in your abdomen or over your bladder
— **YES** — SEE DOCTOR

NO

Have you been vomiting for more than 12 hours without getting better? — **YES** — CALL DOCTOR

NO

In a small child, has the vomiting lasted two to six hours? — **YES** — CALL DOCTOR

NO

Are you vomiting medicine that is necessary for you to take? (Birth control pills and high blood pressure pills are examples.) — **YES** — CALL DOCTOR

NO

PROVIDE SELF-CARE

Self-Care Procedures

- Don't eat solid food until you stop vomiting.
- Drink clear liquids at room temperature (not too cold or too hot). Take small sips. Drink only one to two ounces at a time. Water, "flat" cola and ginger ale are good. Stir any carbonated beverages to get all the bubbles out before sipping them. Don't drink alcohol. Suck on ice chips if nothing else will go down.
- After you stop vomiting, you can go from clear liquid foods like Jell-O (any color but red) and broth to liquids like milk. Try soft foods after that (e.g., bananas, rice, apple-sauce and toast).
- Over-the-counter medications like Emetrol may help.
- Don't smoke.
- Don't take aspirin.
- Call your doctor if you don't get better or if the vomiting comes back.

CHAPTER 14

MUSCLE AND BONE PROBLEMS

Backaches

Most backaches come from strained muscles in the lower back. Other causes include back injuries such as a slipped or herniated disc, arthritis, osteoporosis and urinary tract infection. The goals of treatment are to treat the cause of the backache, relieve the pain, promote healing and avoid reinjury.

How to Avoid Back Pain

Lifting causes a lot of backaches. Here are some lifting Do's and Don'ts to help you avoid straining your back.

Do's:
- Wear good shoes with low heels, not sandals or high heels.
- Stand close to the thing you want to lift.
- Plant your feet squarely, shoulder width apart.
- Bend at the knees, not at the waist. Keep your knees bent as you lift.
- Pull in your stomach and buttocks.
- Keep your back as straight as you can.
- Hold the object close to your body.
- Lift slowly.
- Let your legs carry the weight.
- Get help or use a dolly to move something very heavy.

Don'ts:
- Don't lift if your back hurts.
- Don't lift if you have a history of back trouble.
- Don't lift something that's too heavy.
- Don't lift heavy things over your head.
- Don't lift anything heavy if you're not steady on your feet.

- Don't bend at the waist to pick something up.
- Don't arch your back when you lift or carry.
- Don't lift too fast or with a jerk.
- Don't twist your back when you are holding something. Turn your whole body, from head to toe.
- Don't lift something heavy with one hand and something light with the other. Balance the load.
- Don't try to lift one thing while you hold something else. For example, don't try to pick up a child while you are holding a grocery bag. Put the bag down, or lift the bag and the child at the same time.

Questions to Ask

Is the back pain *extreme* and felt across the upper back (not just on one side) and did it come on suddenly (within about 15 minutes) with no apparent reason such as an injury or back strain? *(Note: These may be symptoms of a dissecting aortic aneurysm.)* → **YES**

SEEK EMERGENCY CARE

NO ↓

Did the pain start inside your chest and move to the upper back? *(Note: You may be having a heart attack. The pain can be dull, and you may not feel it in the chest at all.)* → **YES**

SEEK EMERGENCY CARE

NO ↓

flowchart continued on next page

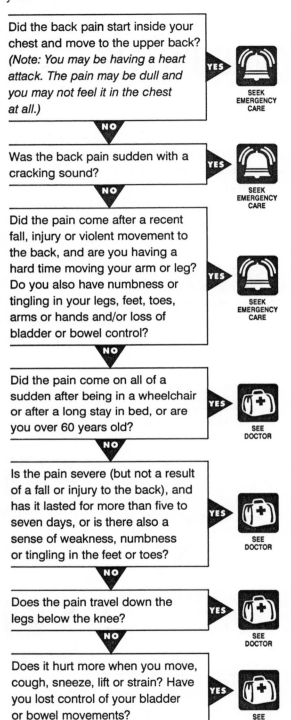

Did the back pain start inside your chest and move to the upper back? *(Note: You may be having a heart attack. The pain may be dull and you may not feel it in the chest at all.)* **YES** → **SEEK EMERGENCY CARE**

NO ↓

Was the back pain sudden with a cracking sound? **YES** → **SEEK EMERGENCY CARE**

NO ↓

Did the pain come after a recent fall, injury or violent movement to the back, and are you having a hard time moving your arm or leg? Do you also have numbness or tingling in your legs, feet, toes, arms or hands and/or loss of bladder or bowel control? **YES** → **SEEK EMERGENCY CARE**

NO ↓

Did the pain come on all of a sudden after being in a wheelchair or after a long stay in bed, or are you over 60 years old? **YES** → **SEE DOCTOR**

NO ↓

Is the pain severe (but not a result of a fall or injury to the back), and has it lasted for more than five to seven days, or is there also a sense of weakness, numbness or tingling in the feet or toes? **YES** → **SEE DOCTOR**

NO ↓

Does the pain travel down the legs below the knee? **YES** → **SEE DOCTOR**

NO ↓

Does it hurt more when you move, cough, sneeze, lift or strain? Have you lost control of your bladder or bowel movements? **YES** → **SEE DOCTOR**

NO ↓

flowchart continued in next column

Does it hurt, burn or itch when you pass urine? Do you have fever or vomiting with the pain? Do you have to go to the bathroom more often? Does your urine smell or have blood in it? **YES** → **SEE DOCTOR**

NO ↓

Is the pain felt on one side of the small of your back, just above the waist, and do you feel sick and have a fever of 101°F or higher? **YES** → **SEE DOCTOR**

NO ↓

Do you also have any of the following:
• Joint stiffness and pain
• Redness, heat or swelling in affected joints
• Cracking or grating sounds with joint movement

YES → **SEE DOCTOR**

NO ↓

 PROVIDE SELF-CARE

Self-Care Procedures

Rest - Resting the back can help treat the pain and avoid reinjury. Resting doesn't have to be in bed, but lying down takes pressure off your back so it can heal faster. Up to three days of bed rest is usually recommended. Your back muscles can get weak if you stay in bed longer than that. To make the most of rest:
• When you need to get up from bed, move slowly, roll on your side and swing your legs to the floor. Push off the bed with your arms.
• Get comfortable when you are lying, standing and sitting. For example, when you lie on your back, keep your upper back flat but your hips and knees bent. Keep your feet flat on the bed. Tip your hips down and up until you find the best spot.
• Take pressure off your lower back. Put a pillow under your knees or lie on your side with your knees bent.

Cold treatment - Cold helps with bruises and swelling. You can make a cold pack by wrapping ice in a towel. Use the cold pack for 20 minutes, then take it off for 20 minutes. Do this over and over for two to three hours a day. Lie on your back with your knees bent and put the ice pack under your lower back. Start as soon as you hurt your back. Keep doing it for three to four days.

Heat treatment - Heat makes blood flow, which helps healing. But don't use heat on a back strain until three to four days after you get hurt. If you use heat sooner, it can make the pain and swelling worse. Use a moist heating pad, a hot-water bottle, hot compresses, a heat lamp, a hot tub, hot baths or hot showers. Use heat for 20 minutes, then take the heat off for 20 minutes. Do this up to three hours a day. Be careful not to burn yourself.

Massage - Massage won't cure a backache, but it can loosen tight muscles.

Braces or corsets - Braces and corsets support your back and keep you from moving it too much. They do what strong back muscles do, but they won't make your back stronger.

Pain relief - Take aspirin, ibuprofen or naproxen sodium for pain. *Note: Do not give aspirin or any medication containing salicylates to anyone 19 years of age or younger, unless directed by a physician, due to its association with Reye's syndrome, a potentially fatal condition.* Acetaminophen will help the pain but not the swelling.

Don't overdo it after taking a painkiller. You can hurt your back more and then it will take longer to heal.

More tips:
- After two to three days of resting your back, try some mild stretching exercises to make stomach and back muscles stronger. Exercise in the morning and afternoon. (Always ask your doctor before starting an exercise program.)
- Don't sit in one place longer than you need to. It strains your lower back.

- Sleep on a firm mattress.
- Never sleep on your stomach. Sleep on your back or side, with your knees bent.
- If your back pain is chronic or doesn't get better on its own, see your doctor. He or she can evaluate your needs. A referral may be given to a physical therapist, a physiatrist (a doctor schooled in physical therapy) or a chiropractor.

Broken Bones

Bones break when stressed. An arm, leg or finger, like a tree limb twisted in the wrong direction, hit too hard or crushed by accident, can splinter and snap.

You may think that the body's 206 bones are as dry and lifeless as dead tree branches. Not so. Bones are made up of living tissue. New bone is added and old bone is broken down daily. This nonstop process continues from our first year until we hit 35 years. At about this age, our bones gradually start to thin as the building process slows down.

There are different kinds of broken bones. Some are called "greenstick" fractures because on the X-ray, the barely visible fracture resembles the pattern of a very young splintered twig. Other breaks are more complicated. Sometimes the bone protrudes through the skin and is called a compound fracture. Other times, the bone may separate partially or completely from the other half. Bones can also break in more than one place.

Bones in children are more pliable and resilient than those in adults. In most cases, children's bones are still growing, especially the long bones of their arms and legs. Damage to the ends of these bones should be monitored carefully because of the risk of stunting the bone's growth.

Bones in some senior citizens become dangerously thin with age. Many postmenopausal women and some elderly men suffer from osteoporosis, a condition in which the bones after age 35 begin losing their ability to absorb calcium from the blood. The bones in people with osteoporosis become brittle and break easily. The female hormone estrogen protects women from osteoporosis until they pass through menopause. Hormone replacement therapy (HRT) can help after menopause.

Broken bones need immediate treatment. Not only are they intensely painful, but unless properly cared for, broken bones may cause future deformities and limited movement.

Prevention

Make sure you and your child wear appropriate protective gear such as shoulder pads, knee pads and a helmet during sporting and recreation events.

Check that everyone in the car is wearing a seat belt. Don't start the engine until everyone has buckled up.

If you or your child likes to roller-blade, these tips may prevent injury:
- Always wear a helmet, elbow and knee pads and wrist guards.
- Skate on smooth, paved surfaces.
- Avoid skating at night.
- Learn how to stop.

If you are a postmenopausal woman, talk to your physician about hormone replacement therapy and:
- Exercise. Moderate, weight-bearing exercise such as walking, aerobics and dancing increases bone mass.
- Eat calcium-rich foods such as low-fat milk products, sardines, broccoli and calcium-fortified foods such as juices, cereals and breads.
- Take calcium supplements if necessary.
- If you smoke, quit. If you drink, limit the amount.

Questions to Ask

Is the person showing these signs of shock:
- Fainting
- Sweating, dizziness, increased thirst, rapid, weak pulse rate
- Cold, pale and clammy skin

YES SEEK EMERGENCY CARE

NO

Does the person have:
- A broken bone in the pelvis or thigh
- Cold, blue skin under the fracture
- Numbness below the fracture

YES SEEK EMERGENCY CARE

NO

If a rib is cracked, is the person also suffering shortness of breath? Is there any deformity at the fracture site? Is the pain so severe the person is unable to bear weight on the injured limb?

YES SEEK EMERGENCY CARE

NO

Is there a lot of bleeding and bruising around the injury?

YES SEE DOCTOR

NO

Is the injury still painful after 48 hours?

YES SEE DOCTOR

NO

 PROVIDE SELF-CARE

Self-Care Procedures

All broken bones require a doctor's attention. Do not try to set a broken bone yourself or try to push a protruding bone back under the skin. However, you may need to immobilize the injured limb until you get medical attention.

- A splint is a good way to immobilize the affected area, reduce pain and prevent shock.
  - Effective splints can be made from rolled-up newspapers and magazines, an umbrella, a stick, a cane and rolled up blankets. Place this type of item around the injury and gently hold it in place with a necktie, strip of cloth or belt. The general rule is to splint a joint above and below the fracture.
  - Lightly tape or tie an injured leg to the uninjured one, putting padding between the legs, if possible. Tape an injured arm to the chest, if the elbow is bent, or to the side if the elbow is straight, placing padding between the body and the arm.
  - For a broken arm, make a sling out of a triangular piece of cloth. Place the forearm in it and tie the ends around the neck so the arm is resting at a 90° angle.
  - Check the pulse in the splinted limb. If you cannot find it, the splint is too tight and must be loosened at once.
  - Check for swelling, numbness, tingling or a blue tinge to the skin. Any of these signs indicate the splint is too tight and must be immediately loosened to prevent permanent injury.
  - Keep the person quiet to avoid moving the injured area.
- Apply ice to the injured area to help reduce swelling and inflammation.
- Take aspirin (avoid if bleeding), ibuprofen or naproxen sodium to reduce pain and swelling. Acetaminophen will help the pain but not the swelling. *Note: Do not give aspirin or any medication containing salicylates to anyone 19 years of age or younger, unless directed by a physician, due to its association with Reye's syndrome, a potentially fatal condition.*

Shoulder and Neck Pain

Shoulder and neck pain is a common condition. Driving a golf ball, cleaning windows or reaching for a jar can strain and injure shoulder muscles and tendons, especially in people who are out of condition. Fortunately, this discomfort rarely suggests a serious condition. Causes of shoulder and neck pain include:

- Poor posture and/or unnatural sleeping positions. Sleeping on a soft mattress can give you a stiff neck the next morning.
- Tension and stress. When you feel tense, the muscles around your neck can go into spasms.
- Tendinitis, inflammation of a tendon, the cordlike tissue that connects muscles to bone. Left untreated, tendinitis can turn into "frozen shoulder," a stiff, painful condition that may limit your ability to use your shoulder.
- Bursitis, inflammation of the sac (bursa) that encases the shoulder joint. Bursitis can be caused by injury, infection, overuse, arthritis or gout.
- Osteoarthritis. Unlike rheumatoid arthritis, osteoarthritis develops from normal wear-and-tear of the joints as we age or from repeated injuries. Aging can cause the joints to wear out, producing bony spurs that can press on nerves and cause pain.
- Accidents and falls. Collarbones can break after falls or auto accidents.
- Motor vehicle accidents. You can develop a whiplash injury when your vehicle is hit from behind.
- Pinched nerve. Arthritis or an injury to your neck can pinch a nerve in your neck. Pain from a pinched nerve usually runs down the arm and one side only.

Sometimes shoulder and neck pain signals serious medical problems, especially with other symptoms such as stiff neck, sudden and severe headache, dizziness, chest pain or pressure and/or loss of consciousness.

Prevention

- Stretching and strengthening routines, especially before exercising, help prevent tendinitis. So can using the right equipment and following the proper technique.
- Avoid injuries to the shoulder by wearing seat belts in cars and trucks and using protective gear during sporting events.
- Avoid vigorous exercise unless you are fit. If you are out of condition, start to strengthen your muscles gradually, and slowly increase exercise intensity.
- Don't sleep on your stomach. You are likely to twist your neck in this position.
- Sleep on a firm mattress. Use a feather, polyester or special neck (cervical) pillow. Use a thinner pillow or none at all if you have pain when you wake up.

Keep the muscles in your shoulders strong and flexible to prevent injury. These exercises can help:

- Stretch the back of your shoulder by reaching with one arm under your chin and across the opposite shoulder, gently push the arm toward your collarbone with the other hand. Hold for 15 seconds. Repeat five times, then switch sides.
- Raise one arm and bend it behind your head to touch the opposite shoulder. Use the other hand to gently pull the elbow toward the opposite shoulder. Hold for 15 seconds. Repeat five times, then switch sides.
- Holding light weights, lift your arms out horizontally and slightly forward. Keeping your thumbs toward the floor, slowly lower your arms halfway, then return to shoulder level. Repeat 10 times.
- Sit straight in a chair. Flex your neck slowly forward and try to touch your chin to your chest. Hold for 10 seconds and go back to the starting position. Repeat five times.
- Sit straight in a chair. Look straight ahead. Slowly tilt your head to the right, trying to touch your right ear to your right shoulder. Do not raise your shoulder to meet your ear. Hold for 10 seconds and straighten your head. Repeat five times on this side and then on your left side.

Questions to Ask

Along with the shoulder and neck pain are you:
- Feeling pressure in your chest, especially on the left side
- Short of breath or having trouble breathing
- Nauseated and/or vomiting
- Sweating
- Anxious
- Having irregular heartbeats

 YES

SEEK EMERGENCY CARE

NO

Did you experience a serious injury that caused shoulder and/or neck pain that is not going away and/or is getting worse?

 YES

SEEK EMERGENCY CARE

NO

Do you have a stiff neck along with a severe headache, fever, nausea and vomiting?

YES

SEEK EMERGENCY CARE

NO

Do you have any of the following:
- Severe or persistent pain, swelling, spasms or a deformity in your shoulder
- A shoulder that is painful and stiff with reduced ability to move it
- Stabbing pain, numbness or tingling
- Pain, tenderness and limited motion in the shoulder

YES

SEE DOCTOR

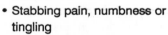 **NO**

Is the shoulder pain severe, interfering with your sleep? Is the shoulder stiff in the morning, swollen, tender or hard to move?

YES

CALL DOCTOR

NO

PROVIDE SELF-CARE

Self-Care Procedures

Unfortunately, no matter how careful people are, injuries do occur. Injured tendons, muscles and ligaments in any part of the body can take a long time to heal. Longer, in fact, than a broken bone. Don't ignore the aches and pains. Studies show that exercising before an injury has healed may not only worsen it, but may greatly increase the chance for reinjury.

Put the arm with the injured shoulder in a sling when you take the person to the doctor.

Treating tendinitis - Taking over-the-counter pain relievers such as aspirin, ibuprofen or naproxen sodium eases the pain and reduces inflammation. Acetaminophen eases muscle soreness but does not help with inflammation. *Note: Do not give aspirin or any medication containing salicylates to anyone 19 years of age or younger, unless directed by a physician, due to its association with Reye's syndrome, a potentially fatal condition.*

R.I.C.E. (rest, ice, compression and elevation) is the accepted treatment for tendinitis. While the pain could linger for weeks, with the proper and immediate treatment, it usually disappears in a few days.

R Rest the injured shoulder. Rest prevents further inflammation, giving the tendon a chance to heal. Resume your activities only after the pain is completely gone.

I Ice the injured area as soon as possible. Immediately putting ice on the injury helps to speed recovery because it not only relieves pain, but also slows blood flow, reducing internal bleeding and swelling.
   - Put ice cubes or crushed ice in a heavy plastic bag with a little water. You can also use a bag of frozen vegetables. Wrap the ice pack in a towel before placing it on the injured areas.
   - Apply the ice pack to the injured shoulder for 10 to 20 minutes. Reapply it every two hours and for the next 48 hours during the times you are not sleeping.

C Compress the shoulder injury. Wear a sling to keep the shoulder from moving, to prevent further damage and to remind yourself to take it easy.

E Elevate the shoulder whenever possible to further reduce the swelling.

The swelling is usually eased within 48 hours. Once the swelling is gone, apply heat to speed up healing, help relieve pain, relax muscles and reduce joint stiffness.
- Use a heating pad set on low or medium or a heat lamp for dry heat. Or use a hot-water bottle, heat pack or hot, damp towel wrapped around the injured area for moist heat. (Damp heat should be no warmer than 105°F.)
- Apply heat to the injured area for 20 to 30 minutes, two to three times a day.

Liniments and balms also relieve the discomfort of sore muscles. They provide a cooling or warming sensation. Although these ointments only mask the pain of sore muscles and do nothing to promote healing, massaging them into the shoulder increases blood flow to help relax the muscles.

Treating bursitis - Arthritis or any prolonged use of a joint can cause the pain and discomfort of bursitis. Fortunately, these flare-ups can be controlled by:
- Applying ice packs to the sore shoulders
- Taking a hot shower, using a heat lamp, applying a hot compress or heating pad to the affected shoulder or rubbing the area with a deep-heating liniment

Treating neck pain from whiplash injuries or pinched nerves - Always see a doctor anytime your motor vehicle is hit from the rear because the accident can cause a whiplash injury. The recommended treatment for whiplash injuries usually consists of using hot and cold packs, massage, exercises, sometimes a neck brace and pain-relieving medications such as aspirin, acetaminophen, ibuprofen and naproxen sodium. Once your symptoms subside, you can resume normal activity.

Note: Do not give aspirin or any medication containing salicylates to anyone 19 years of age or younger, unless directed by a physician, due to its association with Reye's syndrome, a potentially fatal condition.

After first checking with your doctor, you can ease neck discomfort by:

- Resting as much as possible by lying on your back
- Using cold and hot packs. See how to use them in the section on treating tendinitis.
- Improving your posture. When sitting, select a chair with a straight back and push your buttocks into the chair's back. When standing, pull in your chin and stomach.
- Using a cervical (neck) pillow or rolling a hand towel and placing it under your neck
- Avoiding activities that may aggravate your injuries
- Covering your neck with a scarf in cold weather
- Practicing some of the stretching and strengthening exercises listed under Prevention

Dealing with arthritis and osteoporosis -
See the section on arthritis on page 198 and the section on osteoporosis on page 214 for information on these conditions.

Sports Injuries

Common sports injuries include twisted ankles, painful joints and stiff, sore muscles. If you continue to exercise when injured, further damage can leave you laid up for weeks or months. "Break a leg" means good luck only in the theater world. Take care to avoid injury when exercising.

Prevention

Common sense can prevent many sports injuries. The top six typical injuries and ways to prevent them are:

Knee injury
- Avoid looking at your knees when standing or moving.
- Do not bend knees past 90° when doing half knee bends.
- Avoid twisting knees by keeping feet flat as much as possible (during stretches).
- Use softest surface available.
- Wear proper shoes with soft, flexible soles.
- When jumping, land with your knees bent.

Muscle soreness (a symptom of having worked out too hard or too long)
- Do warm-up exercises (e.g., those that stretch the muscles before your activity), not only for vigorous activities like running, but also even for less vigorous ones such as golf.
- Don't overdo it.
- In vigorous activities, go through a cool-down period. Spend five minutes doing the activity at a slower pace. For example, after a run, walk or walk/jog for five minutes so your pulse comes down gradually.

Blisters (due to poor fitting shoes or socks)
- Wear shoes and socks that fit well. (The widest area of your foot should match the widest area of the shoe. You should also be able to wiggle your toes with the shoe on in both a sitting and standing position.) The inner seams of the shoe should not rub against areas of your feet.
- Wear preventive taping, if necessary.

Side stitch (sharp pain felt underneath the rib cage)

- Don't eat or drink two hours prior to exercise.
- Do proper breathing by raising abdominal muscles as you breathe in.
- Don't "work through pain." Stop activity, then walk slowly.

Shin splints (mild to severe ache in front of the lower leg)

- Strengthen muscles in this region.
- Keep calves well-stretched.
- When using an indoor track, don't always run in the same direction.

Achilles tendon pain (caused by a stretch, tear or irritation to the tendon that connects the calf muscles to the back of the heel)

- Do warm-up stretching exercises before the activity. Stretch the Achilles tendon area and hold that position. Don't bounce. Wear proper-fitting shoes that provide shock absorption and stability. Avoid running shoes with a heel counter that is too high.
- Avoid running on hard surfaces like asphalt and concrete. Run on flat surfaces instead of uphill. Running uphill aggravates the stress put on the Achilles tendon.

Questions to Ask

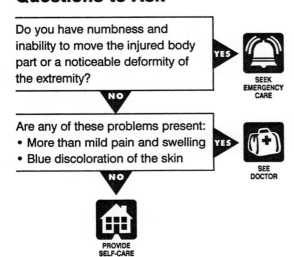

Do you have numbness and inability to move the injured body part or a noticeable deformity of the extremity? **YES** → SEEK EMERGENCY CARE

NO ↓

Are any of these problems present:
- More than mild pain and swelling
- Blue discoloration of the skin

YES → SEE DOCTOR

NO ↓

PROVIDE SELF-CARE

Self-Care Procedures

At the first sign of serious discomfort or pain, stop what you're doing and apply R.I.C.E.: rest, ice, compression and elevation. By following this easy-to-remember formula, you can avoid further injury and speed recovery.

R Rest the injured area for 24 to 48 hours.

I Ice the area for five to 20 minutes every hour for the first 48 to 72 hours, or until the area no longer looks or feels hot.

C Compress the area by wrapping it tightly with an elastic bandage for 30 minutes, then unwrap it for 15 minutes. Begin wrapping from the point farthest from the heart (distally) and wrap toward the center of the body (proximally). Repeat several times.

E Elevate the area to reduce swelling. Prop it up to keep it elevated while you sleep.

Also, doctors recommend taking aspirin, ibuprofen or naproxen sodium to reduce inflammation and pain. (Take these with a full glass of water or milk to prevent stomach irritation.) *Note: Do not give aspirin or any medication containing salicylates to anyone 19 years of age or younger, unless directed by a physician, due to its association with Reye's syndrome, a potentially fatal condition.*

Once the injured area begins to heal, do M.S.A. techniques. M.S.A. stands for movement, strength and alternate activities.

M Movement - Work at establishing a full range of motion as soon as possible after an injury. This will help maintain flexibility during healing and prevent the scar tissue formed by the injury from limiting future performance.

S Strength - Gradually strengthen the injured area once the inflammation is controlled and a range of motion is reestablished.

A Alternate Activities - Do regular exercise using activities that do not strain the injured part. This should be started a few days after the injury, even though the injured part is still healing.

Sprains and Strains

Sprains and strains happen when you over-stretch or tear a tissue between muscles and bones. Sprains and strains hurt and swell up. People often get sprains and strains when they fall, twist an arm or leg, play sports or push their bodies too hard.

How to Avoid Sprains and Strains

Here are some everyday tips:
- Clear ice from porches and sidewalks in winter.
- Wear shoes and boots with nonskid soles.
- Put handrails on stairways at home.
- Use rubber mats or strips in bathtubs and shower stalls. A support bar is a good idea, too.
- Make sure there are light switches near the doors in your house. Make sure outside doors and steps are lit at night.
- Put a night-light in the hallway between the bedroom and bathroom.
- Don't leave shoes, toys, tools or other things where people can trip over them.
- Clean floors with nonskid wax. Secure carpet to the floor.
- Make sure rugs have nonskid backing.
- Be careful when you use a ladder. Make sure it's steady. The ladder should be tall enough that you don't have to stand on the top three steps.

Here are some tips for preventing sports injuries:
- Start slowly. Begin an exercise program doing things that are easy for you. Build up gradually.
- Warm up your muscles with slow, easy stretches before you exercise. You should do this even for all sports. Don't overdo it. If muscles or joints start to hurt, ease up. Cool down after hard exercise. Slow down for about five minutes (e.g., five minutes of walking after running).

- Wear shoes that fit you and the exercise you do.

For more tips to avoid strains and sprains, see "The Do's and Don'ts of Lifting" on page 103.

What to Do for a Sprain or Strain

What should you do for a sprain or strain? That depends on how bad it is. Self-care may work. But you may need a doctor's help for a very bad sprain. The sprain may require a cast or even surgery.

Questions to Ask

Did you hurt yourself in a vehicular accident or fall from a high place?	YES	SEEK EMERGENCY CARE

 NO

Do you note any of these signs: • A bone sticking out • A crookedness or wrong shape to the injured body part • A grating sound from the bones in that part • A loss of feeling in the injured body part • An inability to move the injured body part or put weight on it	YES	SEEK EMERGENCY CARE

 NO

Do you note any of these signs: • The skin around the injury turns blue and/or feels cold and numb. • There is bad pain and swelling. • It hurts to press along the bone. • The pain is getting worse.	YES	SEE DOCTOR

 NO

PROVIDE SELF-CARE

Self-Care Procedures

Stop what you're doing as soon as you feel the sprain or strain. Then use R.I.C.E. to get better. (See R.I.C.E. in the section "Sports Injuries" on page 111.)

More tips:

- Take aspirin, ibuprofen or naproxen sodium every four hours for pain and swelling. Take it with food or milk so it won't bother your stomach. *Note: Do not give aspirin or any medication containing salicylates to anyone 19 years of age or younger, unless directed by a physician, due to its association with Reye's syndrome, a potentially fatal condition.*
- Remove your rings right away if you sprain your finger or hand. (If you don't and your fingers swell up, someone may have to cut the rings off.)
- Use crutches if you have a badly sprained ankle. They help keep the weight off of it so it can heal.

Call your doctor if the sprain or strain doesn't start to get better after four days.

CHAPTER 15

OTHER HEALTH PROBLEMS

Anemia

Are you tired and weak? Do the linings of your lower eyelids look pale? You may be anemic. But what does that mean?

It means that either your red blood cells or the amount of hemoglobin (oxygen-carrying protein) in your red blood cells is low.

Iron-deficiency anemia is the most common form of anemia. In the United States, 20 percent of all women of childbearing age have iron-deficiency anemia (compared to 2 percent of adult men). The primary cause is blood lost during menstruation. But eating too few iron-rich foods or not absorbing enough iron can make the problem worse.

The recommended dietary allowance for iron ranges from 6 milligrams (infants) to 30 milligrams (pregnant women). Yet one government source found that females between the ages of 12 and 50 (those at highest risk for iron-deficiency anemia) get about half of what they need. Pregnancy, breast-feeding a baby, and blood loss from the gastrointestinal tract (either due to ulcers or cancer) can also deplete iron stores. Anyone, older or younger, who has a poor diet is at risk for iron-deficiency anemia.

Folic-acid-deficiency anemia, another type of anemia, occurs when folic acid levels are low, usually due to inadequate dietary intake or faulty absorption. (This may often occur during pregnancy.)

Other less-common forms of anemia include pernicious anemia (inability of the body to properly absorb vitamin B_{12}), sickle-cell anemia (an inherited disorder) and thalassemia anemia (also inherited).

Alcohol, certain drugs and some chronic diseases can also cause anemia.

Questions to Ask

Do you have blood in your stools or urine or have black, tarlike stools with these problems:
- Light-headedness
- Weakness
- Shortness of breath
- Severe abdominal pain

 YES

SEEK EMERGENCY CARE

 NO

Are you dizzy when you stand up or when you exert yourself? **YES**

SEE DOCTOR

 NO

Do you have ringing in your ears? **YES**

SEE DOCTOR

 NO

For women:
- Do you have menstrual bleeding between periods?
- Has menstrual bleeding been heavy for several months?
- Do you normally bleed seven days or more every month?
- Do you suspect that you are pregnant?

YES

CALL DOCTOR

 NO

Do symptoms of anemia (paleness, tiredness, listlessness and weakness) persist despite using the Self-Care Procedures for at least two weeks? **YES**

CALL DOCTOR

 NO

PROVIDE SELF-CARE

Self-Care Procedures

The first step in treating iron-deficiency anemia is to pinpoint the cause. If it's due to a poor diet, you're in luck: Iron-deficiency anemia is not only the most common form of anemia, it's the easiest to correct if it's related to menstruation or deficiencies in diet. Folic-acid vitamin supplements may also be necessary.

You may need to:
- Eat more foods that are good sources of iron. Concentrate on green, leafy vegetables; lean, red meat; beef liver; poultry; fish; wheat germ; oysters; dried fruit and iron-fortified cereals.
- Boost your iron absorption. Foods high in vitamin C (e.g., citrus fruits, tomatoes and strawberries help your body absorb iron from food). And red meat not only supplies a good amount of iron, but it also increases absorption of iron from other food sources.
- Don't drink a lot of tea, as it contains tannins, substances that can inhibit iron absorption. (Herbal tea is okay, though.)
- Take an iron supplement. (Consult your health care professional for proper dosage.) While iron is best absorbed when taken on an empty stomach, it can upset your stomach. Taking iron with meals is less upsetting to the stomach. *(Note: Recent research is suggesting that high levels of iron in the blood may increase the risk for heart attacks. Check with your doctor before taking iron supplements.)*
- Avoid antacids, phosphates (which are found in soft drinks, beer, ice cream, etc.) and the food additive EDTA. These block iron absorption.

Chest Pain

Chest pain can result from a lot of things, including:
- Heart attack
- Lung problems like pneumonia, bronchitis or an injury
- Hiatal hernia
- Heartburn
- Shingles
- Pulled muscle
- Mitral valve prolapse. A common disorder, especially in women, in which the mitral valve of the heart fails to close properly. In most people this is not a serious problem.
- Anxiety
- Swallowing too much air

How do you know when you need medical help for chest pain? It's not always easy to tell. If you're not sure why your chest hurts, it's best to check it out. Getting help for a heart attack or lung injury could save your life.

Questions to Ask

Do you have any of these problems along with the chest pain:
- Pain that spreads to the arm, neck or jaw
- Pressure, especially on your left side
- Shortness of breath or trouble breathing
- Nausea and/or vomiting
- Sweating
- Uneven pulse or heartbeat
- Sense of doom

YES → SEEK EMERGENCY CARE

NO ↓

Did the chest pain come because you were injured badly? Does it hurt all the time and/or is it getting worse?

YES → SEEK EMERGENCY CARE

NO ↓

Do you have a history of heart problems or angina? Has your prescribed medicine stopped working? Have you had an operation or illness that has kept you in bed recently?

YES → SEEK EMERGENCY CARE

NO ↓

flowchart continued on next page

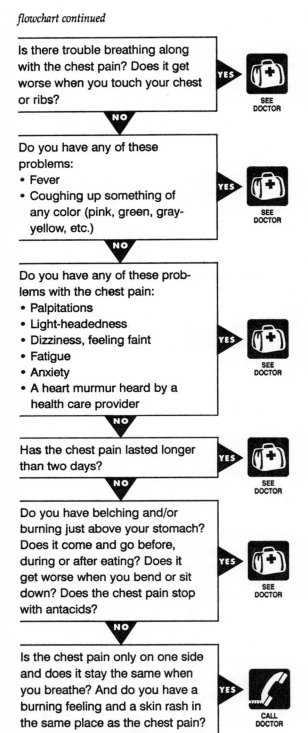

Is there trouble breathing along with the chest pain? Does it get worse when you touch your chest or ribs? **YES** → SEE DOCTOR

NO ↓

Do you have any of these problems:
• Fever
• Coughing up something of any color (pink, green, gray-yellow, etc.) **YES** → SEE DOCTOR

NO ↓

Do you have any of these problems with the chest pain:
• Palpitations
• Light-headedness
• Dizziness, feeling faint
• Fatigue
• Anxiety
• A heart murmur heard by a health care provider **YES** → SEE DOCTOR

NO ↓

Has the chest pain lasted longer than two days? **YES** → SEE DOCTOR

NO ↓

Do you have belching and/or burning just above your stomach? Does it come and go before, during or after eating? Does it get worse when you bend or sit down? Does the chest pain stop with antacids? **YES** → SEE DOCTOR

NO ↓

Is the chest pain only on one side and does it stay the same when you breathe? And do you have a burning feeling and a skin rash in the same place as the chest pain? **YES** → CALL DOCTOR

NO ↓

PROVIDE SELF-CARE

Self-Care Procedures

For a pulled muscle or small injury to your ribs:
• Don't strain the muscle or ribs when they hurt.
• Rest.
• Take aspirin, acetaminophen, ibuprofen or naproxen sodium for the pain. *Note: Do not give aspirin or any medication containing salicylates to anyone 19 years of age or younger, unless directed by a physician, due to its association with Reye's syndrome, a potentially fatal condition.*
• Call your doctor if the pain lasts more than two days.

For a hiatal hernia (a condition in which part of your stomach pushes up through your diaphragm):
• Lose weight if you are overweight.
• Eat five or six small meals a day instead of three large ones.
• Avoid tobacco, alcohol, coffee, spicy foods, peppermint, chocolate, citrus juices and carbonated beverages.
• Take antacids when you have heartburn and before you go to bed.
• Don't eat foods or drink milk two hours before going to bed.
• Don't bend over or lie down after eating.
• Don't wear tight clothes, tight belts or girdles.
• Raise the upper half of your bed three to four inches.

For anxiety and hyperventilation: Some people get chest pain when they feel anxious. Hyperventilation is when you breathe too much air into your lungs.
• Try to stay away from people and things that upset you.
• Talk about your anxiety with family, friends or clergy. (You may want to see a counselor or psychiatrist if this doesn't help.)
• Don't take too much aspirin or other drugs that have salicylates.
• Cover your mouth and nose loosely with a paper bag when you hyperventilate. Breathe in and out at least 10 times. Take the bag away and try breathing normally. Repeat breathing in and out of the bag if you need to.

Fainting

Just before fainting, you may feel a sense of dread followed by the sense that everything around you is swaying. You may see spots before your eyes. Then you go into a cold sweat, your face turns pale and you topple over.

A common cause of fainting is a sudden reduction of blood flow to the brain which results from a temporary drop in blood pressure and pulse rate. These lead to a brief loss of consciousness. A fainting victim may pass out for several seconds or up to 30 minutes.

There are many reasons people faint. Medical reasons include:
- Low blood sugar (hypoglycemia), which is common in early pregnancy
- Anemia
- Any condition in which there is a rapid loss of blood. This can be from internal bleeding such as with a peptic ulcer or a tubal pregnancy or ruptured ovarian cyst in females.
- Heart and circulatory problems such as abnormal heart rhythm, heart attack or stroke
- Eating disorders such as anorexia and bulimia
- Toxic shock syndrome

Other situations that can lead to feeling faint or fainting include:
- Any procedure in women that stretches the cervix such as having an IUD inserted, especially in women who have never been pregnant
- Extreme pain
- A sudden change in body position such as standing up too quickly (postural hypotension)
- Sudden emotional stress or fright
- Taking some prescription medications (e.g., some of the medicines that lower high blood pressure, tranquilizers, antidepressants and even some nonprescription medicines when taken in excessive amounts)

Know, also, that the risk for fainting increases if you are in hot, humid weather, are in a stuffy room or have consumed excessive amounts of alcohol.

Here are some do's and don'ts to remember if someone faints:

Do's:
- Catch the person before he or she falls.
- Place the person in a horizontal position with the head below the level of the heart and the legs raised to promote blood flow to the brain. If a potential fainting victim can lie down right away, he or she may not lose consciousness.
- Turn the victim's head to the side so the tongue doesn't fall back into the throat.
- Loosen any tight clothing.
- Apply moist towels to the person's face and neck.
- Keep the victim warm, especially if the surroundings are chilly.

Don'ts:
- Don't slap or shake anyone who's just fainted.
- Don't try to give the person anything to eat or drink, not even water, until he or she is fully conscious.
- Don't allow the person who has fainted to get up until the sense of physical weakness passes and then be watchful for a few minutes to be sure he or she doesn't faint again.

Questions to Ask

Is the person who fainted not breathing and does he or she not have a pulse? (See "CPR" on page 226.)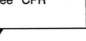

SEEK EMERGENCY CARE

flowchart continued on next page

Are signs of a heart attack also present with the fainting:
- Chest pain or pressure
- Pain that spreads to the arm, neck or jaw
- Shortness of breath or difficulty breathing
- Nausea and/or vomiting
- Sweating
- Rapid, slow or irregular heartbeat
- Anxiety

YES → SEEK EMERGENCY CARE

NO ↓

Are signs of a stroke also present with the fainting:
- Numbness or weakness in the face, arm or leg
- Temporary loss of vision or speech, double vision
- Sudden, severe headache

YES → SEEK EMERGENCY CARE

NO ↓

Did the fainting come after an injury to the head?

YES → SEEK EMERGENCY CARE

NO ↓

Do you have any of these with the fainting:
- Pelvic pain
- Black stools

YES → SEE DOCTOR

NO ↓

Have you fainted more than once?

YES → CALL DOCTOR

NO ↓

Are you taking high blood pressure medication or have you recently taken a new or increased dose of prescription medicine?

YES → CALL DOCTOR

NO ↓

PROVIDE SELF-CARE

Self-Care Procedures

Do these things when you feel faint:
- Lie down and elevate both legs.
- Sit down, bend forward and put your head between your knees.

If you faint easily:
- Get up slowly from bed or from a sitting position.
- Follow your doctor's advice to treat any medical condition which may lead to fainting. Take medicines as prescribed, but let your doctor know about any side effects so he or she can monitor your condition.
- Don't wear tight-fitting clothing around your neck.
- Avoid turning your head suddenly.
- Stay out of stuffy rooms and hot, humid places. If you can't, use a fan.
- Avoid activities that can put your life in danger if you have frequent fainting spells (e.g., driving and climbing high places).
- Drink alcoholic beverages in moderation.

For women who are pregnant:
- Get out of bed slowly.
- Keep crackers at your bedside and eat a few before getting out of bed. Try other foods such as dry toast, graham crackers and bananas.
- Eat small, frequent meals instead of a few large ones. Have a good food source of protein (e.g., lean meat, low-fat cheese and milk) with each meal. Avoid sweets. Don't skip meals or go a long time without eating.
- Don't sit for long periods of time.
- Keep your legs elevated when you sit.
- When you stand, as in a line, don't stand still. Move your legs to pump blood up to your heart.
- Take vitamin and mineral supplements as your doctor prescribes.
- Never lie on your back during the third trimester of pregnancy. It is best to lie on your left side. If you can't, lie on your right side.

Fatigue

Fatigue is feeling tired, drained of energy and exhausted. Fatigue makes it hard for you to do normal daily activities. Feelings of inadequacy, low motivation and little desire for sex can also be symptoms of fatigue. There are many causes of fatigue.

Possible physical causes that need medical care include:
- Chronic fatigue syndrome. The fatigue lasts for six months or more.
- Lupus (the systemic type)
- Multiple sclerosis
- Low thyroid
- Leukemia
- Having the AIDS virus
- Anemia
- Alcohol or drug abuse

Other physical causes include:
- PMS (See page 173.)
- Lack of sleep
- "Crash dieting" and poor eating, which result in vitamin and mineral deficiencies
- Migraine headaches
- Side effects from allergies or chemical sensitivities
- Living or working in hot, humid conditions
- Prolonged effects of the flu or a bad cold

Possible emotional causes and effects:
- Burnout (wearing yourself out by doing too much)
- Boredom
- Change (getting divorced, retiring from work, facing a big decision)
- Depression and/or anxiety

Treatment

The first thing to do is find the cause(s) of the fatigue so you know what to treat. It is important to keep track of any other symptoms that take place with the fatigue, so both physical and emotional causes can be identified and dealt with. For example, iron supplements can help with fatigue that results from iron-deficiency anemia.

Questions to Ask

Do any of these problems occur with the fatigue:
- Chest pain or tightness
- Shortness of breath
- Loss of balance or weakness, especially in one part or one side of the body
- Thoughts of suicide

YES → **SEEK EMERGENCY CARE**

 NO

Do you have any of these problems with the fatigue:
- Loss of weight or appetite
- Yellow skin and/or eyes
- Blurry or double vision
- Excessive vomiting
- Feeling anxious, and not being able to calm down

YES → **SEE DOCTOR**

 NO

Do you have two or more of these problems with the fatigue:
- Swollen lymph glands
- Sore throat
- Headache
- Painful swelling in the neck, armpit or groin
- Fever
- Night sweats
- Excessive thirst or urination

YES → **SEE DOCTOR**

 NO

flowchart continued on next page

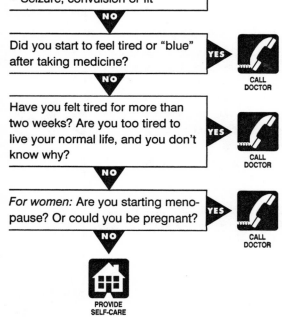

Do you have or have you had any of these problems:
- Arthritis or rheumatism for more than three months
- Fingers that get pale, numb or uncomfortable in the cold
- Mouth sores for more than two weeks
- Low blood counts from anemia, low white cell count or low platelet count
- A rash on your cheeks for more than a month
- Skin rash after being in the sun
- Pain for more than two days when taking deep breaths
- Fainting episode
- Seizure, convulsion or fit

YES → **SEE DOCTOR**

NO ↓

Did you start to feel tired or "blue" after taking medicine?

YES → **CALL DOCTOR**

NO ↓

Have you felt tired for more than two weeks? Are you too tired to live your normal life, and you don't know why?

YES → **CALL DOCTOR**

NO ↓

For women: Are you starting menopause? Or could you be pregnant?

YES → **CALL DOCTOR**

NO ↓

PROVIDE SELF-CARE

Self-Care Procedures

Eat better. Eating too much and "crash dieting" are both hard on your body. Don't skip breakfast. Stay away from rich, sugary snacks. Eat lots of food with iron, whole-grain breads and cereals, and raw fruits and vegetables.

Get more exercise. Exercise can give you more energy, especially if you sit all day at

work, and it can calm you, too. Try taking a walk in the open air if you feel tired. It can help.

Cool off. Working or playing in hot weather can sap you of energy. Living or working in a warm place without fresh air is bad, too. Rest in a cool, dry place as often as you can. Drink lots of water. Open a window when you can.

Rest and relax. A good night's sleep can make you feel much better. But you can relax during the day, too. Take breaks during your work day. Practice deep breathing or meditation.

Change your routine. Try to do something new and interesting every day. If you already do too much, make time for some peace and quiet.

Fever

A body temperature of 98.6°F is average. Many healthy people have temperatures a degree above or below average. Normal body temperature can be from 97° to 100°F.

Body temperature goes up and down during the day, too. Your temperature is usually lower in the morning and higher in the evening. You may think you have a fever when you don't, particularly if you drink something before taking your temperature.

You can take your temperature by mouth or rectum (the opening where you pass solid waste), under the arm or with a special thermometer that you put in your ear. A rectal reading is one degree higher than one by mouth or ear.

Here are some things that can change your body temperature:
- Wearing too many clothes
- Exercise
- Hot, humid weather
- Hormones (The hormones in a woman's body make her temperature go up at certain times of the month.)
- If none of these things is true and your temperature is over 99°F, you may have a fever. If your temperature is over 100°F, you

definitely have a fever. Adults probably don't need to do anything if they feel okay. But be sure to treat a fever if you don't feel good, or if it goes over 104°F (102°F in the elderly).

Questions to Ask

Do any of these problems accompany the fever:
- Seizure
- Listlessness
- Abnormal breathing
- Stiff neck
- Crankiness
- Confusion

 YES

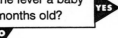
SEEK EMERGENCY CARE

 NO

Is the person with the fever a baby younger than two months old?

YES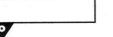
SEE DOCTOR

NO

In a child or adult: Does the person have any of these problems along with the fever:
- Ear pain
- Persistent sore throat
- Vomiting
- Diarrhea
- Pain or burning when passing urine
- Frequent urination

YES
SEE DOCTOR

NO

In an adult: Is the fever higher than 104°F, (102°F in an elderly person)? Has it lasted more than four days even though you have tried to bring it down?

YES
SEE DOCTOR

NO

Has the person had an operation recently? Or does the person have a long-term illness such as:
- Heart disease
- Lung disease
- Kidney disease
- Cancer
- Diabetes

YES
CALL DOCTOR

NO

flowchart continued in next column

---

flowchart continued

Has the fever done any of the following:
- Gone away for more than 24 hours and then returned
- Come soon after a visit to a foreign country
- Come after having a DTP or MMR shot and is present with dizziness

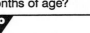 YES
CALL DOCTOR

 NO

Does the fever occur in a baby younger than 6 months of age?

YES
CALL DOCTOR

NO

In a child: Is the fever over 101°F by mouth or 102°F by rectum? Has it stayed there for 48 hours even if you have tried to bring it down?

YES
CALL DOCTOR

NO

PROVIDE SELF-CARE

Self-Care Procedures

- Drink fruit juice, water and other soft drinks.
- Take a sponge bath with warm water. (Don't sponge with alcohol. It doesn't help and the smell makes some people sick.)
- Take aspirin or acetaminophen. *Note: Do not give aspirin or any medication containing salicylates to anyone 19 years of age or younger, unless directed by a physician, due to its association with Reye's syndrome, a potentially fatal condition.*
- Rest in bed.
- Don't wear too many clothes or blankets.
- Don't do heavy exercise.

Headaches

Headaches are one of the most common, but most varied, health problems. Because there are many different reasons behind them, headaches are often difficult to treat without knowing the cause.

Kinds of Headaches

Tension, or muscular, headaches - Most people get this kind of headache. You feel a dull ache in your forehead, above your ears or at the back of your head. You get a tension headache when the muscles in your face, neck or head get tight. This can happen when you:
- Don't get enough sleep
- Feel "stressed out"
- Read
- Do boring work

Migraine headaches - Migraine headaches happen when blood vessels in your head open too wide or close too tight. Women are more prone to migraines than men, and people in the same family often get them. A migraine headache makes your head throb and feels like someone is hitting it with a big hammer. Many people also get these symptoms:
- One side of the head hurting more than the other
- Nausea or vomiting
- Visual problems such as seeing spots
- Light hurting the eyes
- Ringing in the ears

Sinus headaches - Your sinuses are behind your cheeks, around your eyes, and in your nose. You get a sinus headache when your sinuses swell up. Anyone is a candidate for sinus headaches; however, people with allergies often get them.

A sinus headache makes your forehead, cheekbones and nose hurt. It hurts more if you bend over or touch your face. You can get a sinus headache from:
- A cold
- Allergies

- Dirty or polluted air
- Other breathing problems

Headaches can also result from:
- A sensitivity to certain foods and drinks
- Alcohol
- Cigarette smoke
- Exposure to chemicals and/or pollution
- Poison
- Side effects from some medications

A headache can be a symptom of many health conditions, too. Some of these are:
- Allergies
- Depression
- Fever
- High blood pressure
- Low blood sugar
- Infections
- Shingles
- Dental problems

Less often, a headache can be a symptom of a serious health problem that needs immediate medical attention. Examples are:
- Acute glaucoma
- Stroke
- Tumor, blood clot or ruptured blood vessel (aneurysm) in the brain

How to Avoid Headaches

- Keep track of when, where and why you get headaches. If you find out what triggers a headache, try to stay away from it.
- Note early symptoms and try to abort a headache in its earliest stages (e.g., take pain medicine such as acetaminophen right away).
- Exercise at least two or three times a week. This helps keep headaches away.
- Avoids foods and drinks that give you a headache.

Foods That Can Cause Headaches

These foods give some people headaches:
- Alcoholic beverages, especially red wine
- Aspartame (the artificial sweetener in NutraSweet)

- Bananas
- Coffee, tea, cola and other drinks with caffeine
- Chocolate
- Cured meats
- Grapefruits, oranges and other citrus fruit
- Hot dogs, ham and other cured meats
- Food additives (e.g., MSG)
- Hard cheeses such as aged cheddar or provolone
- Nuts
- Onions
- Sour cream
- Vinegar

Questions to Ask

Is the headache associated with any of the following:
- A serious head injury
- A blow to the head that causes severe pain, enlarged pupils, vomiting, confusion or lethargy
- Loss of consciousness

YES 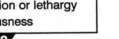 SEEK EMERGENCY CARE

NO

Is the headache associated with any of the following:
- Pain in one eye
- Blurred vision
- Double vision
- Slurring of speech
- Mental confusion
- Personality change
- A problem in moving arms or legs

YES SEEK EMERGENCY CARE

NO

Is the headache associated with fever, drowsiness, nausea, vomiting and a stiff neck?

YES SEEK EMERGENCY CARE

NO

Has the headache been occurring for more than two to three days and increased in frequency and intensity?

YES SEEK EMERGENCY CARE

NO

flowchart continued in next column

flowchart continued

Has the headache come on suddenly, and does it hurt more than others you have had?

YES SEE DOCTOR

NO

Has the headache occurred at the same time of day, week or month?

YES 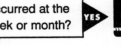 CALL DOCTOR

NO

Have you noticed the headache only after taking newly prescribed or over-the-counter medicines?

YES CALL DOCTOR

NO

PROVIDE SELF-CARE

Self-Care Procedures

When you have a headache:
- Rest in a dark, quiet room with your eyes closed.
- Rub the base of your head with your thumbs. Start under your ears and work back. Rub your temples, too.
- Take a hot bath.
- Put a cold washcloth over your eyes.
- Take aspirin, acetaminophen, ibuprofen or naproxen sodium right away. Painkillers work best when the headache starts. *Note: Do not give aspirin or any medication containing salicylates to anyone 19 years of age or younger, unless directed by a physician, due to its association with Reye's syndrome, a potentially fatal condition.*
- Relax. Try thinking of a calm, happy place. Breathe slowly and deeply.

Insomnia

Do you ever find yourself wide awake long after you go to bed at night? Well, you're not alone. An estimated 40 million Americans are bothered by insomnia. They either have trouble falling asleep at night, wake up in the middle of the night, or wake up too early and can't get back to sleep. And when they're not asleep, insomniacs worry about whether or not they'll be able to sleep. They are also irritable and feel fatigued during the day.

An occasional sleepless night is nothing to lose sleep over. But, if insomnia bothers you for three weeks or longer, it can be a real medical problem. Some medical problems that lead to insomnia include:
• Overactive thyroid gland
• Heart or lung conditions that cause shortness of breath when lying down
• Depression and anxiety disorders
• Allergies and early-morning wheezing
• Any illness, injury or surgery that causes pain and/or discomfort (e.g., arthritis) which interrupts sleep
• Sexual problems (e.g., impotence)
• Hot flashes that interrupt sleep
• Any disorder (urinary, gastrointestinal or neurological) that makes it necessary to urinate or have a bowel movement during the night
• Side effects of certain medications (e.g., decongestants and cortisone drugs)

Other factors that can lead to insomnia:
• Emotional stress
• Too much noise when falling asleep. This includes a snoring partner.
• The use of stimulants such as caffeine from coffee, tea or colas and stay-awake pills (e.g., NoDoz)
• A lack of physical exercise
• Lack of a sex partner

Questions to Ask

Do you have trouble falling or staying asleep because of any of the following:
• Pain or discomfort due to illness or injury
• Waking up to use the bathroom

YES → CALL DOCTOR

NO ↓

Has your sleep been disturbed since you began taking medication of any kind?

YES → CALL DOCTOR

NO ↓

Do you still have trouble sleeping after three weeks, with or without using the Self-Care Procedures listed?

YES → CALL DOCTOR

NO ↓

PROVIDE SELF-CARE

Self-Care Procedures

Many old-fashioned remedies for sleeplessness work for some people. Next time you find yourself unable to sleep, try these time-tested cures.
• Avoid caffeine in all forms after lunchtime. Coffee, tea, chocolate, colas and some other soft drinks contain this stimulant, as do certain over-the-counter and prescription drugs. Check the labels for content.
• Avoid long naps during the day. Naps decrease the quality of nighttime sleep.
• Avoid more than one or two servings of alcoholic beverages at dinnertime and during the rest of the evening. Even though alcohol is a sedative, it can disrupt sleep. Always check with your doctor about using alcohol if you are taking medications.
• Eat foods rich in the amino acid L-tryptophan (e.g., milk, turkey or tuna fish) before you go to bed. Eating carbohydrate-rich foods (e.g., cereal, breads and fruits) may help as well.

(Do not, however, take L-tryptophan supplements.)

- Take a long, warm bath before bedtime. This soothes and unwinds tense muscles, leaving you relaxed enough to fall asleep.
- Read a book or do some repetitive, tedious activity like needlework. Try not to watch TV or listen to the radio. These kinds of distractions may hold your attention and keep you awake.
- Make your bedroom as comfortable as possible. Create a quiet, dark atmosphere. Use clean, fresh sheets and pillows, and keep the room temperature comfortable (neither too warm nor too cool).
- Ban worry from the bedroom. Don't allow yourself to rehash the mistakes of the day as you toss and turn. You're off duty now. The idea is to associate your bed with sleep.
- Develop a regular bedtime routine. Locking or checking doors and windows, brushing your teeth and reading before you turn in every night prime you for sleep.
- Count those sheep! Counting slowly is a soothing, hypnotic activity. By picturing repetitive, monotonous images, you may bore yourself to sleep.
- Try listening to recordings made especially to help promote sleep. Check local bookstores.
- Don't take over-the-counter sleeping pills or the sleeping pills of friends or relatives. Only take sleep medicine with your doctor's permission.

Repetitive Motion Injuries

Repetitive motion injuries (RMIs), also called repetitive strain injuries (RSIs), can occur when you perform the same activity over and over for a long period of time either at work, at home, during sports and/or with hobbies. The types of movements involved include repeated:
- Drilling or hammering
- Lifting
- Pushing or pulling

- Squeezing
- Twisting
- Wrist, finger and hand movements

The injuries that result from RMIs are most often:

- **Tendinitis** - Constant wear and tear on wrists, elbows and shoulders may create tiny tears in the tendons that cause swelling, inflammation and pain. Tendinitis tends to hurt more at night than during the day. Treatment for tendinitis varies with the cause and how severe it is. Tennis elbow is one example of this RMI.

- **Carpal Tunnel Syndrome (CTS)** - Develops when tissues swell inside the carpal tunnel, a narrow tunnel in the wrist. Soft tissue in this tunnel enlarges, pinching the nerves that pass through it. Women are more likely to suffer from CTS than men because their carpal tunnel is usually smaller. Pregnancy can also increase a woman's risk for CTS, though the pain usually disappears after the baby is born. CTS is easier to treat and less likely to cause future problems if it is diagnosed early. (See "Preventing Wrist and Hand Injuries" on page 126.) Once diagnosed, CTS can be treated with:
  - Physical therapy
  - Wearing a splint at night
  - Taking anti-inflammatory medicines such as aspirin, ibuprofen or naproxen sodium
  - Changing the workplace set-up to reduce pressure in the wrist

Sometimes surgery is necessary if these measures aren't enough.

- **Eyestrain** - Results, for example, from working with video display terminals (VDTs). (See "Eye Strain from Computer" on page 57.)

- **Backaches** - Often due to poor posture or improper lifting. (See "Backaches" on page 103.)

Repetitive motion injuries are on the increase. Disability claims for these injuries have more than doubled in the last 10 years. In many cases, computers are the culprits. A writer or busy secretary, for example, often strikes the keys about 200,000 times a day; that's like your fingers taking a 10-mile walk. And chairs without lumbar support can cause back pain. Misplaced monitors can bring on eyestrain and stiff necks. No wonder many keyboard operators experience tendinitis and CTS.

Questions to Ask

Do you have chest pain and any of these problems:
- Pain that spreads to the arm, neck or jaw
- Pressure, especially on the left side
- Shortness of breath or trouble breathing
- Uneven pulse or heartbeat
- Sick stomach and/or throwing up
- Sweating
- Feeling anxious or light-headed

YES

SEEK EMERGENCY CARE

NO

Do you have:
- Severe or persistent pain, swelling or spasm
- Tenderness or stiffness and limited motion in the affected area such as the shoulder, arm or wrist.

YES

SEE DOCTOR

NO

Does pain in your hand, shoulder or wherever wake you from sleep?

YES

CALL DOCTOR

NO

Have you:
- Suffered pain, numbness and tingling in your hand for more than two weeks
- Been unable to make a fist for a couple of weeks

YES

CALL DOCTOR

NO

Do you frequently drop objects and does your thumb feel weak?

YES

CALL DOCTOR

NO

PROVIDE SELF-CARE

Self-Care and Preventive Procedures

For preventing wrist and hand injuries:

Whenever your hands and wrists perform the same activity time and again, you increase your risk for CTS and tendinitis. Change how you do a task and you may avoid some of these injuries.

- Keep your wrists straight when typing. Make sure your fingers are lower than your wrists and don't rest the heels of your hands on the keyboard. Buy a wrist rest for your keyboard to keep your wrists higher than the keyboard. Drop and tip your keyboard or try one of the new ergonomic keyboards.
- Do not hold an object in the same position for a long time. Even simple tasks such as hammering a nail can cause injury when performed over a period of time.
- Give your hands a break by resting them for a few minutes each hour.
- Lift objects with your whole hand or, better yet, with both hands. Gripping or lifting with the thumb and index finger puts stress on your wrist.
- If your line of work causes pain in your hands and wrists, see if you can share different jobs with someone else. Or alternate the stressful tasks with other work.
- Exercise your hands and wrists as often as possible.
  - Stretch your hands. Place them in front, spread your fingers as far apart as possible and hold for five seconds. Relax. Repeat five times with each hand.
  - Turn your wrists in a circle, palms up and then palms down. Relax your fingers and keep your elbows still. Repeat five times.
  - Drop your hands downwards. Shake your hands up and down, then sideways, until the tension is gone.

For carpal tunnel syndrome:
- Lose weight. CTS is linked to obesity; the excess tissue can press on the carpal tunnel.
- Take aspirin, ibuprofen or naproxen sodium, if you can tolerate it, to reduce the pain and

inflammation. *Note: Do not give aspirin or any medication containing salicylates to anyone 19 years of age or younger, unless directed by a physician, due to its association with Reye's syndrome, a potentially fatal condition.*

- Use a wrist splint. Many drug and medical supply stores carry splints that keep the wrist angled slightly back with the thumb parallel to the forearm. This position helps to keep the carpal tunnel open.

For preventing tendinitis:

- Use proper posture, proper equipment and proper technique when doing repetitive tasks.
- Take stretch breaks several times a day.
- Do stretching and strengthening exercises to keep your shoulder, neck and arm muscles strong and flexible.

See also: "Treating Tendinitis" on page 109; "Self-Care Procedures to Prevent Eyestrain" on page 57; "The Do's and Don'ts of Lifting" on page 103 and "Self-Care Procedures for Backaches" on page 104.

Snoring

Snoring is the sound heard when the airway is blocked during sleep. It can result from a number of things, including obesity, enlarged tonsils and adenoids, and deformities in the nasal passages. Smoking, heavy drinking, over-eating (especially before bedtime) and nasal allergies can lead to snoring by swelling the nasal passages and blocking the free flow of air. Also, persons who sleep on their backs are more likely to snore because the tongue falls back toward the throat and partly closes the airway. Nine out of 10 snorers are men, and most of them are age 40 or older.

Snoring can be merely a nuisance or can be a signal of a serious health problem, sleep apnea, which might even require surgery. In sleep apnea, breathing is stopped for a time period of at least 10 seconds, but usually 20 to 30 seconds or even up to one or two minutes during sleep. It is more common in men than in women and typically affects men who are middle-aged and older. It can result from:

- An obstructed airway. This is more common as people age, especially those who are obese or who have smoked for many years.
- A central nervous system disorder such as a stroke, a brain tumor or even a viral brain infection
- A chronic respiratory disease

Questions to Ask

Do you notice the following signs of sleep apnea during your daytime hours:
- Sleepiness or chronic daytime drowsiness
- Poor memory and concentration
- Irritability
- Falling asleep while driving or working
- Loss of sex drive
- Headaches

 YES

SEE DOCTOR

NO

Has your partner ever noticed that your breathing has stopped for 10 seconds or longer in the midst of snoring? YES

SEE DOCTOR

NO

Has snoring persisted despite using the Self-Care Procedures listed? YES

CALL DOCTOR

NO

PROVIDE SELF-CARE

Self-Care Procedures

- Sleep on your side. Prop an extra pillow behind your back so you won't roll over. Try sleeping on a narrow sofa for a few nights to get accustomed to staying on your side.
- Sew a large marble or tennis ball into a pocket on the back of your pajamas. The discomfort it causes will remind you to sleep on your side.

- If you must sleep on your back, raise the head of the bed by putting bricks or blocks between the mattress and box spring. Or buy a wedge especially made to be placed between the mattress and box spring to elevate the head section. Elevating the head prevents the tongue from falling against the back of the throat.
- If you are heavy, lose weight. Excess fatty tissue in the throat can cause snoring.
- Don't drink alcohol or eat a heavy meal within three hours before bedtime. For some reason, both seem to foster snoring.
- If necessary, take an antihistamine or de-congestant before retiring to relieve nasal congestion (which can also contribute to snoring). (Note: Older men should check with their doctors before taking decon-gestants. Decongestants that have ephedrine can cause urinary problems in older men.)
- Get rid of allergens in the bedroom such as dust, down-filled (feathered) pillows and bed linen. This may also relieve nasal congestion.
- Try over-the-counter "nasal strips." These keep the nostrils open and lift them up, keeping nasal passages unobstructed.

Urinary Incontinence

If you have urinary incontinence, you suffer from a loss of bladder control or your body fails to store urine properly. As a result, you can't keep from passing urine, even though you may try to hold it in. Urinary incontinence is not a normal part of aging, but often affects older persons because the sphincter muscles that open the bladder into the urethra become less efficient with aging.

Although you might feel embarrassed if you have urinary incontinence, you should never-theless let your doctor know about it. It could be a symptom of a disorder that could lead to more trouble if not treated and, in most cases, the problem is curable and treatable.

Two categories of urinary incontinence are acute incontinence and persistent incontinence.

The acute form is generally a symptom of a new illness or condition (e.g., bladder infection, inflammation of the prostate, urethra or vagina, and constipation).

Side effects of some medications such as water pills, tranquilizers and antihistamines can also result in acute urinary incontinence.

Acute urinary incontinence comes on suddenly. It is often easily reversed when the condition that caused it is treated.

Persistent incontinence comes on gradually over time. It lingers or remains, even after other conditions or illnesses have been treated. There are many types of persistent incon-tinence. The three types that account for 80 percent of cases are:

- **Stress Incontinence** - Urine leaks out when there is a sudden rise in pressure in the abdomen (belly). The amount ranges from small leaks to large spills. This usually happens with coughing, sneezing, laughing, lifting, jumping or running or with straining to have a bowel movement. Stress incon-tinence is more common in women than in men.

- **Urge Incontinence** - This inability to control the bladder when the urge to urinate occurs comes on suddenly, so there is often not enough time to make it to the toilet. This type typically results in large accidents. It can be caused by a number of things, including an enlarged prostate gland, a spinal cord in-jury, multiple sclerosis or Parkinson's disease.

- **Mixed Incontinence** - This type has ele-ments of both stress and urge incontinence.

Other types of persistent incontinence are:

- **Overflow Incontinence** - Constant dribbling of urine occurs because the bladder overfills. This may be due to an enlarged prostate, diabetes or multiple sclerosis.

- **Functional Incontinence** - With this, a person has trouble getting to the bathroom fast enough, even though he or she has bladder control. This can happen in a person who is physically challenged.

- **Total Incontinence** - In this rare type, with complete loss of bladder control, urine leakage can be continual.

Care and treatment for urinary incontinence will depend on the type and cause(s). The first step is to find out if there is an underlying problem and to correct it. Treatment can also include pelvic floor exercises, also called Kegel exercises, and other Self-Care Procedures, along with medication, collagen injections (for a certain type of stress incontinence) or surgery to correct the specific problem.

Your primary doctor may evaluate and treat your incontinence or send you to a urologist, a doctor who specializes in treating problems of the bladder and urinary tract.

Questions to Ask

Have you lost control of your bladder after an injury to your spine or back?

 YES
SEEK EMERGENCY CARE

 NO

Does your loss of bladder control come with any of these symptoms:
- Loss of consciousness
- Inability to speak or slurred speech
- Loss of sight, double or blurred vision
- Sudden, severe headaches
- Paralysis, weakness or loss of sensation in an arm, or leg and/or the face on the same side of the body
- Change in personality, behavior and/or emotions
- Confusion and dizziness

YES
SEEK EMERGENCY CARE

NO

flowchart continued in next column

flowchart continued

Is the loss of bladder control more than temporary after surgery or an abdominal injury?

 YES
SEE DOCTOR

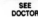 NO

Do you have any of these problems with loss of bladder control:
- Fever and shaking chills
- Back pain (sometimes severe) in one or both sides of the lower back or just at your midline
- Burning, frequent urination
- Blood in the urine or cloudy urine
- Abdominal pain
- Nausea or vomiting

YES
SEE DOCTOR

 NO

With the loss of bladder control, do you have diabetes or symptoms of diabetes such as:
- Extreme thirst
- Unusual hunger
- Excessive loss or gain in weight
- Blurred vision
- Easy fatigue, drowsiness
- Slow healing of cuts and/or infections

YES
SEE DOCTOR

 NO

If you are a man, do you:
- Dribble urine and/or feel the need to urinate again after you have finished urinating
- Void small amounts of urine often during the day
- Have to urinate while sleeping
- Have an intense and sudden need to urinate often
- Have a slow, weak or interrupted stream of urine

YES
SEE DOCTOR

 NO

Do you leak urine when you cough, sneeze, laugh, jump, run or lift heavy objects?

YES
CALL DOCTOR

 NO

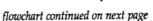

flowchart continued on next page

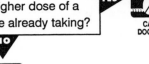

CALL DOCTOR

Did you lose some bladder control only after taking a new medicine or after taking a higher dose of a medicine you were already taking?

YES

NO

PROVIDE SELF-CARE

Self-Care Procedures

- Do Kegel exercises to strengthen your pelvic floor muscles. They can help treat or cure stress incontinence. Even elderly women who have leaked urine for years can benefit greatly from these exercises. Here's how to do them:
  - First, identify where your pelvic floor muscles are. One way to do this is to start to urinate, then hold back and try to stop. If you can slow the stream of urine, even a little, you are using the right muscles. You should feel muscles squeezing around your urethra and anus.
  - Next, relax your body, close your eyes and just imagine that you going to urinate and then hold back from doing so. You should feel the muscles squeeze like you did in the step before this one.
  - Squeeze the muscles for three seconds and then relax them for three seconds. When you squeeze and relax, count slowly. Start out doing this three times a day. Gradually work up to three sets of 10 contractions, holding each one for 10 seconds at a time. You can do them in lying, sitting and/or standing positions.
  - Women can also use pelvic weights prescribed by their doctor. A women inserts a weighted cone into the vagina and squeezes the correct muscles to keep the weight from falling out.
  - When you do these exercises:
    —Do not tense the muscles in your belly or buttocks.

—Do not hold your breath, clench your fists or teeth or make a face.
    —If you are not sure you're doing the exercise right, consult your doctor.
- Squeeze your pelvic floor muscles right before and during whatever it is (coughing, sneezing, jumping, etc.) that causes you to lose urine. Relax the muscles once the activity is over.
- It may take several months to benefit from pelvic floor exercises and you have to keep doing them daily to maintain their benefit.

Other Self-Care Procedures

- Avoid or limit drinks and medicines that have caffeine (e.g., coffee, tea, colas, chocolate and No-Doz).
- Limit carbonated drinks, alcohol, citrus juices, greasy and spicy foods and items that have artificial sweeteners. These can irritate the bladder.
- Drink one to two quarts of water throughout the day.
- Go to the bathroom often, even if you don't feel the urge. When you urinate, empty your bladder as much as you can. Relax for a minute or two and then try to go again. Keep a diary of when you have episodes of incontinence. If you find that you have accidents every three hours, for example, empty your bladder every 2½ hours. Use an alarm clock or wristwatch with an alarm to remind you.
- Wear clothes you can remove quickly and easily when you use the bathroom. Examples are elastic-waist bottoms and items with velcro closures or snaps instead of buttons and zippers. Also, look for belts that are easy to undo or don't wear belts at all.
- Wear absorbent pads or briefs. Ask your doctor if you would benefit from using self-catheters. A self-catheter is a clear, straw-like device, usually made of flexible plastic, that you insert into the opening of the urethra; it helps you empty your bladder completely. Your doctor will need to show you how to use one. You need a prescription for a self-catheter.

To reduce the chances of accidents:

- Empty your bladder before you leave the house, take a nap and go to bed.
- Keep the pathway to your bathroom free of clutter and well lit. Make sure the bathroom door is left open until you use it.
- Use an elevated toilet seat and grab bars if these will make it easier for you to get on and off the toilet.
- Keep a bedpan, plastic urinal (for men) or portable commode chair near your bed. You can get these at medical supply stores and drugstores.

Urinary Tract Infections (UTIs)

About one out of five women will get a urinary tract infection (UTI) during the course of her lifetime. Some women get many UTIs. Men get UTIs, too, but not as often as women do.

What is the urinary tract? Your urinary tract is made up of these parts:

- Kidneys
- Bladder
- Ureters (tubes that connect the kidneys to the bladder)
- Urethra (the opening where urine comes out)

How do we get UTIs? Usually, bacteria enter through the urethra and go to the bladder. They grow in the bladder and move to other parts of the urinary tract.

Bacteria can get into a woman's urethra during sex. You should go to the bathroom right after sex to flush the bacteria out. Women who use a diaphragm for birth control have twice the risk of getting a UTI. Changes that happen during pregnancy and after menopause can also make a woman prone to UTIs.

Also, any irritation to the opening of the urethra can lead to a bladder infection. If you have signs of a vaginal infection (discharge, foul odor, etc.), get treatment for it to help prevent a bladder infection.

Some people are born with urinary tract problems that pave the way for UTIs. Anything that keeps you from passing urine freely can lead to UTIs. Kidney stones or an enlarged prostate gland are two examples. You are also more likely to get a UTI if you have had such infections before.

Sometimes you don't even know you have a UTI. Most often you will have symptoms, though. They come suddenly, with no warning. Here are some of them:

- A strong need to urinate
- More frequent urination than usual
- A sharp pain or burning in the urethra when you pass urine
- Blood in the urine
- Feeling like your bladder is still full after you pass urine
- Soreness in your belly, back or sides
- Chills, fever, nausea

See a doctor if you have any of these symptoms. A UTI can be serious if you don't treat it. The doctor will test a sample of your urine to find the problem. An antibiotic to treat the infection and pain relievers, if necessary, are the usual course of treatment.

How to Avoid Urinary Tract Infections

Here are some things you can do to keep from getting UTIs:

- If you're a woman, wipe from front to back after using the toilet. This keeps bacteria away from the urethra.
- Drink plenty of liquids to flush out your body. Drink fruit juices, especially cranberry juice.
- Empty your bladder as soon as you feel the urge. Don't give bacteria a chance to grow.
- Drink a glass of water before you have sex. Urinate as soon as you can after sex, even if you don't have the urge to.
- If you use a lubricant when you have sex, use a water-soluble one like K-Y Jelly.
- Wear cotton underpants. Bacteria like a warm, wet environment. Cotton helps keep you cool and dry because it lets air flow through.

- Don't take bubble baths if you have had UTIs before. Take showers instead of baths.
- Don't wear tight jeans, pants or underpants.
- If you use a diaphragm, clean it after each use and have your doctor check every once in a while to make sure it still fits. The size may need to be changed if you gain or lose weight or if you have a baby. Replace your diaphragm according to your doctor's advice.

Questions to Ask

Do you have these symptoms:
- Fever and shaking chills
- Back pain in one or both sides of your lower back
- Vomiting and nausea

YES
SEEK EMERGENCY CARE

NO

Do you have these problems:
- Burning when you pass urine
- Passing urine a lot more often than usual
- Bloody or cloudy urine
- Pain in your abdomen or over your bladder
- Nausea or a feeling like you're going to vomit

YES
SEE DOCTOR

NO

Do you have of these problems:
- You urinate a lot, even at night.
- You feel like you have an urgent need to urinate.
- You feel like your bladder is still full after you urinate.
- It stings when you pass urine.
- Your urine smells bad.
- It hurts to have sexual intercourse.

YES
SEE DOCTOR

NO

flowchart continued in next column

flowchart continued

Have you had symptoms for more than three days, without getting better? Did medication the doctor prescribed give you side effects (e.g., skin rash or nausea)?

 YES
CALL DOCTOR

NO

Do you get UTIs a lot?

YES
CALL DOCTOR

NO

PROVIDE SELF-CARE

Self-Care Procedures

- Avoid alcohol, spicy foods and coffee.
- Drink at least eight glasses of water a day. Liquids help wash out the infection.
- Get plenty of rest.
- Check for fever twice a day. Take your temperature in the morning and then in the afternoon or evening.
- Take aspirin, acetaminophen, ibuprofen or naproxen sodium. *Note: Do not give aspirin or any medication containing salicylates to anyone 19 years of age or younger, unless directed by a physician, due to its association with Reye's syndrome, a potentially fatal condition.*
- Go to the bathroom as soon as you feel the need.
- Empty your bladder every time you pass urine. If you have a condition that keeps you from doing this, such as that which occurs in some people with multiple sclerosis, ask your doctor about using intermittent self-catheters.
- Empty your bladder after sex.

See your doctor if you don't feel better in three days.

CHAPTER 16

MENTAL HEALTH CONDITIONS

Alcoholism

Alcoholism is the most common drug abuse problem in the United States. About 11 million Americans suffer from it. Abuse occurs in one of several ways: getting drunk daily, drinking a lot at certain times such as every weekend, binges of heavy drinking for weeks or months with long periods of not drinking and infrequent drinking with loss of control over drinking.

Alcoholism is a disease which affects the alcoholic's physical health, emotional well-being and behavior.

Physical Effects

- Impairs mental/physical reflexes
- Increases the risk of diseases such as cancer of the brain, tongue, mouth, esophagus, larynx, liver and bladder; cirrhosis of the liver and hepatitis; ulcers and gastritis, and irreversible brain damage when used heavily. It can also cause heart and blood pressure problems.
- Can lead to malnutrition
- Is known to cause birth defects

Emotional and Behavioral Effects

- Alters inhibitions and, therefore, may cause someone to do things he or she might not do otherwise (e.g., driving at high speeds or other daredevil acts)
- Alters mood, resulting in anger, violent behavior, depression or even suicide—effects that can intensify as more alcohol is consumed
- May result in memory loss

- Makes family life chaotic. The divorce rate is seven times higher among alcoholics, and children of alcoholics may have long-lasting emotional problems.
- Often results in decreased work attendance and performance as well as problems in dealing with employees and co-workers

Treatment

Alcoholism has a biological basis. The tendency to become alcoholic is inherited. Both men and women are four times more likely to become alcoholics if their parents were.

Treating alcoholism as an illness is important and one thing is certain: The only way to beat a drinking problem is to stop drinking. This can be done through self-help groups such as Alcoholics Anonymous and Rational Recovery, alcohol rehabilitation centers and psychotherapy. Two prescription drugs are available to help in treatment. One, called Antabuse, causes violent physical reactions if a person drinks alcohol while taking the medication. Another one, Naltrexone, blocks the craving for alcohol and the pleasure of getting high.

Questions to Ask

Have you had memory lapses or blackouts due to drinking? **YES** → **SEE DOCTOR**

NO ↓

Do you continue to drink even though you have health problems caused by alcohol? **YES** → **SEE DOCTOR**

NO ↓

flowchart continued on next page

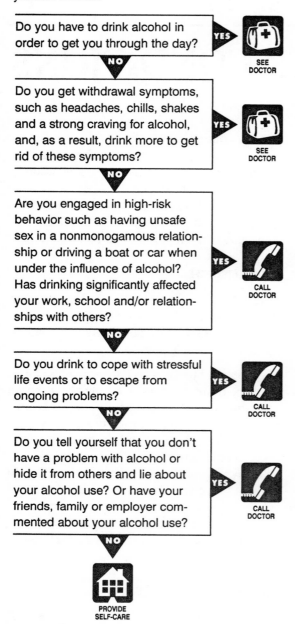

Do you have to drink alcohol in order to get you through the day? **YES** → SEE DOCTOR

NO ↓

Do you get withdrawal symptoms, such as headaches, chills, shakes and a strong craving for alcohol, and, as a result, drink more to get rid of these symptoms? **YES** → SEE DOCTOR

NO ↓

Are you engaged in high-risk behavior such as having unsafe sex in a nonmonogamous relationship or driving a boat or car when under the influence of alcohol? Has drinking significantly affected your work, school and/or relationships with others? **YES** → CALL DOCTOR

NO ↓

Do you drink to cope with stressful life events or to escape from ongoing problems? **YES** → CALL DOCTOR

NO ↓

Do you tell yourself that you don't have a problem with alcohol or hide it from others and lie about your alcohol use? Or have your friends, family or employer commented about your alcohol use? **YES** → CALL DOCTOR

NO ↓

PROVIDE SELF-CARE

Self-Care Procedures

If you are an alcohol user but are not yet abusing it, the sooner you stop using alcohol, the better your chances of avoiding the serious physical and psychological effects.

- Admit to your drinking. This is the first and most important step to avoid becoming an alcohol abuser.
- Change your lifestyle. Try to stay out of situations where alcohol is prominent (e.g., nightclubs, dances and parties) until you can get control over your drinking. Once you've done this, order juice, club soda or coffee if you attend these parties.
- If your friends insist you drink alcohol in order to socialize with them, make it clear that you're serious about stopping. If this is unacceptable to them, find new friends.
- Attend self-help group meetings for alcoholics. Examples include Alcoholics Anonymous (AA), Rational Recovery (RR), Women for Sobriety (WFS) and Men for Sobriety (MFS).
- Contact your Employee Assistance Program representative at work for information and suggestions.

To avoid becoming alcohol dependent:
- Know your limit and stick to it.
- Drink slowly. You are apt to drink less.
- Pour less alcohol and more mixer in each drink.
- Alternate an alcoholic beverage with a nonalcoholic one.
- Eat while drinking. Food helps absorb alcohol in the system.
- Talk to persons who will listen to your feelings and concerns without judging you. You will be less likely to turn to alcohol to "drown your sorrows."
- Find ways to calm yourself other than with alcohol (e.g., hobbies, relaxation exercises, physical activities and movies).
- Realize that you are a role model for your children. They learn what they see. When you drink, do so responsibly.
- Don't mix drinking with driving, drugs or operating machines. These combinations can be fatal.

Anxiety

Anxiety is a sense of dread, fear or distress over a real or imagined threat to your mental or physical well-being. Symptoms of anxiety include:

- Rapid pulse and/or breathing rate
- Racing or pounding heart
- Dry mouth
- Sweating
- Trembling
- Shortness of breath
- Faintness
- Numbness/tingling of the hands, feet or other body part
- Feeling a "lump in the throat"
- Stomach problems

A certain amount of anxiety is normal. It can prompt you to study for a test or alert you to seek safety when you are in physical danger. Anxiety is not normal, though, when there is no apparent reason for it or when it is overwhelming and interferes with day-to-day living.

Anxiety can be a symptom of medical conditions such as:

- Heart attack
- Overactive thyroid gland (hyperthyroidism)
- Low blood sugar (hypoglycemia)
- Excess of hormones made by the glands located above the kidneys called the adrenal glands (Cushing's syndrome)
- Side effect of some medications
- Withdrawal symptoms from nicotine, alcohol or drugs or medicines such as sleeping pills

Anxiety can even be a symptom of a number of illnesses known as anxiety disorders. These include:

- **Phobias** - Disorders from which terror, dread or panic results when a person is faced with a feared object, situation or activity. Examples include specific phobias (such as fear of snakes), social phobias (such as the fear of speaking in front of other people) and complex phobias (such as agoraphobia, the fear of being in places or situations from which escape might be difficult or embarrassing). Agoraphobia can occur with or without panic disorder, defined below.

- **Panic Attacks** - Brief periods of acute anxiety that can occur without warning. Symptoms include shortness of breath, chest discomfort, heart palpitations, sweating and choking. A person having a panic attack for the first time may think he or she is having a heart attack. Panic attacks may or may not be associated with agoraphobia.

Panic disorder is thought to exist when panic attacks:

- Occur without warning
- Take place for one month, and
- Are followed by: the ongoing fear that another panic attack will occur; worry about implications of the attack or its consequences; or a significant change in behavior

- **Obsessive-Compulsive Disorder** - An anxiety disorder where the sufferer has persistent, involuntary thoughts or images (obsessions) and engages in ritualistic acts such as washing their hands according to certain self-imposed rules (compulsions)

- **Post-Traumatic Stress Disorder** - A condition where a person reexperiences a traumatic past event like a wartime situation, hostage taking or rape. Symptoms include nightmares, flashbacks of the event, excessive alertness and emotional numbness to people and activities.

- **Critical Incident Stress Syndrome** - Is similar to post-traumatic stress disorder. With this, a person who has experienced a critical event such as a workplace trauma, threatened or actual acts of violence and/or injury suffers from anxiety, depression and a feeling of being out of control.

When anxiety is mild and/or does not interfere with daily living, it can be dealt with using the listed Self-Care Procedures. Treatment for anxiety disorders includes:

- Treatment of the medical condition, if one exists, which causes the anxiety

- Psychotherapies
- Medication

Self-help groups such as Agoraphobics in Motion (AIM) can also be helpful.

Questions to Ask

Do you have thoughts of suicide that don't go away? Are you planning ways to commit suicide? **YES** →

SEEK EMERGENCY CARE

NO ↓

Are any of these problems present with the anxiety:
- Chest pain (note if it spreads, or radiates, to the arm, neck or jaw)
- Feeling of pressure, especially on the left side of the chest
- Shortness of breath or difficulty in breathing
- Nausea, vomiting, belching
- Sweating
- Irregular heartbeat
- Irregular pulse

YES →

SEEK EMERGENCY CARE

NO ↓

Are these problems present with the anxiety:
- Accumulation of fat on the neck, face and trunk
- Excessive hair growth
- Round face and puffy eyes
- Skin changes (e.g., reddening, thinning and stretch marks)
- High blood pressure

YES →

SEE DOCTOR

NO ↓

Do you have these problems with the anxiety:
- Rapid heartbeat
- Hyperactivity
- Weight loss
- Muscle weakness, tremors
- Bulging eyes
- Feeling hot or warm all the time

YES →

SEE DOCTOR

NO ↓

flowchart continued in next column

flowchart continued

Does the anxiety take place only at these times:
- When you don't eat or when you physically tax yourself too much, especially if you have diabetes
- Premenstrually, for women

YES →

CALL DOCTOR

NO ↓

Did you get the anxiety only after:
- Taking an over-the-counter (OTC) or prescription medicine
- Withdrawing from medication, nicotine, alcohol or drugs

YES →

CALL DOCTOR

NO ↓

Have you had any of these:
- Panic attacks followed for one month by fears of getting another one
- Worry about the implications of the attack or its consequences

or
- A significant change in behavior related to the attacks

YES →

CALL DOCTOR

NO ↓

If you have been through or seen a traumatic event, do you suffer from any of these problems:
- Nightmares, night terrors and/or flashbacks of the event
- Lack of concentration, poor memory, unable to sleep
- Feelings of guilt for surviving the event
- Easily startled by loud noises or anything that reminds you of the event
- Lack of interest in the activities and people you once enjoyed

YES →

CALL DOCTOR

NO ↓

flowchart continued on next page

Do any of these keep you from doing your daily activities:
- Fear of having a panic attack
- Fear of leaving the house or of being left alone
- Checking something over and over again (e.g., seeing if you've locked the door even though it is locked)
- Repeated, unwanted thoughts such as worrying you could harm someone
- Repeated, senseless acts such as washing your hands constantly

YES CALL DOCTOR

NO

Is anxiety in general keeping you from doing the things you need to do every day?

YES CALL DOCTOR

NO

 PROVIDE SELF-CARE

Self-Care Procedures

- Look for the cause of the stress that results in anxiety and deal with it directly.
- Lessen your exposure to things that cause you distress.
- Eat healthy and at regular times. Don't skip meals.
- If you are prone to low blood sugar episodes, eat five to six small meals per day instead of three larger ones. Avoid sweets on a regular basis, but carry a quick source of sugar with you at all times (e.g., a small can of orange juice) if you do get a low blood sugar reaction).
- Exercise regularly.
- Avoid caffeine, nicotine and alcohol.
- Do some form of relaxation exercise daily (e.g., biofeedback, deep muscle relaxation, meditation and deep breathing exercises).

- Don't "bite off more than you can chew." Plan your schedule for what you can handle both physically and mentally.
- Rehearse for events that are coming up in which you have felt anxious in the past or think will cause anxiety. Several times before it really occurs, imagine yourself feeling calm and in control during the event.
- Be prepared to deal with symptoms of anxiety if you anticipate they will happen. For example, if you have hyperventilated in the past, carry a paper bag with you. If you do hyperventilate, cover your mouth and nose with the paper bag. Breathe into the paper bag slowly and rebreathe the air. Do this in and out at least 10 times. Remove the bag and breathe normally a few minutes. Repeat breathing in and out of the paper bag as needed.
- Help others. The positive feelings this can create can help you overcome or forget about your anxiety.

Depression

Life changes, such as the birth of a baby, divorce, death of a loved one or loss of a job, can leave a person feeling depressed. So can worrying about financial problems or illness. And sometimes you may feel empty and depressed for no apparent reason. Some depression is normal and is a part of almost every person's life. Depression can, however, be a side effect of certain medicines, illnesses, or alcoholism, or be a disease in and of itself. Even the lack of natural, unfiltered sunlight between late fall and spring can lead to a type of depression in some sensitive people. This is commonly called seasonal affective disorder (SAD).

Whatever the cause, depression can be treated. Treatment includes medicines, psychotherapy and other therapies specific to the cause of the depression, such as exposure to bright light (similar to sunlight) for depression that results from SAD.

Symptoms of depression include:
- Persistent feelings of sadness or emptiness
- Feelings of helplessness, hopelessness, guilt and worthlessness
- Loss of interest in pleasurable activities, including sex
- Sleep disturbances
- Fatigue
- Loss of energy or enthusiasm
- Difficulty in concentrating or making decisions
- Ongoing physical symptoms such as headaches or digestive disorders that don't respond to treatment
- Crying, tearfulness
- Poor appetite with weight loss, or overeating and weight gain

Questions to Ask

Have you attempted suicide? Are you planning ways to commit suicide? **YES**

NO

SEEK EMERGENCY CARE

flowchart continued in next column

flowchart continued

Have you had markedly diminished interest or pleasure in almost all activities most of the day, nearly every day for at least two weeks? Or have you been in a depressed mood most of the day, nearly every day, and have you experienced any of the following, for at least two weeks:
- Feeling slowed down or restless and unable to sit still
- Feeling worthless or guilty
- Changes in appetite or weight loss or gain
- Thoughts of death or suicide
- Problems concentrating, thinking, remembering, or making decisions
- Trouble sleeping or sleeping too much
- Loss of energy or feeling tired all of the time
- Headaches
- Other aches and pains
- Digestive problems
- Sexual problems
- Feelings of pessimism or hopelessness
- Anxious feelings or worry

YES

SEE DOCTOR

NO

Has depression interfered with daily activities for more than three weeks? Have you withdrawn from normal activities during this time? **YES**

CALL DOCTOR

NO

Has the depression appeared after taking over-the-counter or prescription medicine? **YES**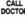

CALL DOCTOR

NO

flowchart continued on next page

Is the depression associated with dark, cloudy weather or winter months, and does it lift when spring comes? **YES**

CALL DOCTOR

NO

PROVIDE SELF-CARE

Self-Care Procedures

To overcome mild, hard-to-explain depression, try these approaches:

- Substitute a positive thought for every negative thought that pops into your head.
- Associate with congenial people, not negative people. They'll lift your morale.
- To focus your attention away from yourself, do something to help someone else.
- Get some physical exercise every day, even if it's just taking the dog for a walk. If you can do something more exhilarating (e.g., biking, playing tennis or chopping firewood), that's even better.
- Do something different. Walk or drive to somewhere new, or try a new restaurant.
- Challenge yourself with a new project. It doesn't have to be difficult, but it should be enjoyable. Do something that you enjoy and allows you to express yourself (e.g., writing and painting).
- Do something that will make you relax. Listen to soft music, read a good book, take a warm bath or shower, do relaxation exercises.
- Talk to a friend, relative, co-worker or anyone who will allow you to vent the tensions and frustrations that you are experiencing.
- Avoid drugs and alcohol. Drinking too much alcohol and the use of drugs can cause or worsen depression.

Stress

Stress is the way our bodies react both physically and emotionally to any change in the status quo—good, bad, real or even imagined. Some physical symptoms created by stress include an increased heart rate, rapid breathing, tense muscles and increased blood pressure. Emotional reactions include irritability, anger, losing one's temper, yelling, lack of concentration and being jumpy. When left unchecked, stress can lead to a variety of health problems, including insomnia, ulcers, back pain, colitis, high blood pressure, heart disease and a lowering of the body's immune system. In fact, the American Academy of Family Physicians states that approximately two-thirds of all visits to the family doctor are for stress-related disorders.

Questions to Ask

Are you so distressed that you have recurrent thoughts of suicide or death? Do you have impulses or plans to commit violence? **YES**

SEEK EMERGENCY CARE

NO

Are you experiencing frequent anxiety, nervousness, crying spells and confusion about how to handle your problems? **YES**

SEE DOCTOR

NO

Are you abusing alcohol, drugs (illegal or prescription) to deal with stress? **YES**

SEE DOCTOR

NO

flowchart continued on next page

Have you been a part of a traumatic event in the past (e.g., armed combat, airplane crash, rape or assault), and do you now experience any of the following:

- Flashbacks (reliving the stressful event), painful memories, nightmares
- Feeling easily startled and/or irritable
- Feeling "emotionally numb" and detached from others and the outside world
- Having a hard time falling asleep and/or staying asleep
- Anxiety and/or depression

YES

SEE DOCTOR

NO

Do you find yourself withdrawing from friends, relatives and co-workers and/or blowing up at them at the slightest provocation?

YES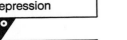

CALL DOCTOR

NO

Do you suffer from a medical illness that you are unable to cope with? Is this leading you to neglect proper treatment?

YES

CALL DOCTOR

NO

PROVIDE SELF-CARE

Self-Care Procedures

Being able to manage stress is important in living a healthy, happy and productive life. Here are some techniques and strategies to effectively deal with stress:

- Maintain a regular program of healthy eating, good health habits, and adequate sleep.
- Exercise regularly. This promotes physical fitness as well as emotional well-being.

- Balance work and play. All work and no play can make you feel stressed. Plan some time for hobbies and recreation. These activities relax your mind and are a good respite from life's worries.
- Help others. We concentrate on ourselves when we're distressed. Sometimes helping others is the perfect remedy for whatever is troubling us.
- Take a shower or bath with warm water. This will soothe and calm your nerves and relax your muscles.
- Have a good cry. Tears of sadness, joy or grief can help cleanse the body of substances that accumulate under stress and also release a natural pain-relieving substance from the brain.
- Laugh a lot. When events seem too overwhelming, keep a sense of humor. Laughter makes our muscles go limp and releases tension. It's difficult to feel stress in the middle of a belly laugh. Learn to laugh as a relaxation technique.
- Learn acceptance. Sometimes a difficult problem is out of your control. When this happens, accept it until changes can be made. This is better than worrying and getting nowhere.
- Talk out troubles. It sometimes helps to talk with a friend, relative or member of the clergy. Another person can help you see a problem from a different point of view.
- Escape for a little while. When you feel you are getting nowhere with a problem, a temporary diversion can help. Going to a movie, reading a book, visiting a museum or taking a drive can help you out of a rut. Temporarily leaving a difficult situation can help you develop new attitudes.
- Reward yourself. Starting today, reward yourself with little things that make you feel good. Treat yourself to a bubble bath, buy the hardcover edition of a book, call an old friend long distance, buy a flower, picnic in the park during lunchtime, try a new perfume or cologne or give yourself some "me" time.

- Do relaxation exercises daily. Good ones include visualization (imagining a soothing, restful scene), deep muscle relaxation (tensing and relaxing muscle fibers), meditation and deep breathing.
- Budget your time. Make a "to-do" list. Rank in priority your daily tasks. Avoid committing yourself to doing too much.
- Develop and maintain a positive attitude. View changes as positive challenges, opportunities or blessings.
- Rehearse for stressful events. Imagine yourself feeling calm and confident in an anticipated stressful situation. You will be able to relax more easily when the situation arises.
- Modify your environment to get rid of or manage your exposure to things that cause stress.

CHAPTER 17

CHILDREN'S HEALTH

Bed-Wetting

Wetting the bed is not only uncomfortable, it is also embarrassing, especially for a child older than three years. And that's not all. Afraid of waking up in a soaked bed, children who wet their beds may avoid going to pajama parties, friends' houses or summer camp.

Three out of four toddlers stay dry all night by age 3½. By age 5, one in five still wets the bed and at age 6, the numbers drop to one in 10. Just about all bed-wetting stops by the time children reach puberty. Boys are more likely than girls to wet their beds. Bed-wetting may start again during stressful times.

No one really knows what causes enuresis, the medical term for bed-wetting. From the 1930s through the 1960s, it was commonly believed that children who wet their beds had psychological problems. Today, it is suspected that bed-wetting may be caused by slow development of the nerves that control the bladder.

Even a small bladder unable to hold the urine produced during the night can result in bed-wetting. Bed-wetting can be a symptom of a serious illness (e.g., diabetes or a urinary tract infection), especially if it starts in a child who has previously been dry through the night.

Questions to Ask

Does your child drink an excessive amount of fluids, urinate more than usual during the day and night and/or show other signs such as fatigue, increased appetite and weight gain and itching around the genitals? **YES**

SEE DOCTOR

NO

Does your child have a fever, abdominal pain or burning when urinating? **YES**

SEE DOCTOR

NO

Is your child older than 6 years and has never been dry at night, or has he or she been dry at night for an extended time and is now wetting again? **YES**

CALL DOCTOR

NO

PROVIDE SELF-CARE

Self-Care Procedures

Your patience and love will go a long way to help a child who wets the bed. Children have no control over this condition; they don't wet the bed on purpose. Making the child feel guilty, getting angry or acting disgusted will only delay solving this problem. Try to be understanding and supportive.

Psychologists recommend that you simply wait it out. Don't praise the child for a dry bed or punish him or her when it's wet. To help make life easier for your child and yourself, consider the following:

- Have your child change the bed as well as his or her bed clothes during the night, if he or she is able to do so. Or keep a flannel-covered rubber sheet nearby so your child can put it over the wet sheets.
- Set an alarm clock two to three hours after your child falls asleep so he or she can be awakened to go to the bathroom.
- Make sure your child urinates before getting into bed.
- Encourage your child to follow instructions, if any, that the doctor suggests, such as bladder-stretching or stream-interruption exercises or behavior modification devices.
- Obtain a bed-wetting alarm. (This is best suited for children 5 years and older.) Modern enuresis alarms have moisture sensors that attach directly on the underwear. At the first drop of liquid, a buzzer sounds, waking up the child. Eventually, kids learn to wake up whenever they feel the urge to urinate. Newer models of these alarms can help prevent wet beds about 85 to 90 percent of the time.

Bed-wetting alarms and information can be obtained from:

- Nite Train'r Alarm: Koregon Enterprises, 9735 S.W. Sunshine Court, Beaverton, OR 97005; 800-544-4240.
- Nytone Alarm: Nytone Medical Products, 2424 South 900 West, Salt Lake City, UT 84119; 801-973-4090.
- Wet-Stop Alarm: Palco Laboratories, 8030 Soquel Ave., Santa Cruz, CA 95062; 800-346-4488.

Also, check with local home medical supply companies and local pharmacies that carry or can provide home medical equipment.

Chicken Pox

Chicken pox is a very contagious disease caused by a virus (varicella/herpes zoster). It is spread from child to child, and sometimes to adults, by sneezing, coughing, contaminated clothing and direct contact with open blisters. Children exposed to the virus get chicken pox seven to 21 days later.

Most of the time there are no symptoms before the rash appears. Some children, though, may be tired, have a fever and complain of a stomach ache a day or two before a flat, red rash appears. The rash generally begins on the scalp, face and back, but can spread to any body surface. It is rarely seen, though, on the palms of hands or soles of feet. Sores smaller than a pencil eraser, and which are sometimes encrusted, can also be found in the mouth, on the eyelids and in the genital area.

Within hours, these flat, red spots turn into tiny clear blisters that itch a lot. As your child scratches the blisters, serum spills out, dries and forms hard crusts that loosen and drop off about two weeks later. Since the rash continues to break out for the first two to six days, new red spots are often seen alongside old dried scabs. Some children have very few spots while others are covered.

Most children recover from chicken pox uneventfully in less than two weeks. Complications are rare, although chicken pox can occasionally lead to encephalitis (inflammation of the brain), meningitis or pneumonia. Children who have cancer and those who take medications that affect the immune system are at a higher risk of complications from chicken pox. The biggest problem parents face with chicken pox, though, is infected blisters.

There is prescription medication available that can decrease the length and severity of chicken pox; however, it is not recommended for routine cases. Also, it is only effective if started within 24 hours of the onset of the infection.

It does not interfere with the child's developing immunity to chicken pox. Ask your doctor for more information.

One attack of chicken pox usually gives your child lifelong immunity. Children rarely have a second round of chicken pox, but if it does occur, the attacks are usually very mild.

Prevention

A vaccine (Varivax) has been developed for chicken pox. It has been given Food and Drug Administration approval. Ask your child's health care provider about it.

Questions to Ask

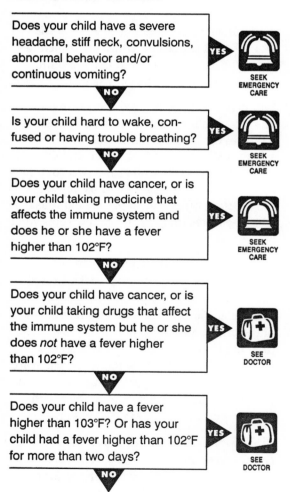

Does your child have a severe headache, stiff neck, convulsions, abnormal behavior and/or continuous vomiting? **YES** → SEEK EMERGENCY CARE

NO

Is your child hard to wake, confused or having trouble breathing? **YES** → SEEK EMERGENCY CARE

NO

Does your child have cancer, or is your child taking medicine that affects the immune system and does he or she have a fever higher than 102°F? **YES** → SEEK EMERGENCY CARE

NO

Does your child have cancer, or is your child taking drugs that affect the immune system but he or she does *not* have a fever higher than 102°F? **YES** → SEE DOCTOR

NO

Does your child have a fever higher than 103°F? Or has your child had a fever higher than 102°F for more than two days? **YES** → SEE DOCTOR

NO

flowchart continued in next column

flowchart continued

Does your child have any scabs that are red, oozing pus or bleeding, or has he or she developed a red rash with tiny pink dots? **YES** → CALL DOCTOR

NO → PROVIDE SELF-CARE

Self-Care Procedures

The goals are to make your child comfortable and to reduce and relieve the itching so your child does not scratch off the scabs (this could start a secondary infection and/or leave scars).

- Encourage your child not to scratch the scabs. Keep him or her busy with other activities.
- Give your child a cool bath without soap every three to four hours for the first couple of days (15 to 20 minutes at a time). Add ½ cup of baking soda or a colloidal oatmeal bath packet (e.g., Aveeno) to the bath water. Pat, do not rub, your child dry.
- Dip a washcloth in cool water and place it on the itchy areas.
- Apply calamine (not Caladryl) lotion for temporary relief. Trim your child's fingernails to prevent infection caused by opened blisters. Scratching off the crusty scabs may leave permanent scars.
- Cover the hands of infants with cotton socks if they are scratching their sores.
- Wash your child's hands three times a day with an antibacterial soap (e.g., Safeguard or Dial) to avoid infecting the open blisters.
- Keep your child cool and calm. Heat and sweating make the itching worse. Also, keep your child out of the sun. Extra chicken pox will occur on parts of the skin exposed to the sun.
- Give your child Benadryl, an over-the-counter antihistamine, if the itching is severe or stops your child from sleeping. (See label for proper dosage.)

- Give your child acetaminophen (children's versions of the following: Tylenol, Tempra, Liquiprin, Datril, Anacin 3 or Panadol) for the fever. *Note: Do not give aspirin or any medication containing salicylates to anyone 19 years of age or younger, unless directed by a physician, due to its association with Reye's syndrome, a potentially fatal condition.*
- Give your child soft foods and cold fluids if he or she has sores in the mouth. Do not offer salty foods or citrus fruits that may irritate the sores.
- Have your child gargle with salt water (¼ teaspoon salt in four ounces of water) to help ease itching in the mouth, if necessary.
- Reassure your child that the "bumps" are not serious and will go away in a week or so.

Colic

Colic is one of the most frustrating conditions parents deal with. Your baby cries for hours on end for no apparent reason, tucking those tiny knees close to the stomach as if in severe pain. Typically, the attacks start in the evening when you may be most tired and your patience thin.

Nothing seems to stop the screaming of a colicky infant—not even feeding, changing the diaper or cuddling. Take comfort, though. Colic is rarely dangerous and doesn't last a long time. It usually begins after an infant is two weeks old, peaks at about three months of age and most often ends by the fourth month.

The cause of colic is a mystery. Some pediatricians think it is due to an underdeveloped digestive tract. Others blame food allergies, abdominal gas, not enough sleep or oversensitivity to a busy and noisy home. Still others think it is a combination of these factors. An attack of colic may end with the passage of gas or stool.

Once in a while, colic may be an early sign of a serious medical problem. For example, in the medical condition called intussusception, the bowel becomes obstructed. A doctor can examine your baby and run laboratory tests to check for this and other medical conditions.

Prevention

- Have your infant sit up rather than lie down at feeding time to avoid swallowing air.
- If breast-feeding, watch your intake of caffeine drinks like colas, coffee, cocoa and tea.
- Stop eating milk products on a one-week trial basis. One study showed that when the mother stopped eating dairy foods, her baby's colic often disappeared. (If you do this, check with your doctor about taking calcium supplements.)
- Do not overheat the milk or formula.
- Make sure the bottle's nipple holes are not too small. Tiny holes cause babies to swallow air as they suck on the nipples.
- Try a different type of formula (e.g., a soy-based one instead of one made with cow's milk).
- Make mealtime a quiet, calm time.
- Feed more frequently. Burp your baby more often.

Questions to Ask

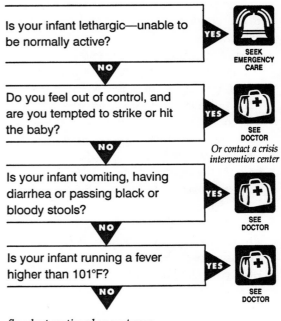

Is your infant lethargic—unable to be normally active? **YES** → SEEK EMERGENCY CARE

NO

Do you feel out of control, and are you tempted to strike or hit the baby? **YES** → SEE DOCTOR *Or contact a crisis intervention center*

NO

Is your infant vomiting, having diarrhea or passing black or bloody stools? **YES** → SEE DOCTOR

NO

Is your infant running a fever higher than 101°F? **YES** → SEE DOCTOR

NO

flowchart continued on next page

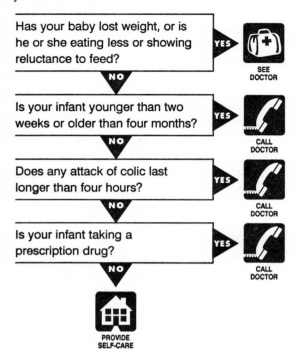

Has your baby lost weight, or is he or she eating less or showing reluctance to feed? **YES** → SEE DOCTOR

NO ↓

Is your infant younger than two weeks or older than four months? **YES** → CALL DOCTOR

NO ↓

Does any attack of colic last longer than four hours? **YES** → CALL DOCTOR

NO ↓

Is your infant taking a prescription drug? **YES** → CALL DOCTOR

NO ↓

PROVIDE SELF-CARE

Self-Care Procedures

First, stay calm and try to relax. It takes a lot of patience and tolerance to deal with a screaming baby, especially when nothing seems wrong. While none of these Self-Care Procedures will cure colic, they may bring you and your baby some relief.

- Be sure your baby is getting enough to eat. Hunger, not colic, may be causing the crying.
- Try different types of purchased nipples. If the nipple hole is too small, enlarge it.
  - To check the hole size, put cold formula in the bottle and turn it upside down. Shake or squeeze the bottle.
  - Count the number of drops of formula. The right-size hole delivers about one drop per second.
  - If there are fewer drops per second, make the hole bigger by using a knife to make a crosscut over the existing hole.
- Hold your child up for feeding and for a short while afterwards.
- Burp your baby after each ounce of formula or every few minutes when breast-feeding.

- Use a pacifier. (Never, however, put a pacifier on a string around your baby's neck.)
- Wrap your infant in a cozy blanket and gently rock him or her, or use an automatic swing. The back-and-forth motion tends to quiet a wailing baby.
- Try what is called the "colic carry." Carefully place your baby facedown, with his or her face on your open hand and his or her legs straddling your inner elbow. Support your baby by holding his or her back with your other hand and walk around the house for a while.
- Vacuum while carrying your infant in a "baby carrier" worn on your chest. Apparently, the noise of a running vacuum soothes a colicky baby.
- Play soothing music. This may benefit you as well as the baby.
- Take your baby for a ride outdoors in the stroller or in the car.
- Run the dryer or dishwasher. Put your baby in an infant seat and lean it against the side of the dryer or on the counter close to the dishwasher. (Stay with your baby and make sure the baby will not be harmed by the heat or steam given off by these appliances.) The vibration may put your child to sleep.
- Do not give the baby liquid antacids (e.g., Maalox) or simethicone drops. These have not been shown to be helpful.
- Let your baby cry himself or herself to sleep if none of the Self-Care Procedures work. (Don't let your baby cry, however, for more than four hours.)

Croup

What could be more frightening than to awaken during the night to the sound of your child gasping for air and "barking like a seal"? Yet these are the classical signs of croup, a respiratory infection that typically affects children between the ages of three months and three years. While it may sound frightening, croup is rarely cause for concern. Croup usually lasts from three to seven days. Generally, it worsens at night and tends to improve during the day. Sometimes steroid medication that is prescribed early in the illness helps to ease the severity of the symptoms.

A virus is the most common cause of croup. Infected by a virus, cells in the voice box and windpipe react by secreting mucus that narrow these air passages. The secretions dry and thicken, making it even more difficult for your child to breathe. Dissolving the dried secretions with steam is often all that is needed to relieve your child's discomfort. Children usually outgrow croup as they get older and the windpipe becomes wider.

Sometimes croup is confused with another condition called epiglottitis (inflammation of the structure behind the root of the tongue). Typically seen in children older than three years, epiglottitis is often more serious than croup because it can completely block the airway and cause meningitis (inflammation of the lining of the brain and spinal cord) or respiratory arrest. Children with epiglottitis tend to drool, tilt their heads forward, have a fever and jut their jaw out as they try to breathe.

Sometimes what sounds like croup may instead indicate that your child has inhaled a foreign object. If the object blocks the windpipe, your child will have trouble breathing and will need immediate emergency care.

Prevention

- Use a humidifier near your child's bed for several nights after the first attack. Use a cool-mist vaporizer if your child has a fever because warm moist air can raise body temperature. Clean the vaporizer after each use.
- Purchase a humidifier for your furnace if croup is a recurring problem. Change the filter often.

Questions to Ask

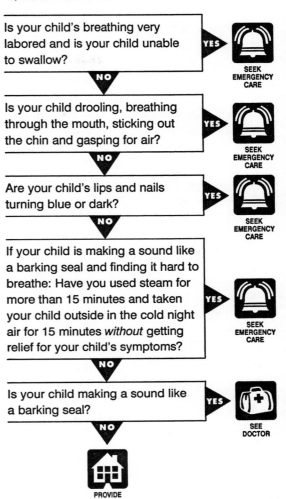

Is your child's breathing very labored and is your child unable to swallow? **YES** → SEEK EMERGENCY CARE

NO

Is your child drooling, breathing through the mouth, sticking out the chin and gasping for air? **YES** → SEEK EMERGENCY CARE

NO

Are your child's lips and nails turning blue or dark? **YES** → SEEK EMERGENCY CARE

NO

If your child is making a sound like a barking seal and finding it hard to breathe: Have you used steam for more than 15 minutes and taken your child outside in the cold night air for 15 minutes *without* getting relief for your child's symptoms? **YES** → SEEK EMERGENCY CARE

NO

Is your child making a sound like a barking seal? **YES** → SEE DOCTOR

NO

→ PROVIDE SELF-CARE

Self-Care Procedures

- Try not to panic. While wheezing and barking sounds are frightening, remaining calm will lessen your child's fear and anxiety.
  - Hold your child to comfort him or her. Helping your child to relax may help stop the windpipe from constricting and make breathing easier.
- Use a hot bath or shower to help relieve the congestion:
  - Take your child to the bathroom and close the door.
  - Turn on the hot water in the sink and shower to fill the room with steam.

- Do not put your child in the shower. Instead, sit your child on the toilet or a chair, but not on the floor. Try reading a book to your child to pass the time and ease any fears.
- Open the window to let in cool air. This helps to create more steam.
- Allow at least 15 minutes for the steam to ease the symptoms. If the symptoms continue, carry your child outdoors to breathe the cold night air. If this doesn't ease the breathing difficulties, seek emergency care.
- Use a vaporizer in your child's room. Cool-mist vaporizers are preferred because they give off cool air and avoid the risk of scalding with hot water. Clean the vaporizer after each use.
  - Make a "croup tent" by placing the vaporizer under the crib or bed. Drape a blanket over the crib near the child's head or over an umbrella if your child now sleeps in a bed, to trap the steam. Never leave your child alone while he or she is in a croup tent. Stay awake to monitor your child.
- Crying is a good sign. It means that your child's symptoms are subsiding. A crying child is able to breathe.

Lice

Head lice are tiny parasites about the size of a sesame seed. These flat, wingless "bugs" survive by sucking human blood. Louse bites cause an intense itching and red spots on the skin that look like mosquito bites. The adult lice are rarely seen. Instead, you see what are called nits, clusters of lice eggs deposited on hair strands that are often mistaken for dandruff.

Lice spread quickly from person to person. No matter how well-groomed and clean your child is, he or she can get them in school, from toilet seats or from anyone who already has them. Female lice lay about six eggs a day. The eggs hatch in eight to 10 days, after which they soon begin their annoying biting.

There are three types of lice: head lice, pubic lice and body lice. All are very attracted to body heat. Head lice are the most common type, especially among children in day-care centers, camps and schools. Pubic lice, found on the pubic hair, are called "crabs" because the lice look like crabs. Body lice live in the seams of dirty clothes and bedding.

Prevention

To prevent head lice, children should be told:
- Do not share hats, brushes or combs.
- Do not lie on a pillow shared with another child.
- Shampoo hair and bathe frequently.

You should:
- Change bed linens often and wash them in hot water and dry them in a dryer, especially during an epidemic of lice at school.
- Vacuum furniture, mattresses, rugs, stuffed animals and car seats if anyone in your family is infected with lice. Do not use insecticidal sprays for lice.
- Immediately notify anyone who may have been in close contact with your child to help prevent infecting others with lice. Be sure to contact:
  - Your child's school
  - Your child-care provider
  - Parents of your child's friends
  - Neighbors
- Wash combs and brushes. Then soak them in hot, not boiling, water for 10 minutes.
- Check your children for head lice and nits at least once a week. Check more often if your child is scratching his or her head. Look for nits around the nape of the neck and behind the ears. Use two round toothpicks to spread hairs apart to look for nits.

Questions to Ask

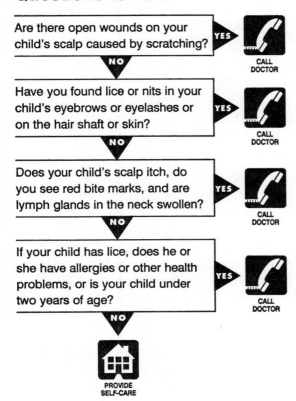

Are there open wounds on your child's scalp caused by scratching? **YES** → CALL DOCTOR

NO ↓

Have you found lice or nits in your child's eyebrows or eyelashes or on the hair shaft or skin? **YES** → CALL DOCTOR

NO ↓

Does your child's scalp itch, do you see red bite marks, and are lymph glands in the neck swollen? **YES** → CALL DOCTOR

NO ↓

If your child has lice, does he or she have allergies or other health problems, or is your child under two years of age? **YES** → CALL DOCTOR

NO ↓

PROVIDE SELF-CARE

Self-Care Procedures

Only insecticidal shampoos, lotions and creams kill lice. You can buy these products without a prescription at a drugstore. Your doctor can also prescribe medication to treat lice and kill the nits. All lice-killing products are pesticides; consequently, they must be used with caution and only as directed.

Everyone in your household should be checked for lice and nits. However, only treat those who are infested. Lice-killing products are not to be used to prevent infestation.

When using an insecticidal shampoo:
- Follow the directions exactly as given, and:
  - Remove your child's shirt.
  - Give your child a towel to cover his or her eyes. Do not use the shampoo around your child's eyes.
  - Lean your child over the sink as you apply the shampoo. Do not put your child in the shower or bathtub; the shampoo should only be applied to the head and neck.
- Don't use too much shampoo or you'll make your child's scalp too dry.
- If you have open sores on your hands, wear gloves or have someone else shampoo your child's hair.

To remove the nits:
- Shine a flashlight into the scalp, or other infected body part. Nits may be gray and hard to see. If your child has blonde hair, check your child's scalp carefully because the nits will be harder to find.
- Begin in one part of the scalp and move row-by-row, even strand-by-strand, when necessary.
- Remove nits from the hair strands with tweezers, safety manicure scissors, a nit-comb (available at the drugstore) or your fingernails. Some products come with a fine-toothed comb you can use to dislodge the nits.
  - Before using the comb, dip it in hot vinegar. This will help loosen the nits.
  - Comb the hair from the scalp toward the ends. After each pass, check the comb for nits.
  - Or, using hair clips to hold the hair, separate it into four or five sections. Starting in one section, lift about an inch of hair upward and outward. Place the comb on the scalp and comb the hair from the scalp to its tip. Repeat for each section of hair.
  - Soak all combs, brushes and barrettes for several hours in the insecticidal shampoo or for 10 minutes in hot water.
- Check for nits every day for about 10 days.
- If necessary, shampoo again a week later to kill any newly hatched nits. It is not necessary to remove nits after treatment is completed, except for cosmetic purposes.

You should also:

- Immediately wash bedding and clothing in water hotter than 125°F. Heat kills the lice and destroys the nits. If an item cannot be washed, put it in an airtight plastic bag and seal. Do not open it for at least two weeks. Deprived of blood, the lice will die.
- Dry-clean clothing and hats that cannot be washed.
- Vacuum all mattresses, pillows, rugs and upholstered furniture, especially in areas where children play. Using the long, narrow attachment, suck lice or nits out of car seats, toys, stuffed animals and other small areas. Dispose of the vacuum cleaner bags.

Measles

Measles is a very contagious disease caused by the rubeola virus. Also called red or seven-day measles, it mostly occurs in children, but can affect older persons, too. With proper immunization, though, the disease is preventable. The American Academy of Pediatrics recommends two measles, mumps, rubella (MMR) vaccinations: the first to be given between 12 and 15 months of age and the second to be given between the ages of four and six (when a child enters school) or between the ages of 11 and 12 (when a child enters middle school or junior high). A child who receives immunizations will probably never get the measles. So make sure your child gets these shots.

When a child does get the measles, he or she has probably been exposed to someone else who had them 10 to 12 days earlier. The symptoms of measles usually take place in this order:

- Temperature of 102°F or higher
- Fatigue
- Loss of appetite
- Runny nose and sneezing
- Cough
- Red eyes and sensitivity to light
- Tiny white spots (called Koplik spots) in the mouth and throat

- Blotchy red rash that starts on the face and spreads to the rest of the body: to the chest and abdomen and then to the arms and legs. The rash usually lasts for up to seven days.

The measles virus is spread by nose, mouth or throat secretions, either on soiled articles or through coughing, sneezing and so on. It can be picked up three to six days before the rash appears as well as up to several days after the rash starts.

If your child has been exposed to measles, but hasn't been immunized, contact his or her doctor or the public health department. If done early enough, a measles vaccine may prevent him or her from getting measles. An injection of gamma globulin can help protect your child against measles for three months. Let your child's school know if your child has measles. All cases of measles must be reported to the public health department.

When your child gets the measles, not much can be done to shorten the illness. Your child will probably start feeling better by the fourth day of the rash unless other problems occur. Possible complications include eye or ear infections, pneumonia and meningitis.

Questions to Ask

Are any of these problems present:
- Blue or purple lips or nails
- Convulsion
- Extreme difficulty in breathing
- Inability to speak more than three or four words between breaths
- Confusion or excessive drowsiness
- Severe headache and stiff neck
- Bleeding from the nose or mouth or into the skin
- Dark purple splotches on the skin

 YES

SEEK EMERGENCY CARE

 NO

flowchart continued on next page

Are any of these problems present:
- Sore throat
- Earache or tugging at the ears
- A yellow discharge from the eyes or nose
- Breathing that is labored, but not due to a stuffy nose
- Fever that comes back after temperature has been normal for a day or more or fever that is still present beyond the fourth day of the rash

YES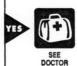

SEE
DOCTOR

NO

PROVIDE
SELF-CARE

Self-Care Procedures

- Keep a record of your child's temperature. Take it in the morning and the evening. Give the recommended dose of acetaminophen for fever and/or aches and pains. *Note: Do not give aspirin or any medication containing salicylates to anyone 19 years of age or younger, unless directed by a physician, due to its association with Reye's syndrome, a potentially fatal condition.*
- Isolate your child from other people who have not had measles or a measles immunization. Any child who has come in contact with your child should be taken for a measles immunization unless he or she has already been immunized or had the measles.
- Because your child's eyes may be sensitive:
  - Keep the lighting in the house dim. Draw the drapes, pull the shades down and use low-wattage light bulbs.
  - If your child must go outdoors, have him or her wear sunglasses.
  - Keep the TV and video games turned off.
  - Urge your child not to read or do close-up work.
  - Wipe your child's closed eyes with a clean wet cloth or wet cotton ball several times a day.

- For a cough:
  - Use a cool-mist vaporizer, especially at night. Use distilled, not tap, water in the vaporizer and change the water daily.
  - Have your child—if he or she is five years of age or older—suck on cough drops, lozenges or hard candy.
  - Give your child plenty of fluids. Water is helpful in loosening mucus and also soothes an irritated throat. Fruit juices and even tea and soda are also good.
  - Give your child cough medicines as recommended by his or her doctor or pharmacist.
  - You can make your own cough medicine at home by mixing one part lemon juice and two parts honey or corn syrup. (Do not give to children under one year of age.)
- Have your child rest until the fever and rash go away.
- Keep your child home from school until seven to 10 days after the fever and rash disappear and until his or her appetite, strength and feeling of well-being are back to normal.

Seizures

A seizure is an out-of-control misfire between nerve cells in the brain. When these nerve cells short-circuit, normal brain functions are disrupted.

Sometimes the cause of a seizure is not known. There are several things, however, that are known to cause seizures. Fever fits are seizures that occur when a child has a high fever. In fact, high fevers are the most common cause of seizures in children ages six months to four years. A temperature higher than 102°F can set off a fever fit. Illnesses that cause a rapid rise in temperature, such as roseola, are often linked to fever fits. Spiking high temperatures seem to confuse the brain's normal electrical impulses. Seizures can also occur in normal, healthy children whose internal thermometer has not fully developed.

Seizures also may be triggered by poisons, infections, reactions to medications and drugs, Reye's syndrome, snakebites and vaccinations. Even breath-holding can set off a seizure. And seizure is the most common symptom of epilepsy, a disorder of the brain.

Types of seizures fall into two general groups: general and partial. A general seizure affects the whole brain and can cause loss of consciousness and/or convulsions. Damage is confined to small areas of the brain with a partial seizure.

Types of general seizures are:
- **Nonconvulsive ones.** These are also called absence or petit mal seizures. Symptoms include staring into space and repeated blinking. The child is unaware of the seizure, but someone else may think he or she is daydreaming or not paying attention. These can occur once a day or more than a hundred times a day and can result in learning problems.
- **Convulsive.** These are also called tonic-clonic or grand mal seizures. There can be many symptoms, including crying out, falling down, losing consciousness, entire body stiffening, then uncontrollable jerks and twitches. The child's muscles relax after the seizure. He or she may lose bowel and bladder control and may be confused, sleepy and have a headache.

Types of partial seizures are:
- Simple ones in which symptoms include tingling feelings, twitching, seeing flashing lights, hallucination of smell and/or taste
- Complex ones involving episodes (e.g., sitting motionless or moving or behaving in strange or repetitive ways) called automatisms. Examples include lip smacking, chewing and fidgeting with the hands. There is usually no loss of consciousness, but the child who has this type of seizure may be confused and not remember details of it.

Most seizures are brief, lasting from one to five minutes. Short-lasting seizures do not cause permanent damage unless they are associated with lack of breathing and turning blue. Seizures that have not stopped after 30 minutes, though, may signal a more serious condition. Any child who experiences a seizure should be evaluated by a doctor. Less than half of children who have a seizure ever have another one.

Prevention

The best way to prevent a fever fit is to rapidly reduce the fever. This is especially important for a child who has had a fever fit in the past. He or she is more likely to have another one with future fevers. Also:
- Dress your child in loose clothes to avoid overheating.
- Rinse your child with tepid water or give acetaminophen if the fever rises above 103°F. Continue trying to reduce the fever in this way until it is 101°F or less. *Note: Do not give aspirin or any medication containing salicylates to anyone 19 years of age or younger, unless directed by a physician, due to its association with Reye's syndrome, a potentially fatal condition.*
- Discuss using fever-lowering suppositories with your doctor. Using one at the first sign of a fever may prevent a seizure.

Questions to Ask

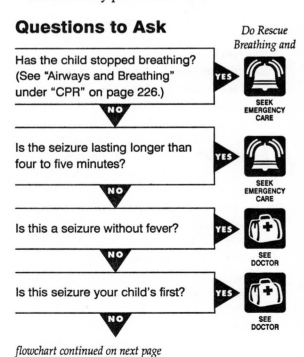

Do Rescue Breathing and

Has the child stopped breathing? (See "Airways and Breathing" under "CPR" on page 226.) **YES** → SEEK EMERGENCY CARE

NO ↓

Is the seizure lasting longer than four to five minutes? **YES** → SEEK EMERGENCY CARE

NO ↓

Is this a seizure without fever? **YES** → SEE DOCTOR

NO ↓

Is this seizure your child's first? **YES** → SEE DOCTOR

NO ↓

flowchart continued on next page

Is your child younger than six months or older than four years? **YES**

SEE
DOCTOR

NO

PROVIDE
SELF-CARE

Self-Care Procedures

It is easy to panic while watching a child have a seizure. Try to remember, though, that if it is a fever seizure, it will stop within a few minutes by itself. The primary concern should be preventing injury to the child during the seizure and lowering his or her temperature.

- During the seizure, protect the child from falling and hitting his or her head on a table edge or any sharp object. Move furniture, toys and such out of the way.
- Make sure his or her air passage is open.
  - Gently pull on the jaw as you extend the neck backwards.
  - Roll the child on the side to allow saliva to drain from the mouth.
  - Clear the mouth of vomit, if there is any, so the child can breathe.
- Do not force anything into a child's mouth to prevent him or her from biting the tongue. Children rarely bite their tongues during a fever seizure.
- If the seizure is due to a fever, start lowering your child's temperature as soon as the seizure subsides by sponging the body with room temperature water. Do not put the child in a bathtub. Do not use an ice pack because it drops the temperature too quickly.
- Do not give medication, foods or fluids by mouth during a seizure.
- Note how many minutes the seizure lasts and observe the symptoms that take place so you can report these to the doctor.
- Following the seizure, the child will likely be sleepy and not remember what has happened. This is normal.
- Dress the child in light, loose-fitting clothing and put him or her to sleep in a cool room.

Skin Rashes

Skin rashes come in all forms and sizes. Some are raised bumps; others are flat red blotches. Some are itchy blisters; others are patches of rough skin. Most rashes are harmless and clear up on their own within a few days, but a few may need medical attention.

The chart on page 92 lists information on some common skin rashes.

Questions to Ask

Is the child having trouble breathing or swallowing or is the tongue swollen? If yes, give shot and follow other instructions from emergency "bee sting" kit if the child carries one with him or her for severe reactions to insect stings. **YES**

SEEK
EMERGENCY
CARE

NO

Does your child have a purple, blotchy rash with cool extremities? **YES**

SEEK
EMERGENCY
CARE

NO

Does the child have any of the following:
- Fever
- Headache
- Sore throat
- A fine red rash that feels rough like sandpaper
- Joint pain along with a target-like rash

YES

SEE
DOCTOR

NO

Are there any large, fluid-filled blisters present or pus or swelling around the rash lesions? **YES**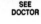

SEE
DOCTOR

NO

Has your child recently been exposed to someone with a "strep" infection? **YES**

SEE
DOCTOR

NO

flowchart continued on next page

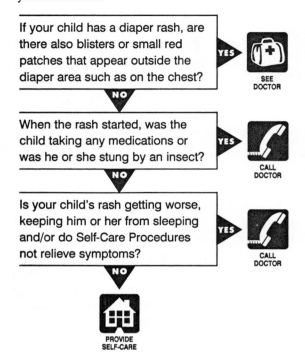

If your child has a diaper rash, are there also blisters or small red patches that appear outside the diaper area such as on the chest? **YES** → **SEE DOCTOR**

NO ↓

When the rash started, was the child taking any medications or was he or she stung by an insect? **YES** → **CALL DOCTOR**

NO ↓

Is your child's rash getting worse, keeping him or her from sleeping and/or do Self-Care Procedures not relieve symptoms? **YES** → **CALL DOCTOR**

NO ↓

PROVIDE SELF-CARE

Self-Care Procedures

Diaper rash is best treated by:
- Changing diapers as soon as they become wet or soiled (even at night if the rash is extensive)
- Washing your baby with plenty of warm water, not disposable wipes, to prevent irritating the skin. If the skin appears irritated, apply a light coat of zinc oxide ointment after the skin is completely dry.
- Keeping the skin dry and exposed to air
- Keeping your baby naked, on a soft, fluffy towel, for 10 to 15 minutes before putting on a fresh diaper
- Putting diapers on loosely so air can circulate under them. If disposable diapers are used, punch a few holes in them. Avoid ones with tight leg bands.
- Not using plastic pants until the rash is gone
- Washing cloth diapers in mild soap. Add ½ cup of vinegar to your rinse water to help remove what's left of the soap.

Cradle cap can be treated by using an antidandruff shampoo. Use it once a day, massaging your baby's scalp with a soft brush or washcloth for five minutes. You can soften the hard crusts of this rash by applying mineral oil on the scalp before washing your child's hair. Be sure to thoroughly wash the oil out; otherwise, the cradle cap condition may worsen.

Heat rash is best treated by keeping your child in a cool, dry area. It will usually disappear within two to three days if you keep the skin cool. You can ease your child's discomfort by:
- Giving him or her a bath in cool water, without soap, every couple of hours
- Letting your child's skin air dry
- Applying calamine (not Caladryl) lotion to the very itchy spots
- Putting corn starch in body creases (e.g., inside elbows)
- Avoiding ointments and creams that can block the sweat gland pores

Hives can be eased by:
- Giving your child an antihistamine such as Benadryl. Check the labels of cold medications. Those that contain diphenhydramine or chlorpheniramine are good choices, too. Remember, though, that most antihistamines are likely to make your child drowsy.
- Cooling off your child. Rub an ice cube over the hives, drape a washcloth dipped in cool water over the affected areas or give a cool-water bath.
- Applying calamine lotion, witch hazel or zinc oxide to the rash.
- Finding and eliminating the cause of the allergic reaction.

To relieve the itchy rash typical of poison ivy, oak and sumac:
- As soon as possible, remove your child's clothes and shoes. Wash him or her with soap and water to remove the plant oil from his or her skin. Rub the affected skin area with alcohol or alcohol wipes, then rinse with water. Wash all clothes and shoes your child has on.

- Trim your child's nails. Encourage your child not to scratch. Keep your child busy with other activities.
- Soak the rash area in cool water, or give your child baths with Aveeno (an over-the-counter colloidal oatmeal product) or put one cup of oatmeal in a tub full of water.
- Give your child a hot shower if he or she can tolerate it. At first the itching will get worse, but after a while it stops and the relief can last for hours. Repeat as soon as the itching starts again.
- Use calamine lotion every three to four hours.
- Apply a hydrocortisone cream. Put a very small dab of cream on the rash. Be careful not to rub and spread the poison. If you can see the cream on the skin, you've used too much. Repeat as needed every two to four hours. Do not use these creams near the eyes.
- Teach your child to recognize poison ivy, oak and sumac. Tell your child to stay away from them.

Protect your child from Lyme disease by:
- Having him or her wear long pants tucked into socks and long-sleeve shirts when walking through fields and forests. (Light-colored, tightly woven clothing is best.)
- Inspecting or having your child examined for ticks after these activities. Remove any ticks found on the skin. Use tweezers to grasp the tick as close to the skin as possible. Pull gently and carefully in a steady upward motion at the point where the tick's mouth-part enters the skin. Try not to crush the tick because the secretions released may spread disease. Wash the wound area and your hands with soap and water after removing ticks. Save the tick in a closed jar of alcohol. It could help in diagnosing Lyme disease.

Swollen Glands

Running throughout the body is a powerful military-like network ready to protect the body against an invasion of foreign agents. This network, called the lymphatic system, is made up of bean-sized lymph glands (also called nodes) and the road-like lymph channels that connect them. When a virus or other organism invades the body, the lymph glands set to work, cranking out a type of white blood cell ready to kill the invaders. Lymph glands also act as filters, trapping viruses, bacteria and cancer cells.

Normally, you cannot feel your child's lymph glands except when they swell in response to an infection or other invader. As a general rule, infections cause swollen lymph glands that are tender to the touch. The nodes often stay enlarged long after the infection is gone. In fact, most visits to the doctor's office for swollen glands occur after parents notice a neck node that has been present for a while. These nodes are generally painless and harmless. Be aware, though, that when the nodes are hard and rubbery and are increasing in size, they may be caused by a more serious disease such as lymphoma (cancer of the lymph glands), leukemia or other type of cancer.

The salivary glands are another type of gland. They are found under the tongue, on the floor of the mouth and just below the ear lobe. They are not lymph glands. It is the salivary glands located under the ear lobe, close to the jaw line, that swell when invaded by the virus that causes mumps.

Causes of Swollen Glands

- Infections in the throat and/or ear are the most common causes of swollen glands in the neck. Infections in the feet, legs and genital area cause lymph glands to swell in the groin.
- Infectious mononucleosis, known among high school and college students as "the kissing disease" or "mono"
- Mumps

- German measles
- Cat scratch fever (caused by an infection carried on a cat's claws and transmitted to the child through a scratch)
- Insect bites
- Medications such as Dilantin (taken for epilepsy)
- Recent dental work
- Lymphoma, a cancer of the lymph glands, or leukemia
- Tuberculosis (TB)

Prevention

- Make sure your children's immunizations against measles, mumps and rubella (MMR) are up-to-date.
- Keep your child away from other people who you know have contagious conditions.

Questions to Ask

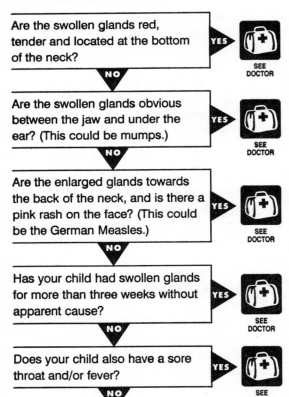

Are the swollen glands red, tender and located at the bottom of the neck? **YES** — SEE DOCTOR

NO

Are the swollen glands obvious between the jaw and under the ear? (This could be mumps.) **YES** — SEE DOCTOR

NO

Are the enlarged glands towards the back of the neck, and is there a pink rash on the face? (This could be the German Measles.) **YES** — SEE DOCTOR

NO

Has your child had swollen glands for more than three weeks without apparent cause? **YES** — SEE DOCTOR

NO

Does your child also have a sore throat and/or fever? **YES** — SEE DOCTOR

NO

flowchart continued in next column

flowchart continued

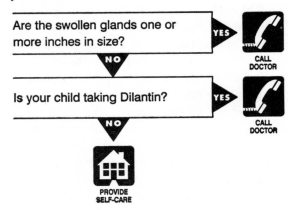

Are the swollen glands one or more inches in size? **YES** — CALL DOCTOR

NO

Is your child taking Dilantin? **YES** — CALL DOCTOR

NO

PROVIDE SELF-CARE

Self-Care Procedures

There is little you can do for swollen glands except to treat the underlying cause. Watch to see if the glands enlarge or if others swell as well. If the swollen glands continue to enlarge or last more than three or four weeks, it's a good idea to consult your doctor.

You can, however, make your child more comfortable by:
- Encouraging him or her to rest when tired and to avoid activities that may cause more fatigue.
- Giving your child lots of liquids to drink.
- Applying warm compresses and antiseptic creams to any scratches or other injuries.

See also: "Self-Care Procedures for Measles" on page 151, for "Sore Throats" on page 66 and for "Tonsillitis" on page 157.

Tonsillitis

The tonsils are masses of tissue at the back of the throat. They act as a filter to help prevent infections in the throat, mouth and sinuses from spreading to other parts of the body. They also produce antibodies that fight throat and nose infections. Tonsillitis occurs when the tonsils get inflamed, the cause for which is a bacterial or viral infection.

Symptoms of tonsillitis include:
- Mild to severe throat pain
- Swollen lymph glands on either side of the neck or jaw
- Ear pain
- Difficulty in swallowing
- Chills and fever
- Headache

A throat culture is necessary to diagnose the cause of tonsillitis. Antibiotics are prescribed for strep or other bacterial infections, but not for viral ones.

More often than not, having tonsillitis, even when it recurs up to seven times a year, does not mean that the tonsils should be removed (in a surgical procedure called a tonsillectomy). Don't pressure your child's doctor to remove your child's tonsils just because this was commonly done years ago. Only under certain medical conditions should a tonsillectomy be done.

Questions to Ask

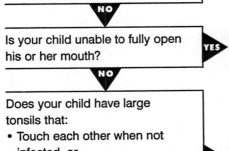

Is the tonsillitis severe and/or are these problems present?
- Extreme difficulty in swallowing
- Inability to swallow saliva
- Difficulty in breathing
- Inability to say more than three to four words between breaths
- Drooling

YES → SEEK EMERGENCY CARE

NO ↓

Is your child unable to fully open his or her mouth?

YES → SEE DOCTOR

NO ↓

Does your child have large tonsils that:
- Touch each other when not infected, or
- Result in continued mouth breathing, or
- Muffle speech, which is due to no other cause

YES → SEE DOCTOR

NO ↓

flowchart continued in next column

flowchart continued

Do any of the following accompany your child's tonsillitis:
- Fever
- Swollen, enlarged or tender neck glands
- Headache
- Ear pain or tugging at the ears
- Bad breath
- Loss of appetite
- Vomiting or abdominal pain

YES → SEE DOCTOR

NO ↓

Do the tonsils or back of the throat look bright red or have visible pus deposits?

YES → SEE DOCTOR

NO ↓

Does someone else in the family have a strep throat or does your child get strep throat often?

YES → CALL DOCTOR

NO ↓

Has your child's sore throat lasted more than two weeks even though it is mild?

YES → CALL DOCTOR

NO ↓

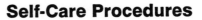

PROVIDE SELF-CARE

Self-Care Procedures

You can take some steps to relieve your child's discomfort from tonsillitis. Have him or her:
- Gargle every few hours with a solution of ¼ teaspoon of salt dissolved in four ounces of warm water, if your child is older than eight years.
- Drink plenty of warm beverages such as tea (with or without honey) and soup, if tolerated. (Do not give honey to a child under one year of age.)
- Use a cool-mist vaporizer or humidifier in the room where he or she spends most of his or her time. (Use distilled water in it and clean after each use.)

- Eat foods that are soft and/or cold and easy to swallow (e.g., juices, popsicles and ice cream). Avoid spicy foods.
- Suck on a piece of hard candy or medicated lozenge occasionally (if your child is five years of age or older). Corn syrup can be used periodically for younger children.
- Take the recommended dosage of acetaminophen for pain and/or fever. *Note: Do not give aspirin or any medication containing salicylates to anyone 19 years of age or younger, unless directed by a physician, due to its association with Reye's syndrome, a potentially fatal condition.*
- Avoid throat sprays. These may contain benzocaine, which could cause an adverse reaction.
- Avoid secondhand cigarette smoke.

Wheezing

Wheezing is a high-pitched purring or whistling sound. It is heard more on breathing out than on breathing in. The wheezing sound is usually caused by air flowing through swollen and narrowed breathing tubes that are in spasm. Muscle spasms in the airways make breathing even more difficult.

Wheezing is sometimes confused with other respiratory sounds. The sounds of croup, for example, resemble a harsh, raspy noise on breathing in and are sometimes accompanied by a high-pitched cough. A stuffed nose, though, emits a snorting sound. And a rattling sound is often due to mucus in the windpipe.

Consider wheezing as a warning sign that your child is having trouble breathing. It is a good idea to check with your physician if your child wheezes.

Causes of Wheezing

- Asthma, which is often a disease of childhood. More than half of the affected youngsters outgrow asthma by the time they become adults, though it can recur later in life. Asthma attacks can be frightening for

parent and child alike. However, while they can be quite serious, they are not often fatal. Many things can trigger an asthma attack such as:
- Exposure to something your child is allergic to, including dust mites, pollen, mold, food, animal dander and perfume
- Exercise
- Medications
- Stressful event
- Change in the weather, especially a rapid rise or fall in barometric pressure and temperature
- Noxious fumes from wet paint, disinfectants, pesticides, tobacco smoke, burning coals, vehicle exhaust, wood smoke and similar smells, to name a few
- Ice cold drinks or cold air. Breathing tubes sometimes constrict when exposed to extreme cold.
- Respiratory infection (bacterial or viral, especially in infants)
- Foreign objects caught in the airway
- Severe allergic reaction
- Pneumonia, acute bronchitis or congestive heart failure
- Genetic disorders that affect the lungs

Questions to Ask

(Note: You may need to do the Heimlich maneuver [for choking], rescue breathing or CPR, and call 911 or your local rescue squad if your child is turning blue and/or not breathing. Take an emergency first aid class for children to learn when and how to do each of these procedures.)

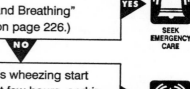

Is your child turning blue and/or not breathing?
(See "Airway and Breathing" under "CPR" on page 226.)

YES → Do Rescue Breathing and **SEEK EMERGENCY CARE**

NO

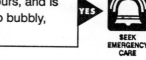

Did your child's wheezing start during the past few hours, and is he or she coughing up bubbly, pink or white phlegm?

YES → **SEEK EMERGENCY CARE**

NO

flowchart continued on next page

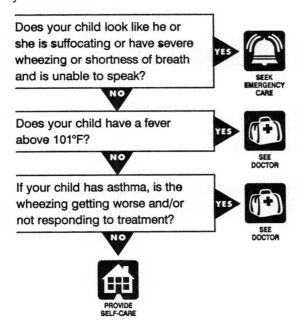

Does your child look like he or she is suffocating or have severe wheezing or shortness of breath and is unable to speak? **YES** → SEEK EMERGENCY CARE

NO

Does your child have a fever above 101°F? **YES** → SEE DOCTOR

NO

If your child has asthma, is the wheezing getting worse and/or not responding to treatment? **YES** → SEE DOCTOR

NO

PROVIDE SELF-CARE

Self-Care Procedures

While there is no cure for viral infections, allergic reactions and asthma, you can ease your child's wheezing in many ways:

- Encourage your child to drink lots of fluids to thin the mucus. Coax your child to slowly sip juice, water, broth or weak tea. Do not give your child ice cold drinks.
- Set up a vaporizer, preferably a cold-mist model, or carry your child to the bathroom and turn on the hot water faucets in the sink and shower. (See "Self-Care Procedures for Croup" on page 147.) Clean vaporizer after each use.

For a child suffering from asthma, follow the home treatment regimen recommended by your doctor. You may be told to:

- Remain calm. Have your child use the bronchodilator as instructed by his or her doctor.
- If the asthma attack is caused by an allergic reaction, find ways to reduce your child's exposure to the allergens that trigger the attack.
- Prepare a solution of bleach (¾ cup of bleach per gallon of water) and wipe bathroom tiles and floors, kitchen appliances, woodwork

and anywhere else fungus and mold may be growing. Then air out the room.

- Pet dander sets off allergic reactions in many children. If your child is allergic to cats or dogs, try to keep the animal outside or away from your child, but especially out of the bedroom.
- Vacuum often to suck up dust mites, pollen and pet dander. But first put a dust and pollen filter mask on your child to prevent his or her breathing the disturbed dust.
- Cover your child's mattress and pillow in plastic to avoid exposure to dust mites that like to hide in the creases. And wash mattress pads in hot water every week.
- If you smoke, quit. Even residual smoke in a room can trigger an attack.
- Use washable throw rugs instead of carpeting. Carpeting is like a magnet to pollen, pet dander, mold and dust mites; its fibers attract these allergens.
- Install an air conditioner or electronic air filter on your furnace.
- Change and/or wash furnace and air conditioner filters frequently.
- Use a medically approved portable air purifier in your child's room.
- Use pillows with polyester fibers, not feathers.

If the asthma attack is caused by exercise, have your child:

- Avoid exercising in cold weather.
- Swim, because pool areas are usually humid.
- Start out slowly and pace him- or herself during the activity to avoid an attack.
- Take prescribed medication about 15 minutes before exercising.
- Shower, wash his or her hair and put on clean clothes after coming in contact with grass, pollen, animals or other substances he or she is allergic to.

(Note: Keep small objects, such as detachable toy parts and foods like peanuts and popcorn, out of the reach of small children, to prevent them from inhaling them.)

CHAPTER 18

WOMEN'S HEALTH

Breast Cancer and Breast Self-Examination

Breast cancer is the most common form of cancer among women, accounting for 30 percent of cancers women get. Over the course of her lifetime, a woman's risk for breast cancer is one in eight. Each year, there are approximately 180,000 new cases of breast cancer and 45,000 deaths from it. Only lung cancer causes more cancer deaths among women.

The chance of developing breast cancer increases dramatically with age. The National Cancer Institute has given the following statistics for a woman's chances of developing breast cancer:

By Age	Chances
25	1 in 19,608
30	1 in 2,525
35	1 in 622
40	1 in 217
45	1 in 93
50	1 in 50
55	1 in 33
60	1 in 24
65	1 in 17
70	1 in 14
75	1 in 11
80	1 in 10
85	1 in 9
Ever	1 in 8

Men can also develop breast cancer, but it is very unusual. About 300 men die each year from the disease.

Breast cancer results from malignant tumors which invade and destroy normal tissue. When these tumors break away and spread to other parts of the body, it is called metastasis. Breast cancers can spread to the lymph nodes, lungs, liver, bone and brain.

The risk of breast cancer increases above the normal risk with these factors:
- Having had cancer in one breast, which increases the risk for cancer in the other breast
- Never giving birth or giving birth after age 30
- Early onset of menstruation (before age 12)
- Late menopause (after age 55)
- Family history of breast cancer, especially for mothers, daughters and sisters of women with breast cancer prior to menopause
- Exposure to radiation
- Diet high in fat
- Obesity
- Diabetes
- Recent trauma

Detection

Recommendations for mammograms vary among government and health organizations. Some favor screening before age 50. All suggest a mammogram every year or at least every two years after age 50. Any woman who notices a lump in her breast or any of the other symptoms mentioned previously should see her doctor as soon as possible. Tests can be done to tell if cancerous cells are present. Also, make sure you have mammograms at facilities that are accredited by the American College of

Radiology. Call the National Cancer Institute hotline at 800-4-CANCER to find ones in your area.

Treatment

There are a variety of treatments for breast cancer. The main treatment is surgery. The removal of the cancerous area is most often recommended along with taking a sample of the lymph nodes in the armpit to see if cancer has spread there. Other treatments are radiation therapy, chemotherapy and hormonal therapy.

It is important to find out the type of cancer cell that is involved. If the cancer is a type that spreads quickly, a more extensive surgical treatment may be chosen.

Types of surgical procedures:

Lumpectomy - The lump and a border of surrounding tissue are removed.

Partial or segmental mastectomy - The tumor and up to one-fourth of the breast tissue are removed.

Simple or total mastectomy - The entire breast is removed.

Modified radical mastectomy - The entire breast, the underarm lymph nodes and the lining covering the chest muscles, but not the muscles themselves, are removed.

Radical mastectomy - The breast, lymph nodes in the armpit and the chest muscles under the breast are removed.

Ask your doctor about the benefits and risks for each surgical option and decide together which option is best for you.

Questions to Ask

Do you see or feel any lumps, thickening or changes of any kind when you examine your breasts? For example, is there dimpling, puckering or retraction of the skin or a change in the shape or contour of the breast?

YES SEE DOCTOR

NO

Do you have breast pain or a constant tenderness that lasts throughout the menstrual cycle?

YES SEE DOCTOR

NO

If you normally have lumpy breasts (already diagnosed as being benign by your doctor), do you notice any new lumps or have any lumps changed in size? Or are you concerned about having benign lumps?

YES SEE DOCTOR

NO

Do the nipples become drawn into the chest or inverted totally, change shape or become crusty from a discharge?

YES SEE DOCTOR

NO

Is there any nonmilky discharge when you squeeze the nipple of either breast or both breasts?

YES SEE DOCTOR

NO

Do you have a family history of breast cancer which leads you to be concerned even in the absence of noticeable problems when you examine your breasts?

YES CALL DOCTOR

NO

Have you had a recent trauma that resulted in a breast lump being formed?

YES CALL DOCTOR

NO

PROVIDE SELF-CARE

Self-Care Procedures

How to Examine Your Breasts

It is normal to have some lumpiness or thickening in the breasts. By examining your breasts once each month, you will learn what is normal for you and when any changes do occur. Some women find that doing a daily or weekly self-exam works better for them. They learn their breasts at all phases of their menstrual cycle. The more you examine your breasts, the better you can learn what is normal for you. Your "job" isn't just to find lumps, but also to notice if there are any changes.

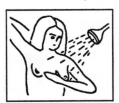 **In the shower** - With your fingers flat, move gently over every part of each breast. Use your right hand to examine the left breast and your left hand to examine the right breast. Check for any thickening, hard lump or knot.

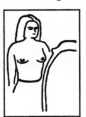 **In front of a mirror** - Check your breasts with your arms at your sides. Then raise your arms overhead. Look for 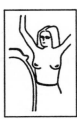 any changes in the shape of each breast, swelling, dimpling or changes in the nipples.

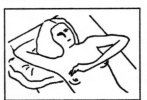 **Lying down** - To examine your right breast, put a pillow under your right shoulder. Place your right hand behind your head. Keeping the fingers of your left hand flat, press gently in small circular motions around an imaginary clock face. Begin at the outermost top of your right breast for 12 o'clock, then move to 10 o'clock, and so on, until you get back to 12 o'clock. Each breast will have a normal ridge of firm tissue. Then move in one inch toward the nipple. Keep circling to examine every part of your breast, including the nipple.

Repeat the procedure on the left breast with a pillow under the left shoulder and your left hand behind your head. Finally, squeeze the  nipple of each breast gently between the thumb and index finger. Any discharge, clear or bloody, should be reported to your physician immediately. Continue to perform breast self-examination monthly.

Self-Care and Preventive Procedures

- Eat a low-fat diet of 25 percent or less of total calories as fat. Focus on fresh fruits and vegetables, whole grains and so on.
- Eat vegetables that contain a substance called sulforaphane, which may help protect against breast cancer. Examples are broccoli, cabbage, cauliflower and brussels sprouts.
- Avoid unnecessary X-rays. Wear a lead apron when you have dental X-rays and other X-rays not of the chest.
- Don't smoke. Stop smoking if you do.
- Breast-feed your babies. This may reduce your risk for breast cancer, especially before menopause.
- Limit foods that are salt-cured, smoked and preserved with nitrites and nitrates. Examples are hot dogs, bacon, smoked sausage and ham.
- Limit alcohol.

Eating Disorders: Anorexia Nervosa and Bulimia

An eating disorder may be defined, in a sense, as self-abuse. It can be just as harmful to your health as substance abuse involving alcohol or drugs. Two of these disorders, anorexia and bulimia, result from the fear of overeating and of gaining weight. They also share other common traits that reflect the mental and physical health of the sufferer:

- Depression
- Low self-esteem, poor body image
- Self-destructive outlook, self-punishment for some imagined wrong
- Disturbed family relationships
- Increased rate of illness due to low weight, frequent weight gain/loss and/or poor nutrition
- Abnormal preoccupation with food and with feeling out of control

In addition, anorexia and bulimia have factors specific to each. Anorexia nervosa sufferers:

- Are females of pre- or teenage
- Grow up in "overachieving" families who establish unusually high expectations for their children
- Place exaggerated emphasis on body image and perfection
- Have parents who are very busy and involved in their own lives. The anorexic may feel the need to be perfect to gain parental attention.
- Have marked physical effects: loss of head hair, stoppage of ovulation/menstruation, slowed heart rate, low blood pressure and intolerance to cold
- Have depression more extreme than in bulimia patients
- Develop osteoporosis later in life due to lack of calcium and decreased production of estrogen if menstruation stops. Excessive exercise can contribute to this as well.
- Have severe damage to heart and vital organs if weight drops sufficiently

Approximately 1 percent of American females have anorexia.

Bulimia sufferers:

- Can be overweight, underweight or normal weight
- Are mostly female, older teen or young adult
- Are characterized by binge eating and then vomiting (purging) and/or taking laxatives and/or water pills (diuretics) to "undo" the binge

- Have severe health problems that arise from a binge-purge cycle of eating. These include tears and ruptures in the stomach lining, irregular heartbeat, kidney damage from low potassium levels, damage to tooth enamel from acids produced in vomiting and cessation of menstruation.
- Repress anger from inability to express emotions in an assertive way. They fear upsetting important people in their lives.

Approximately 2 percent of college students and 1 percent of U.S. women overall have bulimia. Bulimia can follow anorexia and vice versa.

There is no one cause for these eating disorders. Many factors contribute to them:

- A possible genetic predisposition
- Metabolic and biochemical problems or abnormalities
- Social pressure to be thin
- Personal or family pressures

Treatment for anorexia and/or bulimia includes:

- Medical diagnosis and care, the earlier the better
- Psychotherapy, individual, family and/or group
- Behavior therapy
- Medication. Antidepressant medicine is sometimes used.
- Nutrition therapy, including vitamin and mineral supplements
- Hospitalization, if necessary, especially in anorexia, if weight has dropped about 25 percent or more below normal weight and/or has affected vital functions

Questions to Ask

Have you gotten to a weight that is 15 percent less than what is standard for your age and height by intentionally dieting and exercising (not due to any known illness)?

YES

SEE DOCTOR

 NO

flowchart continued on next page

Do you have any of these problems:

- Irregular heartbeat
- Slow pulse, low blood pressure
- Low body temperature, cold hands and feet
- Thin hair (or hair loss) on the head, baby-like hair on the body (lanugo)
- Dry skin, fingernails that split, peel or crack
- Problems with digestion, bloating, constipation
- Three or more missed periods (in a row), delayed onset of menstruation, infertility
- Sometimes depression and lethargy, sometimes euphoria and hyperactivity
- Tiredness, weakness, muscle cramps, tremors
- Lack of concentration

YES

SEE DOCTOR

NO

Do you have an intense fear of gaining weight or of getting fat, or do you see yourself as fat even though you are of normal weight, or are underweight? Do you continue to diet and exercise excessively even though you have reached your goal weight?

YES

SEE DOCTOR

NO

Are you aware that your eating pattern is not normal, and are you afraid that you will not be able to stop binge eating? Are you depressed after bingeing on food?

YES

SEE DOCTOR

NO

flowchart continued in next column

Do you:
- Hoard food
- Leave the table right after meals to "go to the bathroom" to induce vomiting and/or spend long periods of time in the bathroom as a result of taking laxatives and/or water pills

YES

SEE DOCTOR

NO

Do you have recurrent episodes when you eat a large amount of food in less than two hours and at a very fast pace, and do you do at least three of the following:

- Eat high calorie, easily consumed food during a binge
- Binge eat with no one watching
- Stop the binge eating when you get abdominal pain, go to sleep, interact socially or induce vomiting
- Attempt to lose weight repeatedly with severe diets, self-induced vomiting and/or laxatives or water pills
- Have weight changes of more than 10 pounds due to bingeing and fasting

YES

SEE DOCTOR

NO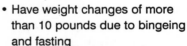

PROVIDE SELF-CARE

Self-Care Procedures

Eating disorders are too complicated and physically hazardous to be treated with self-care procedures. Experts agree that experienced professionals should treat people who have eating disorders.

But to avoid succumbing to an eating disorder, follow these suggestions:

- Accept yourself and your body. You don't need to be or look like anyone else. Spend time with people who accept you as you are, not people who focus exclusively on thinness.

- Eat a wholesome, nutritious diet. Focus on complex carbohydrates (e.g., whole grains and beans), fresh fruits and vegetables, low-fat dairy foods and low-fat meats.
- Eat at regular times during the day. Don't skip meals. If you do so, you are more likely to binge when you do eat.
- Avoid refined foods (e.g., white flour and sugar) and "junk" foods high in calories, fat and sugar (e.g., cakes, cookies or pastry). Bulimics tend to binge on junk food. The more they eat, the more they want.
- Get regular moderate exercise. If you find that you are exercising excessively, make an effort to get involved in nonexercise activities with friends and family.
- Find success in things that you do. Your work, hobbies and volunteer activities will promote self-esteem.
- Educate yourself. Learn as much as you can about eating disorders from books and organizations that deal with them.
- Parents who want to help daughters avoid eating disorders should promote a balance between their daughters' competing needs for both independence and family involvement.

Endometriosis

Endometriosis is an abnormal condition that occurs when growth of the tissue that lines the inside of the uterus (endometrium) is found outside of the uterus in other areas of the body. Endometriosis can only occur after menstruation begins in a woman. Women in their 20s, 30s and 40s are most likely to get endometriosis.

The most common symptoms of endometriosis are:
- Pain before and during menstrual periods (usually worse than the pain in normal menstrual cramps)
- Pain during or after sexual intercourse
- Painful urination

- Lower back pain and/or painful bowel movements with menstrual periods
- Pelvic soreness/tenderness

Pain, however, is not always present. Other symptoms include:
- Premenstrual vaginal spotting of blood
- Abnormally heavy or long menstrual periods
- Infertility

The exact cause of endometriosis is unknown. One theory suggests that some of the lining of the uterus during menstruation moves backward through the fallopian tubes into the abdominal cavity, where it attaches and grows. Other theories point to problems with the immune system and/or hormones. There is also some evidence that the condition may be inherited. Places where endometriosis is commonly found are:
- Outside surface of the uterus
- Fallopian tubes
- Ovaries
- Lining of the pelvic cavity
- Area between the vagina and the rectum

An accurate diagnosis of endometriosis must be made by your gynecologist. He or she may perform a laparoscopy, which is an outpatient surgical procedure in which a slim telescope is inserted through a very small opening made in the navel. This allows your doctor to examine the abdominal organs and evaluate the extent of the disease.

The management of endometriosis is aimed at suppressing levels of the hormones estrogen and progesterone. These hormones cause endometriosis to grow. Mild to moderate endometriosis may be relieved at menopause.

Treatment for endometriosis can include surgery or medication therapy. Surgical treatment can be a conservative approach, such as removing areas of endometriosis through a laparoscope using laser, cautery or small surgical instruments to destroy the growths. These treatments are used to reduce pain and allow pregnancy to occur in some women.

A less conservative approach is removal of the ovaries. The fallopian tubes and uterus can also be removed. Surgeries of this kind would likely eliminate pain, but leave a woman unable to conceive.

Medication therapy consists of:
- Painkillers, as well as antiprostaglandins (e.g., ibuprofen and naproxen sodium)
- Oral contraceptives, which temporarily stop ovulation and menstruation. They are more likely to be used for very mild cases of endometriosis.
- Antiestrogens, which suppress a woman's production of estrogen. This will stop the menstrual cycle and prevent further growth of endometriosis since endometriosis needs estrogen to grow. These can have side effects such as acne, hair growth on the face and changes in the libido.
- Progesterone, used to cast off the endometrial cells and thus destroy them
- Gonadotropin-releasing hormone (GnRH) agonist drugs, which will stop the production of estrogen. This therapy causes a medically induced menopause that is temporary.

Questions to Ask

Do you have a lot of pain:
- During sex
- When you menstruate and the pain has gotten worse over time
- When you urinate

YES → CALL DOCTOR

NO ↓

Have you tried to get pregnant, but have not been able to in 12 or more months?

YES → CALL DOCTOR

NO ↓

PROVIDE SELF-CARE

Self-Care Procedures

Self-Care Procedures are very limited for endometriosis. It needs medical treatment. Things you can do to enhance medical treatment include:
- Exercise regularly.
- Eat a diet high in nutrients and low in fat, especially saturated fat, mostly found in coconut and palm oils, animal sources of fat and hydrogenated vegetable fats.
- Take aspirin, acetaminophen, ibuprofen or naproxen sodium for pain. Check with your doctor for his or her preference. *Note: Do not give aspirin or any medication containing salicylates to anyone 19 years of age of younger, unless directed by a physician, due to its association with Reye's syndrome, a potentially fatal condition.*
- Consider using oral contraceptives for birth control. Women who take the Pill have a reduced incidence of endometriosis.

Fibroids

Fibroids are benign (not cancerous) tumors made mostly of muscle tissue. They are found in the wall of the uterus and sometimes on the cervix. They can range in size from as small as a pea to as large as a cantaloupe or even a basketball! With larger fibroids, a woman's uterus can grow to the size of a pregnancy that is more than 20 weeks along. About 20 to 25 percent of women over 35 get fibroids. A woman is more likely to get fibroids if:
- She has not been pregnant.
- She has a close relative who also had or has them.
- She is African American. The risk is three to five times higher than it is for Caucasian women.

Why fibroids occur is not really known. They do, however, depend on estrogen for their growth. They may shrink or even disappear after menopause.

Symptoms of Fibroids

Some women with uterine fibroids do not have any symptoms or problems from them. When symptoms or problems occur, they vary due to the number, size and locations of the fibroid(s). These include:

- Abdominal swelling, especially if the fibroids are large
- Heavy menstrual bleeding
- Bleeding between periods or after intercourse
- Pain (backache, during sex, during periods), from pressure on the internal organs
- Bleeding after menopause
- Anemia from excessive bleeding
- Frequent urination, from pressure on the bladder
- Chronic constipation, from pressure on the rectum
- Infertility, because the fallopian tubes may be blocked or the uterus may be distorted
- Miscarriage, because if the fibroid is inside the uterus, the placenta may not implant the way it should

You can find out if you have fibroids when your doctor takes a medical history and does a pelvic exam. The doctor can also do other tests such as an ultrasound or a D & C to confirm their presence, location and size. The ultrasound is the most common test for diagnosing fibroids.

Treatment for fibroids include:

- "Watchful waiting" if they are small, harmless and painless or not causing any problems. Your doctor will "watch" for any changes and may suggest "waiting" for menopause, since fibroids often shrink or disappear after that time. If you have problems during this "waiting" period (e.g., too much pain, too much bleeding, your abdomen gets too big, you have to take daily iron supplements to prevent anemia or you have gastrointestinal problems), you may decide that you do not want to "wait" for menopause, but instead choose to have something done to treat your fibroids.

- Medication. One type, called gonadotropin-releasing hormone (GnRH) agonists, blocks the production of estrogen by the ovaries. This shrinks fibroids in some cases, but is not a cure. The fibroids return promptly when the medicine is stopped. Shrinking the fibroids might allow a minor surgery to be done instead of a major one. (See surgical methods listed.) GnRh agonists are taken for a few months, but not more than six, because their side effects mimic menopause.

There are two basic surgical methods:

- **Myomectomy** - The fibroids are removed, but the uterus is not. There are three approaches.
  - Laparoscopic - A laparoscope is used with a laser to remove the fibroids.
  - Hysteroscopic - The fibroids are cut out and the uterine lining is destroyed by laser (ablation). This makes a woman sterile. Laser ablation can also be done with a small electrocautery ball known as a "rollerball."
  - Laparotomic - Surgery in which the abdomen is opened and the fibroids are removed under direct vision.

- **Hysterectomy** - Surgery that removes the uterus and the fibroids with it. Depending on the size of the fibroids, this can be done:
  - Vaginally
  - Through abdominal surgery

A hysterectomy is recommended when the fibroid is very large or when there is severe bleeding that can't be stopped by other treatments. A hysterectomy leaves a women sterile and is the only certain way, according to many experts, to get rid of fibroids. Myomectomy methods may allow fibroids to grow back. The more fibroids there are to begin with, the greater the chance they will grow back.

A hysterectomy may also be done in the rare occasion that the fibroid becomes cancerous.

Questions to Ask

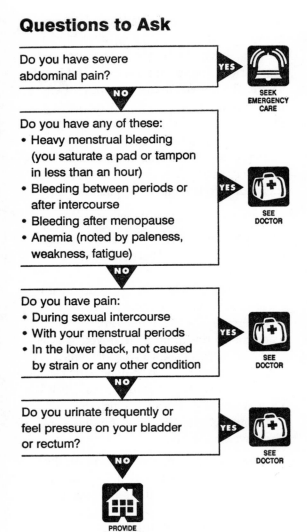

Do you have severe abdominal pain? **YES** → SEEK EMERGENCY CARE

NO ↓

Do you have any of these:
- Heavy menstrual bleeding (you saturate a pad or tampon in less than an hour)
- Bleeding between periods or after intercourse
- Bleeding after menopause
- Anemia (noted by paleness, weakness, fatigue)

YES → SEE DOCTOR

NO ↓

Do you have pain:
- During sexual intercourse
- With your menstrual periods
- In the lower back, not caused by strain or any other condition

YES → SEE DOCTOR

NO ↓

Do you urinate frequently or feel pressure on your bladder or rectum?

YES → SEE DOCTOR

NO ↓

PROVIDE SELF-CARE

Self-Care and Preventive Procedures

- Maintain a healthy body weight. The more body fat you have, the more estrogen your body is likely to have, which enhances fibroid growth.
- Exercise regularly. This may reduce your body's fat and estrogen levels.
- Eat a diet low in fat.

Menopause

Menopause is when a woman's menstrual periods stop altogether. It signals the end of fertility. A woman is said to have gone through menopause when her menstrual periods have stopped for an entire year. "The change," as menopause is often called, generally occurs between the ages of 45 and 55. It can, though, take place as early as 35 or as late as 65 years of age. It can also result from the surgical removal of both ovaries. The physical and emotional signs and symptoms that go with "the change" usually span one to two years or more (peri-menopause). They vary from woman to woman. The changes, themselves, are a result of a number of factors. These include hormone changes such as estrogen decline, the aging process itself and stress.

Physical signs and symptoms associated with menopause are:
- Hot flashes, which are sudden waves of heat that can start in the waist or chest and work their way to the neck and face and some-times the rest of the body. They are more common in the evening and during hot weather. They can hit as often as every 90 minutes. Each one can last from 15 seconds to 30 minutes—five minutes is average. Seventy-five to 80 percent of women going through menopause experience hot flashes; some are more bothered by them than others. Sometimes heart palpitations accompany hot flashes.
- Irregular periods that vary and can include:
  - Periods that get shorter and lighter for two or more years
  - Periods that stop for a few months and then start up again and are more widely spaced
  - Periods that bring heavy bleeding and/or the passage of many or large blood clots. (This can lead to anemia.)
- Vaginal dryness resulting from hormonal changes. The vaginal wall also becomes thinner. This drying and thinning can make sexual intercourse painful or uncomfortable

and can lead to irritation and increased risk for infection.

- Loss of bladder tone, which can result in stress incontinence (leaking urine when you cough, sneeze or exercise)
- Headaches, dizziness
- Skin and hair changes. Skin is more likely to wrinkle, and there may be a growth of facial hair but a thinning of hair in the temple region.
- Breast tenderness
- Bloating in upper abdomen
- Loss of some strength and tone of muscles
- Bones becoming more brittle, increasing the risk for osteoporosis
- Increased risk for heart attack when estrogen levels drop

Emotional changes associated with menopause are:

- Irritability
- Mood changes
- Lack of concentration, difficulty with memory
- Tension, anxiety, depression
- Insomnia (may result from hot flashes that interrupt sleep)

Treatment for the symptoms of menopause varies from woman to woman. If symptoms cause little or no distress, medical treatment is not needed. The Self-Care Procedures listed may be all that is required. Hormone replacement therapy (HRT) can reduce many of the symptoms of menopause. It also offers significant protection against osteoporosis and heart disease. Each woman should discuss the benefits and risks of HRT with her doctor. (See "Osteoporosis" on page 214 and "Chest Pain" on page 115.)

Medication to treat depression and/or anxiety may be warranted in some women. Also, certain sedative medicines can help with hot flashes.

Questions to Ask

Do you have any of these:
- Extreme pain during intercourse
- Pain or burning when urinating
- Thick, white or colored vaginal discharge
- Fever, chills

YES

SEE DOCTOR

 NO

Do you have heavy bleeding with your periods or pass many or large blood clots which leave you pale and very tired?

YES

CALL DOCTOR

NO

Have you begun having menstrual periods again after going without any for six months?

YES

CALL DOCTOR

NO

Are hot flashes severe, frequent or persistent enough that they interfere with normal activities?

YES

CALL DOCTOR

NO

Do you have risk factors for osteoporosis:
- Family history of osteoporosis
- Small bone frame
- Thin
- Fair skin (Caucasian or Asian race)
- Had surgery to remove ovaries before natural menopause or menopause before 48 years of age
- Lack of calcium in diet
- Lack of weight-bearing exercise
- Alcohol abuse
- Hyperthyroidism
- Use of steroid medicine

YES

CALL DOCTOR

 NO

flowchart continued on next page

---

flowchart continued

If you're taking hormone replacement therapy, do you have any of the following:
- Side effects
- Return of menopausal symptoms

YES

CALL
DOCTOR

NO

PROVIDE
SELF-CARE

Self-Care Procedures

To reduce the discomfort of hot flashes, try these tactics:
- Wear lightweight clothes made of natural fibers.
- Limit or avoid beverages that contain caffeine or alcohol.
- Avoid rich and spicy foods and heavy meals.
- Take 400 international units (I.U.) of vitamin E daily. (Consult your doctor first, though.)
- Have cool drinks, especially water, when you feel a hot flash coming on and before and after exercising. Avoid hot drinks.
- Keep cool. Open a window. Lower the thermostat when the heat is on. Use air-conditioning and/or fans. Carry a small fan with you (hand- or battery-operated).
- Try to relax when you get a hot flash. Getting stressed over one only makes it worse.
- Use relaxation techniques such as meditation, biofeedback or yoga.
- Take 400 I.U. of vitamin E daily, but consult your doctor first.

If you suffer from night sweats (hot flashes that occur as you sleep):
- Wear loose-fitting cotton nightwear. Have changes of nightwear ready.
- Sleep with only a top sheet, not blankets.
- Keep the room cool.

To deal with vaginal dryness and painful intercourse:
- Don't use deodorant soaps or scented products in the vaginal area.
- Use a water-soluble lubricant (e.g., K-Y Jelly and Replens) to facilitate penetration during intercourse. Avoid oils or petroleum-based products. They encourage infection.
- Ask your doctor about intravaginal estrogen cream.
- Remain sexually active. Having sex often may lessen the chance of having the vagina constrict and helps keep natural lubrication and maintains pelvic muscle tone. (This includes reaching orgasm with a partner or alone.)
- Drink plenty of water daily for healthy vaginal tissues. Avoid using antihistamines unless truly necessary. They dry mucous membranes in the body.

To deal with emotional symptoms:
- Exercise regularly. This will help maintain your body's hormonal balance.
- Talk to other women who have gone through or are going through menopause. You can help each other cope with emotional symptoms.
- Avoid stressful situations as much as possible.
- Use relaxation techniques (e.g., meditation, yoga, listening to soft music, massages).
- Eat healthy. Check with your doctor about taking vitamin/mineral supplements.

Menstrual Cramps

Menstrual cramps are also called dysmenorrhea or painful periods. Most women experience them at some time during their life. They can be very mild or severe enough to leave a woman unable to carry out her normal activities for the first one to three days of her period. They may also differ from month to month, or year to year. The pain felt during menstrual cramps may be accompanied by backache, fatigue, vomiting, diarrhea and headaches. It can be made worse by premenstrual bloating (water retention).

There are two types of dysmenorrhea: primary and secondary. The primary form usually occurs in females who have just begun to menstruate. This form may disappear or become less severe after a woman reaches her mid-20s or gives birth. The cause of menstrual cramps is thought to be related to hormonelike substances called prostaglandins. These are chemicals that occur naturally in the body. Certain prostaglandins cause muscles in the uterus to go into spasm.

Dysmenorrhea occurs much less often in women who do not ovulate. For this reason, oral contraceptives reduce painful periods in 70 to 80 percent of women who take them. When the Pill is stopped, women usually get the same level of pain they had before they took it.

Secondary dysmenorrhea refers to menstrual cramps that are due to other disorders of the reproductive system, such as fibroids, endometriosis, ovarian cysts and, rarely, cancer. Having an intrauterine device (IUD), especially if you've never been pregnant, can also cause menstrual cramps—the exception being the Progestasert IUD. It releases a small amount of progesterone into the uterus that helps with cramps and lightens menstrual flow.

Questions to Ask

Have your menstrual periods been especially painful since having an intrauterine contraceptive device (IUD) inserted? **YES** — SEE DOCTOR

NO

Do you have any signs of infection such as fever and foul-smelling vaginal discharge, or do you have black stools or blood in the stools? **YES** — SEE DOCTOR

NO

Do you have a heavier than usual blood flow and/or a period that is late by one or more weeks (for women who are still capable of bearing children)? **YES** — CALL DOCTOR

NO

flowchart continued in next column

flowchart continued

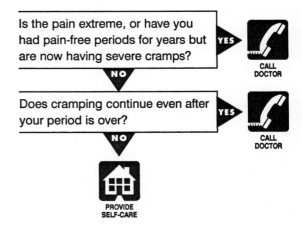

Is the pain extreme, or have you had pain-free periods for years but are now having severe cramps? **YES** — CALL DOCTOR

NO

Does cramping continue even after your period is over? **YES** — CALL DOCTOR

NO

PROVIDE SELF-CARE

Self-Care Procedures

To relieve menstrual cramps:
- Take aspirin, ibuprofen or naproxen sodium around the clock as directed to relieve pain and inhibit the release of prostaglandins. Acetaminophen will help with pain, but not with prostaglandins. Know that most over-the-counter menstrual discomfort products contain acetaminophen and not a pain reliever that also inhibits prostaglandins. Read labels. *Note: Do not give aspirin or any medication containing salicylates to anyone 19 years of age or younger, unless directed by a physician, due to its association with Reye's syndrome, a potentially fatal condition.*
- Drink a hot cup of regular, chamomile or mint tea.
- Whenever possible, lie on your back, supporting your knees with a pillow.
- Hold a heating pad or hot-water bottle on your abdomen or lower back.
- Take a warm bath.
- Gently massage your abdomen.
- Do mild exercises like stretching, walking or biking. Exercise may improve blood flow and reduce pelvic pain.
- Unless you have reasons to avoid alcohol, have a glass of wine or other alcoholic beverage. Alcohol slows down uterine contractions.
- Get plenty of rest and avoid stressful situations as your period approaches.

- For birth control, consider using the Pill, because it blocks the production of prostaglandins, or the Progestasert IUD, because its use lessens menstrual cramps.

If you still feel pain after using Self-Care Procedures, call your doctor.

Ovarian Cysts

The ovaries are two almond-sized organs on either side of the uterus. They produce eggs and female hormones (estrogen, progesterone and others). Growths called cysts can form in, on or near the ovaries. Rarely cancerous, cysts are sacs filled with fluid or semi-solid material. Ovarian cysts are commonly found in women in their reproductive years. Taking hormones does not cause cysts.

Women more likely to get ovarian cysts are:
- Between the ages of 20 and 35
- Those who take a medication for epilepsy called Valporate
- Those who have endometriosis, pelvic inflammatory disease (PID) or the eating disorder bulimia

Signs and Symptoms

Most of the time, ovarian cysts are harmless and cause no symptoms. When symptoms do occur, they include:
- A feeling of fullness or swelling of the abdomen
- Weight gain
- A dull constant ache on either or both sides of the pelvis
- Pain during intercourse
- Delayed, irregular or painful menstrual periods
- Increased facial hair
- Sharp, severe abdominal pain, fever, and/or vomiting. This may be caused by a bleeding cyst or one that breaks or twists.

Ovarian cysts are of three basic types:
- **Functional cysts** - This is the most common type. These cysts are related to variations in the normal function of the ovaries. For example, they form when an egg tries to release as it should during normal ovulation. They can last four to six weeks. Rarely do they secrete hormones.
- **Follicular and corpus luteum cysts** - A follicular cyst is one in which the egg-making follicle of the ovary enlarges and fills with fluid. A corpus luteum cyst is a yellow mass of tissue that forms from the follicle after ovulation. These types of cysts come and go each month and are associated with normal ovarian function.
- **Abnormal cysts or neoplastic cysts** - These result from cell growth and are mostly benign. In rare cases, they can be cancerous. Abnormal cysts require medical treatment by your doctor. Examples include:
  - Dermoid cyst - which consists of a growth filled with various types of tissue such as fatty material, hair, teeth, bits of bone and cartilage.
  - Polycystic ovaries - caused by a buildup of multiple small cysts which cause hormonal imbalances that can result in irregular periods, body hair growth and infertility.

Detection

You can find out if you have ovarian cysts through:
- A pelvic exam, in which your doctor can feel the size of your ovaries and discover abnormalities
- An ultrasound, in which sound waves create pictures of internal organs through a device placed on your abdomen or a probe inserted inside your vagina
- A laparoscopy, a minor surgical procedure which allows your doctor to see the structures inside your abdomen

Treatment

Treatment for ovarian cysts will depend on:
- Size and type of cyst(s)
- Age and whether you are in your reproductive years or have reached menopause
- Desire to have children

- Overall health status
- Severity of symptoms

Some cysts may resolve without any treatment within one to two months. In others, hormone therapy with oral contraceptives may be tried to suppress the cyst(s). If a cyst does not respond to this treatment, surgery may be needed to remove the cyst. If a cyst is found early, the surgery may not have to be extensive and the cyst may be removed leaving the ovary. Sometimes the ovary needs to be removed and surgery may include removal of the fallopian tube and uterus as well.

Questions to Ask

Do you have severe abdominal pain, fever and vomiting?

YES → SEE DOCTOR

NO

Do you have any of the following that are not due to other known reasons:
- Abdominal fullness or swelling
- Delayed, irregular or painful menstrual periods
- Pain during intercourse
- Dull and constant ache on either or both sides of your pelvis

YES → CALL DOCTOR

NO

PROVIDE SELF-CARE

Self-Care and Preventive Procedures

- Reduce caffeine intake.
- Have regular pelvic exams according to your doctor's recommendations.
- Take acetaminophen, aspirin, ibuprofen or naproxen sodium for minor pain. *Note: Do not give aspirin or any medication containing salicylates to anyone 19 years of age or younger, unless directed by a physician, due to its association with Reye's syndrome, a potentially fatal condition.*

Premenstrual Syndrome (PMS)

Four out of 10 menstruating women suffer premenstrual syndrome (PMS). A syndrome is a group of signs and symptoms that indicate a disorder. There have been as many as 150 symptoms associated with PMS. The most common ones are:
- Irritability
- Anxiety
- Depression
- Headache
- Bloating
- Fatigue
- Feelings of hostility and anger
- Food cravings (especially for chocolate, sweet and salty foods)

The exact cause or causes for PMS are not known; however, there are many theories. One points to low levels of the hormone progesterone. Others link it to nutritional or chemical deficiencies. One thing is certain though: To be classified as PMS, symptoms must occur between ovulation and menstruation—i.e., appear anytime within two weeks before the menstrual period, and disappear shortly after the period begins. (PMS is thought to cease with menopause.)

For some women, symptoms are slight and may last only a few days before menstruation. For others, they can be severe and last the whole two weeks before every period. Also worth noting is that other disorders women experience (e.g., arthritis and clinical depression) may be worse during this same premenstrual period. This is known as premenstrual magnification (PMM).

PMS is often confused with depression. An evaluation by your doctor can help with a correct diagnosis.

Treatments for PMS may include:
- Medical management with medicines such as:
  - The prescribed hormone progesterone (suppositories or an oral form)

- Water pills such as spironolactone (Aldactone)
- Dietary changes such as:
  - Eating five to six light meals instead of three large ones; not skipping meals
  - Avoiding caffeine and alcohol
  - Avoiding sweets
  - Limiting salt and fat
  - Vitamin supplements, especially B_6
  - Adequate intake of calcium and magnesium
- Lifestyle changes such as regular exercise that includes 20 minutes of aerobic exercise (e.g., walking or aerobic dance) at least three times a week
- Limiting and learning to deal with stress

Questions to Ask

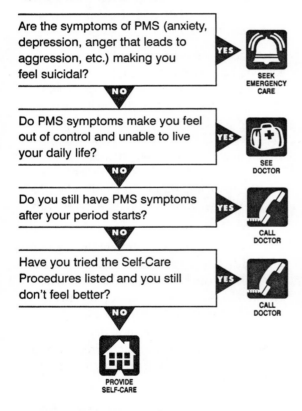

Are the symptoms of PMS (anxiety, depression, anger that leads to aggression, etc.) making you feel suicidal? **YES** → SEEK EMERGENCY CARE

NO ↓

Do PMS symptoms make you feel out of control and unable to live your daily life? **YES** → SEE DOCTOR

NO ↓

Do you still have PMS symptoms after your period starts? **YES** → CALL DOCTOR

NO ↓

Have you tried the Self-Care Procedures listed and you still don't feel better? **YES** → CALL DOCTOR

NO ↓

PROVIDE SELF-CARE

Self-Care Procedures

- Exercise three times a week for 20 minutes. Swimming, walking and bicycling all relax your muscles and help you lose water weight.
- Eat five to six small meals a day instead of three large ones. Chose: whole grains, fruits

and vegetables; good food sources of calcium such as skim milk, nonfat yogurt, collard greens, kale, calcium-fortified cereals and juices; and sources of magnesium such as spinach, other green, leafy vegetables and whole grain cereals.

- Limit salt, fat and sugar. Doing so may help keep your breasts from getting sore. It may also cut down on your body's estrogen. Estrogen is a hormone that is thought to help cause PMS.
- If you need to satisfy a food craving, do so in moderation. For example, if you crave chocolate, have a small chocolate bar or add chocolate syrup to skim milk. If you crave salt, eat a small bag of pretzels.
- Stay away from caffeine, alcohol and cigarettes for two weeks before your period is due.
- The vitamin supplements listed here seem to help some women. Ask your doctor if you should take them and in what amounts:
  - Vitamin E
  - Vitamin B_6
  - Calcium
  - Magnesium
  - L-tyrosine, an amino acid
- Take naps if PMS keeps you up at night.
- Learn to relax. Try deep breathing, meditation, yoga or a hot bath.
- Try to avoid stress when you have PMS.

Toxic Shock Syndrome

Toxic shock syndrome (TSS) is a potentially fatal disease that is caused by bacteria. It is a form of blood poisoning that results when poisons (toxins) are released by the suspect bacteria. It can result from wounds or infection in the throat, lungs, skin or bone. It most often, though, affects women of childbearing age, especially women who use superabsorbent tampons. These tampons may trap the suspect bacteria and provide a breeding ground for them, especially when left in place for a long period of time. Also, the superabsorbent fibers in some tampons may cause microscopic tears in the vagina that allow the transmission of the bacteria's toxin. Though not common, TSS can also occur in persons following surgery, including women who have had cesarean sections. Symptoms come on fast and are often severe:

- High, sudden fever
- Muscle aches
- Vomiting
- Diarrhea
- Sunburn-like rash, including peeling skin on hands and feet
- Rapid pulse
- Extreme fatigue and weakness
- Sore throat
- Dizziness
- Fainting
- Drop in blood pressure

Prevention

Take the following precautions to prevent TSS:

- Never use tampons if you've experienced TSS in the past.
- Use sanitary napkins instead of tampons whenever possible.
- Alternate tampons with sanitary pads or mini-pads during a menstrual period.
- Don't use superabsorbent tampons.
- Don't use tampons with plastic applicators.
- Lubricate the tampon applicator with a water-soluble (nongreasy) lubricant like K-Y Jelly before insertion.
- Change tampons and sanitary pads every four to six hours, or more frequently.

Questions to Ask

Are any of the symptoms of toxic shock syndrome (see list) present during your menstrual period or at any other time? **YES**

SEEK
EMERGENCY
CARE

NO

PROVIDE
SELF-CARE

Self-Care Procedures

Follow the recommendations previously listed to prevent toxic shock syndrome.

Vaginal Yeast Infections

Yeast infections are the most common type of vaginal infections. Other names for this are monilia, candidiasis or fungus infection. Vaginal yeast infections result from the overgrowth of Candida albicans, which is normally present in harmless amounts in the vagina, the digestive tract and the mouth. Some women rarely have a yeast infection; others have them regularly. Certain things may trigger them:

- Hormonal changes that come with pregnancy or even before monthly periods
- Taking hormones, including birth control pills
- Taking antibiotics, especially "broad-spectrum" ones
- Taking steroid medicines such as prednisone
- Having elevated blood sugar such as that found in uncontrolled diabetes
- Vaginal intercourse, especially with inadequate lubrication

Symptoms can range from mild to severe. They include:

- Itching, irritation and redness around the external genitalia
- A thick, white discharge that looks like cottage cheese. (It may smell like yeast.)
- Burning and/or pain when you urinate or have sex

Prevention

- Practice good hygiene. Wash regularly to clean the inside folds of the vulva where germs are likely to grow. Dry the vaginal area thoroughly after you shower or bathe.
- Wipe from front to back after using the toilet.
- Wear all-cotton underpants and panty hose with cotton crotches.

- Don't wear slacks and shorts that are tight in the crotch and thighs or other tight-fitting clothing such as panty girdles.
- Change underwear and workout clothes right away after exercising.
- Use unscented tampons or sanitary pads and change tampons and sanitary pads frequently.
- Don't use bath oils, bubble baths, feminine hygiene sprays and perfumed or deodorant soaps.
- Don't sit around in a wet bathing suit.
- Shower after you swim in a pool to remove the chlorine from your skin. Dry the vaginal area thoroughly.
- Take antibiotics (especially broad-spectrum ones such as Keflex, Ceclor, Bactrim DS, Septra, amoxicillin and ampicillin) only when necessary to treat bacterial (not viral) infections. These promote the growth of yeast. Ask your doctor for an antibiotic that is not broad spectrum if it will treat the specific bacterial infection you have.
- If you tend to get yeast infections whenever you take an antibiotic, ask your doctor to prescribe a vaginal antifungal agent as well, or take an over-the-counter one.
- Eat well. Include yogurt that contains live cultures of lactobacillus acidophilus.
- Make sure your partner is checked for infection and treated, especially if you get recurring infections. This will avoid reinfection.
- Get plenty of rest for your body to fight infections.

Treatment

Treatment for vaginal yeast infections consists mostly of vaginal creams or suppositories that get rid of the Candida overgrowth. These can be over-the-counter ones (e.g., Monistat and Gyne-Lotrimin) or ones prescribed by your doctor (e.g., Terazol and Vagistat). Other treatments include gentian violet (a purple solution applied to the vaginal area) and oral medicines (e.g., Diflucan, Sporanox, Nystatin and Nizoral). Oral medicines are used for chronic yeast infections.

First and foremost, though, is to make sure you have the problem correctly diagnosed. A burning sensation could be a symptom of a urinary tract infection caused by bacteria that require an antibiotic. Antibiotics do not help a yeast infection; they only make them worse. Check with your doctor if you are not sure that your problem is a yeast infection, especially if this is the first time you have symptoms of one and if the infection you treat comes back within two months or does not respond to treatment at all.

Chronic vaginal yeast infections can be one of the first signs of diabetes, sexually transmitted diseases or AIDS in women.

Questions to Ask

Do you have any other symptoms such as vaginal swelling and/or unusual bleeding? Does the discharge have a foul-smelling odor? **YES** SEE DOCTOR

NO

Do symptoms of vaginal yeast infection worsen or continue one week or longer despite Self-Care Procedures, or do they come back within two months after treatment? **YES** SEE DOCTOR

NO

PROVIDE SELF-CARE

Self-Care Procedures

To get rid of a yeast infection, try the following:

- Use an over-the-counter vaginal medication cream or suppositories (e.g., Monistat) as directed. Women who have had yeast infections whenever they take antibiotics in the past should use these preparations during the period of antibiotic treatment.
- Douche with a mild solution of one to three tablespoons of vinegar diluted in a quart of warm water. Repeat once a day until the symptoms subside, but do not use longer than a week.
- Limit your intake of sugar and foods that contain sugar since sugar promotes the growth of yeast.
- Eat yogurt and other foods that contain live cultures of lactobacillus acidophilus several times daily (especially when taking an antibiotic). If you can't tolerate yogurt, ask your pharmacist for an over-the-counter product that contains this beneficial bacteria (lactobacillus acidophilus).

CHAPTER 19

MEN'S HEALTH

Enlarged Prostate

The prostate gland is walnut-shaped and produces seminal fluid. Located below a man's bladder, it actually surrounds a portion of the bladder and the beginning of the urethra (tube that carries urine away from the bladder). If they live long enough, most men will eventually suffer from an enlarged prostate gland—a condition called benign prostatic hypertrophy (BPH).

An enlarged prostate is troublesome but is usually not cancerous or life-threatening. The symptoms are:
- Increased urgency to urinate
- Frequent urination, especially during the night
- Delay in onset of urine flow
- Diminished or slow stream of urine flow
- Incomplete emptying of the bladder

These symptoms indicate that the prostate gland has enlarged enough to partially obstruct the flow of urine. Sometimes BPH causes a urinary tract infection (UTI). Over time, a few men might have bladder or kidney problems or both.

Your doctor can diagnose BPH through a number of methods. These include:
- A physical exam that includes asking questions about your current symptoms and past medical problems, an examination of your prostate gland, a check of your urine for signs of infection and a blood test to determine if the prostate has affected your kidneys.
- Tests that measure urine flow, the amount of urine left in your bladder after you urinate and the pressure in your bladder as you urinate.

- A blood test called a prostate-specific antigen (PSA) test, which can help find prostate cancer. Not all doctors agree that being tested for PSA levels lowers a person's chance of dying from prostate cancer. The PSA test is not always accurate either. You should discuss this test with your doctor.
- Other tests such as X-rays, cystoscopy (in which the doctor directly views the prostate and bladder) and an ultrasound (sound wave pictures of the prostate, kidneys or bladder). Many men do not need these tests. They are costly and are not very helpful for most men with BPH.

Treatment for BPH varies depending on symptoms. Discuss the benefits and possible problems with your doctor for each treatment option. Treatment options include:

- **Watchful waiting** - Get regular exams to see if your BPH is causing problems or getting worse.

- **Medications** - There are two types:
  - Alpha blockers, which help relax muscles in the prostate. Hytrin is the only one approved for BPH treatment by the Food and Drug Administration.
  - Finasteride (brand name Proscar), which causes the prostate to shrink

There is no evidence that these medications reduce the rate of BPH complications or the need for future surgery. They can have side effects, too, so you should see your doctor for monitoring.

- **Balloon dilation** - a surgical procedure done in the operating room or doctor's office. A balloon-tipped catheter is inserted into the penis, through the urethra and into the bladder. The balloon is inflated to stretch the urethra in order to allow urine to flow more easily.
- **Surgery** - There are three types:
  - Transurethral resection of the prostate (TURP), which is the most common type. It relieves symptoms by reducing pressure on the urethra and is a proven way to treat BPH effectively.
  - Transurethral incision of the prostate (TUIP), which also reduces the pressure of the prostate on the urethra, thus making it easier to urinate. TUIP may be used instead of TURP when the prostate is not enlarged as much.
  - Open prostatectomy, which may be used if the prostate is very large. An incision is made in the lower abdomen to remove part of the inside of the prostate.

Prostate surgery can result in problems such as impotence and/or incontinence. Most men, however, who undergo surgery have no major problems. Nonetheless, it is important to discuss the benefits and risks of these procedures with your doctor.

Questions to Ask

Do you have one or more of these problems:
- A feeling that you have to urinate right away, or the need to urinate often, especially at night
- A feeling that you can't empty your bladder completely
- A feeling of hesitancy or delay, or straining to urinate
- A weak or interrupted urinary strain

YES ▶
SEE DOCTOR

NO ▼

flowchart continued in next column

flowchart continued

Do you have one or more of these symptoms of an infection that may result from BPH:
- Burning, frequent or painful urination
- Pain in the lower back, groin or testicles
- Pain in or near the penis
- Pain on ejaculation
- Discharge from the penis (blood or pus)
- Fever and/or chills

YES ▶
SEE DOCTOR

NO ▼

PROVIDE SELF-CARE

Self-Care Procedures

- Remain sexually active.
- Take hot baths.
- Avoid dampness and cold temperatures.
- Do not let the bladder get too full. Urinate as soon as the urge arises. Relax when you urinate.
- When you take long trips, make frequent stops to urinate. Keep a container in the car that you can urinate in when you can't get to a bathroom in time.
- Whenever possible, sit on a hard chair instead of a soft one.
- Limit coffee, tea, alcohol and spicy foods.
- Drink eight or more glasses of water every day, but don't drink liquids too close to bedtime.
- Reduce stress.
- Don't smoke.
- Avoid over-the-counter antihistamines.

Jock Itch

Jock itch is typified by redness, itching and scaliness in the groin and thigh area, and is usually caused by a fungus infection. It can also result from a bacterial infection or be a reaction to chemicals in clothing, irritating garments or medicines that you take.

Jock itch gets its name because an athletic supporter worn during exercise, which is subsequently stored in a dark, poorly ventilated locker, then perhaps worn again without being laundered, provides the ideal environment in which the fungi thrive. (Under similar conditions, women's clothing can develop this problem, too.)

Questions to Ask

Do symptoms of jock itch persist longer than two weeks despite Self-Care Procedures?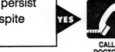

YES

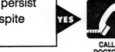

CALL DOCTOR

NO

PROVIDE SELF-CARE

Self-Care Procedures

To relieve jock itch and prevent future attacks:
- Don't wear tight, close-fitting clothing. Boxer shorts are recommended for men.
- Change underwear frequently, especially after work, if you have a job that leaves you hot and sweaty.
- Bathe or shower immediately after exercising.
- Apply talc or other powder to the groin area to help keep it dry.
- Don't store damp clothing in a locker or gym bag. Wash workout clothes after each use.
- Sleep in the nude.
- Avoid antibacterial (deodorant) soaps.

An antifungal cream, powder or lotion like tolnaftate (Tinactin) may also help relieve jock itch. It takes up to two weeks to work.

Testicular Cancer and Testicular Self-Examination

Cancer of the testicles accounts for only about 1 percent of all cancers in men. It is, though, the most common type of cancer in males aged 20 to 40, but can occur anytime after age 15. It strikes about 5,000 males a year. Often only one testicle is affected.

The cause of testicular cancer is not known. However, there are known risk factors, such as:
- Uncorrected undescended testicles in infant and young boys. (Parents should see that their infant boys are checked at birth for undescended testicles.)
- A family history of testicular cancer
- Having an identical twin with testicular cancer
- Viral infections
- Injury to the scrotum

Signs and Symptoms

In the early stages, testicular cancer may have no symptoms. When there are symptoms, they include:
- Small, painless lump in a testicle
- Enlarged testicle
- Feeling of heaviness in the testicle or groin
- Pain in the testicle
- A change in the way the testicle feels
- Enlarged male breasts and nipples
- Blood or fluid suddenly accumulating in the scrotum.

Testicular cancer is curable 90 to 95 percent of the time if found and treated early. The testicle is surgically removed. Other modalities can further treat the disease:
- Chemotherapy
- Radiation therapy
- Surgically removing nearby lymph nodes if necessary

The American Academy of Family Physicians Subcommittee for Male Patients recommends the teaching of testicular self-examination (TSE) between the ages of 13 and 18. The testicles are located behind the penis and contained within the scrotum. They should be about the same size and feel smooth, rubbery and egg-shaped. The left one sometimes hangs lower than the right.

Questions to Ask

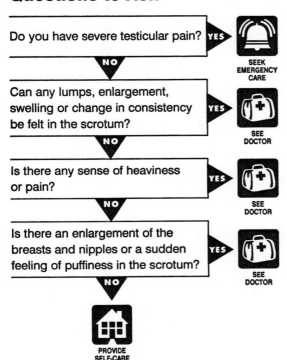

Do you have severe testicular pain? **YES** → **SEEK EMERGENCY CARE**

NO ↓

Can any lumps, enlargement, swelling or change in consistency be felt in the scrotum? **YES** → **SEE DOCTOR**

NO ↓

Is there any sense of heaviness or pain? **YES** → **SEE DOCTOR**

NO ↓

Is there an enlargement of the breasts and nipples or a sudden feeling of puffiness in the scrotum? **YES** → **SEE DOCTOR**

NO ↓

PROVIDE SELF-CARE

Testicular Self-Exam (TSE)

Self-examination of the testicles is best performed when the scrotum is relaxed, after a warm bath or shower. This will also allow the testicles to drop down.

How to do TSE:

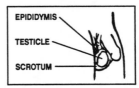
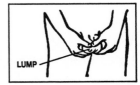

EPIDIDYMIS, TESTICLE, SCROTUM, LUMP

- Examine each testicle gently with both hands. The index and middle fingers should be placed underneath the testicle while the thumbs are placed on the top. Roll the testicle gently between the thumbs and fingers. One testicle may be larger than the other. This is normal.
- The epididymis is a cord-like structure on the top and back of the testicle that stores and transports the sperm. Do not confuse the epididymis with an abnormal lump.
- Feel for any abnormal lumps (about the size of a pea) on the front or the side of the testicle. These lumps are usually painless.

If you do find a lump, you should contact your doctor right away. The lump may be due to an infection, and a doctor can decide the proper treatment. If the lump is not an infection, it is likely to be cancer. Remember, though, that testicular cancer is highly curable, especially when detected and treated early. Testicular cancer almost always occurs in only one testicle, and the other testicle is all that is needed for full sexual function.

Routine testicular self-exams are important, but they cannot substitute for a doctor's examination. Your doctor should examine your testicles when you have a physical exam. You can also ask your doctor to teach you the correct way to do TSE. Continue to perform testicular self-exam monthly, or as recommended by your doctor.

CHAPTER 20

SEXUALLY TRANSMITTED DISEASES (STDs)

Infections that pass from one person to another during sexual contact are known as sexually transmitted diseases (STDs). Sexual contact is defined as vaginal, anal or oral sex.

Sexually transmitted diseases include chlamydia, gonorrhea, syphilis and genital herpes. Acquired immune deficiency syndrome (AIDS) is often classified as a sexually transmitted disease, but it can be passed through means other than sexual contact. So, though mentioned at times, it is not defined here. (See page 194 for information on AIDS.) Note, though, that the Self-Care Preventive Procedures listed can help prevent sexually acquired human immunodeficiency virus (HIV) (see page 187).

Basic Facts About STDs

Signs and Symptoms

STDs are transmitted through intimate sexual contact. Each STD has its own set of symptoms, but a discharge from the penis or vagina, pain when urinating (in males), and open sores or blisters in the genital area are typical of most STDs. Unfortunately, early stages of STDs often have no detectable symptoms. In addition, you can also have more than one STD at the same time. Gonorrhea and chlamydia, for example, are often picked up at the same time.

Fast Response Counts

If you suspect you have an STD, see a doctor as soon as possible. Your sexual partner(s) should also be contacted and treated.

Depending on the infection, STDs can cause serious, long-term problems like birth defects, infertility, diseases of the brain or, in the case of AIDS, death.

Treatment

Some STDs can be treated and cured with antibiotics. For others, such as AIDS, there is no cure. Prevention is the only treatment.

At present, no vaccines exist to prevent STDs. And once you've had an STD, you can get it again. You can't develop an immunity once you've been exposed.

A minor does not need parental consent to receive treatment for an STD, so parents do not have to know.

(Note: Medical treatment, not self-care treatment, is necessary for sexually transmitted diseases. One exception is genital herpes for which many self-care remedies can help alleviate the discomfort that occurs with recurrent attacks. Self-Care Preventive Procedures, however, should be followed to lower the risk for contracting STDs. [See page 187.])

Chlamydia

Chlamydia is now the most common sexually transmitted disease (STD) in the United States. It affects more men and women than syphilis, gonorrhea and genital herpes combined. In fact, chances are that persons who have had these other STDs are playing host to chlamydia as well. Chlamydia can also accelerate the appearance of AIDS symptoms for persons infected with human immunodeficiency virus (HIV).

Symptoms of chlamydia in men include burning or discomfort when urinating, a whitish discharge from the tip of the penis and pain in the scrotum. In women, symptoms include slight yellowish-green vaginal discharge, vaginal irritation, a frequent need to urinate and pain when urinating. There can also be chronic abdominal pain and bleeding between menstrual periods.

These symptoms can, however, be so mild that they often go unnoticed. It is estimated that 75 percent of women and 25 percent of men who have chlamydia have no symptoms until complications set in. If they do appear, they usually do so two to four weeks after being infected.

The only sure way to know whether or not you have chlamydia is to be tested. Doctors recommend that sexually active people who are not involved in a long-term, monogamous relationship should be tested periodically. You should be aware, though, that the most reliable test for chlamydia is a tissue culture that is expensive and not widely available. For that reason, many doctors use a simpler slide test instead. A small amount of fluid is collected from the infected site with a cotton swab. Sometimes the results are available the same day of the test.

Anyone who has chlamydia should be treated with oral antibiotics (e.g., tetracycline or erythromycin) for two to three weeks. Doctors will treat the infected sexual partner even if he or she doesn't show any symptoms. Sex should be avoided until treatment is completed in both the person affected and in his or her sex partners. If left untreated, chlamydia can cause a variety of serious problems, including infection and inflammation of the prostate and surrounding structures in men and pelvic inflammatory disease (PID) and infertility in women. Infants born to mothers who have chlamydia are likely to develop pneumonia or serious eye infections in the first several months of life as well as permanent lung damage later on.

Questions to Ask

For men: Do you have these problems:
- A whitish discharge from the penis
- Burning or discomfort when urinating
- Pain and swelling in the scrotum

 YES
SEE DOCTOR

NO

For women: Do you have these problems:
- A yellowish-green vaginal discharge
- Frequent need to urinate
- Chronic abdominal pain
- Bleeding between menstrual periods

YES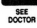
SEE DOCTOR

NO

Does your sexual partner have or do you suspect he or she might have a sexually transmitted disease? Does he or she have multiple sex partners?

 YES
CALL DOCTOR

NO

Do you want to rule out the presence of chlamydia because you are considering a new sexual relationship, planning to get married or pregnant, or for any other reason?

 YES
CALL DOCTOR

NO

See Self-Care Preventive Procedures on page 187.

Genital Herpes

Herpes simplex virus II (HSVII) is spread by direct skin-to-skin contact from the site of infection to the contact site. Once you are infected, the virus remains with you forever. It causes symptoms, though, only during flare-ups.

Symptoms include sores with blisters on the genital area and anus and sometimes on the thighs and buttocks. After a few days, the blisters break open and leave painful, shallow ulcers which can last from five days to three weeks. If infected for the first time, you may experience flu-like symptoms, such as swollen glands, fever and body aches, but subsequent attacks are almost always much milder. These attacks may be triggered by emotional stress, fatigue, menstruation, other illnesses or even by vigorous sexual intercourse. Itching, irritation and tingling in the genital area may occur one to two days before the outbreak of the blisters or sores. (This period is called the prodrome.) Genital herpes is contagious during the prodrome, when blisters are present and up to a week or two after they have disappeared. If a pregnant woman has an outbreak of genital herpes when her baby is due, a cesarean section may need to be done so the baby does not get infected during delivery.

No cure exists for genital herpes. Treatment includes prescription medication (Zovirax, available in oral and topical forms) and self-help measures to treat herpes symptoms. (See Self-Care Procedures for Genital Herpes.) Medical care is especially helpful during the first attack of genital herpes. Self-help remedies may be all that is necessary during recurrent episodes.

In some people herpes-like sores and blisters can be a side effect of taking certain prescription medicine. One example is sulpha drugs, which are often used to treat urinary tract infections. Consult your doctor if you suspect this.

Questions to Ask

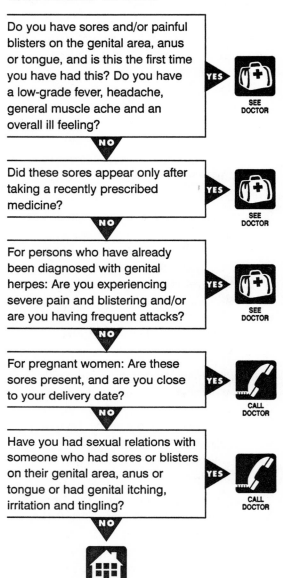

Do you have sores and/or painful blisters on the genital area, anus or tongue, and is this the first time you have had this? Do you have a low-grade fever, headache, general muscle ache and an overall ill feeling? **YES** → SEE DOCTOR

NO

Did these sores appear only after taking a recently prescribed medicine? **YES** → SEE DOCTOR

NO

For persons who have already been diagnosed with genital herpes: Are you experiencing severe pain and blistering and/or are you having frequent attacks? **YES** → SEE DOCTOR

NO

For pregnant women: Are these sores present, and are you close to your delivery date? **YES** → CALL DOCTOR

NO

Have you had sexual relations with someone who had sores or blisters on their genital area, anus or tongue or had genital itching, irritation and tingling? **YES** → CALL DOCTOR

NO

PROVIDE SELF-CARE

Self-Care Procedures for Genital Herpes

- Bathe the affected genital area twice a day with mild soap and water. Gently pat dry with a towel or use a hair dryer set on warm. Using Aveeno (colloidal oatmeal soap or bath treatments) may also be soothing.

- Take a hot bath, if you can tolerate it. This may help to inactivate the virus and promote healing.
- Use sitz baths to soak the affected area. A sitz bath device—which you can buy at a medical supply store or in some drugstores—fits over the toilet.
- Apply ice packs on the genital area for five to 10 minutes. This may help relieve itching and inflammation.
- Wear loose-fitting pants or skirts. Avoid wearing panty hose and tight-fitting clothing. These could irritate the inflamed area. Wear cotton, not nylon underwear.
- Squirt tepid water over the genital area while urinating. This may help decrease the pain.
- Take a mild pain reliever such as aspirin, acetaminophen, ibuprofen or naproxen sodium. *Note: Do not give aspirin or any medication containing salicylates to anyone 19 years of age or younger, unless directed by a physician, due to its association with Reye's syndrome, a potentially fatal condition.*
- A local anesthetic ointment (e.g., Lidocaine) can help during the most painful part of an attack. Check with your doctor before using.
- Ask your doctor about using the antiviral drug acyclovir (Zovirax), available in oral and topical forms.
- To avoid spreading the virus to your eyes, don't touch your eyes during an outbreak.
- Avoid sexual intercourse:
  - At the first sign of a herpes outbreak. (This may be evident by the feeling of tingling and itching in the genital area and takes place before blisters are noticeable.) Note, though, that herpes can be contracted even though there are no visible blisters, because viral lesions may be present on the female's cervix or inside the male's urethra.
  - When active lesions are present
  - One to two weeks after they have disappeared

Gonorrhea

Gonorrhea is one of the most common infectious diseases in the world. Often called "the clap," "dose" or "drip," it is caused by a specific bacterium that is transmitted during vaginal, oral or anal sex. A newborn baby can also get gonorrhea during birth if its mother is infected. Gonorrhea can be symptom-free. In fact, about 60 to 80 percent of infected women have no symptoms.

The signs of gonorrhea can, however, show up within two to 10 days after sexual contact with an infected person. In men, symptoms include pain at the tip of the penis, pain and burning during urination and a thick, yellow, cloudy penile discharge that gradually increases. In women, symptoms include mild itching and burning around the vagina, a thick yellowish-green vaginal discharge, burning on urination and severe lower abdominal pain (usually within a week or so after a menstrual period).

If ignored, gonorrhea can cause widespread infection and/or infertility. But gonorrhea can be cured with specific antibiotics. If you've been infected with a type of gonorrhea that's resistant to penicillin, your doctor will have to use another medicine.

To treat gonorrhea successfully, you should heed the following:
- Take prescribed medications.
- To avoid reinfection, be sure that your sexual partner is also treated.
- Have follow-up cultures to determine if the treatment was effective.

Questions to Ask

For men: Do you have any of these problems:
- A discharge of pus from the penis
- Discomfort or pain when urinating
- Irritation and itching of the penis
- Pain during intercourse

YES

SEE DOCTOR

NO

flowchart continued on next page

For women: Do you have any of these problems:
- Itching and burning around the vagina
- A vaginal discharge (this could be slight, cloudy or yellowish-green in color with a foul odor)
- Burning or pain when urinating
- The need to urinate often
- Discomfort in the lower abdomen
- Abnormal bleeding from the vagina

YES SEE DOCTOR

NO

Are you symptom-free, but may have contracted gonorrhea or another sexually transmitted disease from someone you suspect may be infected?

YES CALL DOCTOR

NO

Do you want to rule out the presence of a sexually transmitted disease because you have had multiple sex partners and you are considering a new sexual relationship or planning to get married or pregnant?

YES 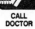 CALL DOCTOR

NO

See Self-Care Preventive Procedures on page 187.

Syphilis

Syphilis is sometimes called "pox" or "bad blood." Left untreated, syphilis is one of the most serious sexually transmitted diseases, leading to heart failure, blindness, insanity or death. Syphilis can progress slowly, through three stages, over a period of many years. When detected early, however, syphilis can be cured. Be alert for the following symptoms.

Primary Stage

A large, painless, ulcer-like sore known as a chancre occurs two to six weeks after infection and generally appears around the area of sexual contact. The chancre disappears within a few weeks.

Secondary Stage

Within a month after the end of the primary stage, a widespread skin rash appears, cropping up on the palms of the hands, soles of the feet and sometimes around the mouth and nose. The rash has small, red, scaling bumps that do not itch. Swollen lymph nodes, fever and flu-like symptoms may also occur. Small patches of hair may fall out of the scalp, beard, eyelashes and eyebrows.

Latent Stage

Once syphilis reaches this stage, it may go unnoticed for years, quietly damaging the heart, central nervous system, muscles and various other organs and tissues. The resulting effects are often fatal.

If you've been exposed to syphilis or have its symptoms, see a doctor or consult your county health department. For syphilis in its early stages, treatment consists of a single injection of long-lasting penicillin. If the disease has progressed further, you'll require three consecutive weekly injections. (If you're allergic to penicillin, you'll receive an alternative antibiotic, taken orally for two to four weeks.) You should have a blood test three, six and 12 months after treatment to be sure the disease is completely cured.

Once treatment is complete, you're no longer contagious. But if syphilis is left untreated, you're contagious for up to one year after you first contract the infection.

Questions to Ask

Do you have a large, painless, ulcer-like sore (chancre) in the genital area, anus or mouth? **YES** → **SEE DOCTOR**

NO ↓

Did you have such a sore two to six weeks ago that healed, but now experience flu-like symptoms (fever, headache, general ill feeling) and/or a skin rash of small, red, scaling bumps that do not itch? **YES** → **SEE DOCTOR**

NO ↓

Are you suspicious of having contracted syphilis or another sexually transmitted disease from someone you suspect may be infected? **YES** → **CALL DOCTOR**

NO ↓

Do you want to rule out the presence of syphilis or another sexually transmitted disease because you or your sex partner has had multiple sex partners and are considering a new sexual relationship, planning to get married or pregnant? **YES** → **CALL DOCTOR**

NO ↓

See Self-Care Preventive Procedures Listed.

Self-Care Preventive Procedures

- There's only one way to guarantee you'll never get a sexually transmitted disease: Never have sex.
- Limiting your sexual activity to one person your entire life is a close second, provided your partner is also monogamous and does not have a sexually transmitted disease.
- Avoid sexual contact with persons whose health status and practices are not known.
- Discuss a new partner's sexual history with him or her before beginning a sexual relationship. (Be aware, though, that persons are not always honest about their sexual history.)

- Latex condoms can reduce the spread of sexually transmitted diseases when used properly and carefully and for every sex act. They do not eliminate the risk entirely.
- Plan ahead for safe sex. Decide what you'll say and be willing to do with a potential sex partner. Both women and men should carry latex condoms and insist that they be used every time they have sex.
- Using spermicidal foams, jellies, creams (especially those that contain Nonoxynol-9) and a diaphragm can offer additional protection when used with a condom. Use water-based lubricants. Don't use oil-based ones (e.g., Vaseline); they can damage latex condoms.
- Don't have sex while under the influence of drugs or alcohol, except in a monogamous relationship in which neither partner is infected with an STD.
- Avoid sex if either partner has signs and symptoms of a genital tract infection.
- Wash the genitals with soap and water before and after sex.
- Seek treatment for a sexually transmitted disease if you know your sex partner is infected.
- Ask your doctor to check for STDs every six months if you have multiple sex partners, even if you don't have any symptoms.

CHAPTER 21

DENTAL HEALTH

Abscess

A tooth abscess is formed when there is inflammation and/or infection in the bone and/or the tooth's canals. This generally occurs in a tooth that has a deep cavity, a very deep filling or one that has been injured. The pain caused by an abscessed tooth can be persistent, throbbing and severe. Other symptoms include fever, earache and swelling of the glands on one side of the face or neck. It can also cause a general ill feeling, bad breath and a foul taste in the mouth.

A tooth abscess is usually treated with either a root canal or by extracting the tooth. A root canal is done if the dentist thinks the tooth can be saved. The infection is first removed either through a hole drilled through the top of the tooth or through an incision made in the gums at the site of the infection. These measures relieve the pain and pressure caused by a tooth abscess. An antibiotic will also be prescribed.

For the most part, tooth abscesses can be prevented with regular dental care. This includes daily brushing (with a fluoride toothpaste) and flossing and regular dental checkups and cleanings.

Questions to Ask

Do you have one or more of these problems with the toothache:
- Continuous or throbbing pain
- Fever
- Earache
- Neck or jaw tenderness or swollen glands in the side where the tooth aches
- General ill feeling
- Bad breath and/or foul taste in the mouth

YES → SEE DOCTOR

 NO

Does the pain come and go or only occur when you are eating or drinking?

YES → CALL DOCTOR

 NO

PROVIDE SELF-CARE

Self-Care Procedures

- To reduce pain, take aspirin, acetaminophen, ibuprofen or naproxen sodium. *Note: Do not give aspirin or any medication containing salicylates to anyone 19 years of age or younger, unless directed by a physician, due to its association with Reye's syndrome, a potentially fatal condition.*
- Hold an ice pack on the jaw. This will relieve some of the pain.
- Never place a crushed aspirin on the tooth. Aspirin burns the gums and destroys tooth enamel.
- Do not drink extremely hot or cold liquids.

- Do not chew gum.
- Avoid sweets and hot and spicy foods. A liquid diet may be necessary for a day or two until the pain subsides.
- Gargle with warm salt water every hour.
- See a dentist even if the pain subsides.

Broken or Knocked-Out Tooth

Your teeth are meant to last a lifetime. They are vulnerable, however, to nicks, chips and strains. To protect your teeth from damage and injury, take these precautions:
- Don't chew ice, pens or pencils.
- Don't use your teeth to open paper clips or otherwise to function as tools.
- If you smoke a pipe, don't bite down on the stem.
- If you grind your teeth at night, ask your dentist if you should be fitted for a bite plate to prevent tooth grinding.
- If you play contact sports like football or hockey, wear a protective mouth guard.
- Always wear a seat belt when riding in a car.
- Avoid sucking on lemons or chewing aspirin or vitamin C tablets. The acid wears away tooth enamel. *Note: Do not give aspirin or any medication containing salicylates to anyone 19 years of age or younger, unless directed by a physician, due to its association with Reye's syndrome, a potentially fatal condition.*

If a tooth does accidentally get knocked out, go to the dentist as soon as possible. (Keep the tooth moist until you get there.) Your dentist may be able to successfully put it back in. If the reimplantation can be accomplished within about half an hour, there is a possibility that the interior pulp will survive. Even up to six hours, the outer tissue of the tooth may survive and allow successful reattachment. There is little chance that the tooth can be put back in 24 hours after it has been knocked out.

Questions to Ask

Have one or more teeth been broken or knocked out? (Note: See a dentist as soon as possible. This is a dental emergency.) **YES**

SEEK EMERGENCY CARE

NO

PROVIDE SELF-CARE

Self-Care Procedures

For a broken tooth:
- To reduce swelling, apply a cold compress to the area.
- Save any broken tooth fragments and take them to the dentist.

If your tooth has been knocked out:
- Rinse the tooth with clear water.
- If possible (and if you're alert), gently put it back in the socket or hold it under your tongue. Otherwise, put the tooth in a glass of milk or a wet cloth.
- If the gum is bleeding, hold a gauze pad, a clean handkerchief or a tissue tightly in place over the wound.
- Try to get to a dentist within 30 minutes of the accident.

Periodontal (Gum) Disease

Plaque buildup, crooked teeth, illness, poorly fitting dentures, trapped food particles and certain medications can irritate or destroy your gums. With good oral hygiene, however, you can prevent periodontal (gum) disease. If caught in the early stages, gum disease is easily treated. If ignored, the gums and supporting tissues wither and your teeth may loosen and fall out.

Knowing the signs and symptoms of periodontal disease is important for early treatment. Pay attention to the following:

- Swollen red gums that bleed easily (a condition called gingivitis)
- Teeth that are exposed at the gum line (a sign that gums have pulled away from the teeth)
- Permanent teeth that are loose or separating from each other
- Bad breath and a foul taste in the mouth
- Pus around the gums and teeth

Periodontal disease should be treated by a periodontist, a dentist who specializes in this area of dentistry. Material called tartar or calculus (which is calcified plaque) can form even when normal brushing and flossing are done. The dentist or dental hygienist should remove tartar at regular intervals. When periodontitis (pockets of infection and areas of weakened bone) are established, the dentist can treat the problem with surgery or with a process known as "deep scaling."

Questions to Ask

Are one or more of the symptoms of gum disease present:
- Swollen gums
- Gums that bleed easily
- Teeth exposed at the gum line
- Loose teeth
- Teeth separating from each other
- Pus around gums and teeth
- Bad breath and/or a foul taste in the mouth

YES
SEE DOCTOR

NO

PROVIDE SELF-CARE

Self-Care Procedures

- Make sure to brush and floss your teeth regularly. Use a soft, rounded bristle toothbrush (unless your dentist has told you otherwise). Have your dentist or hygienist show you how to brush and floss your teeth correctly.
- Eat sugary foods infrequently. When you eat sweets, do so with meals, not in between meals. Finish the meal with cheese because this tends to neutralize acid formation.
- Include foods with good sources of vitamins A and C daily. (These two vitamins promote gum health.) Vitamin A can be found in cantaloupe, broccoli, spinach, winter squash, liver and dairy products fortified with vitamin A. Good vitamin C food sources include oranges, grapefruit, tomatoes, potatoes, green peppers and broccoli.

Temporomandibular Joint Syndrome (TMJ)

Temporomandibular joint syndrome (TMJ) occurs when the muscles, joints and ligaments of the jaw move out of alignment. Resulting symptoms include earaches, headaches, pain in the jaw area radiating to the face or the neck and shoulders, ringing in the ears or pain when opening and closing the mouth. These TMJ symptoms frequently mimic other conditions, so the problem is often misdiagnosed. TMJ has a number of possible causes:

- Bruxism (grinding your teeth in your sleep)
- Sleeping in a way that misaligns the jaw or creates tension in the neck
- Stress-induced muscle tension in the neck and shoulders
- Incorrect or uneven bite

TMJ may or may not require professional treatment. The condition, however, should be evaluated by a dentist. Many dentists specialize in the diagnosis and treatment of TMJ. They may prescribe anti-inflammatory medicine, tranquilizers or muscle relaxants for a short period of time, braces to correct the bite or a bite plate to wear when sleeping. Some doctors recommend surgery to correct TMJ, but you should get more than one opinion before consenting to a surgical remedy.

Questions to Ask

Are you unable to open or close your mouth because of severe pain?	YES →

SEEK EMERGENCY CARE

NO ↓

Do you experience one or more of the following:
- Inability to open the jaw completely
- Pain when you open your mouth widely
- Persistent symptoms of head-ache, earache or pain in the jaw area that is also felt in the face, neck or shoulders
- "Clicking" or "popping" sounds when you open your mouth and when you chew

YES →

SEE DOCTOR

NO ↓

PROVIDE SELF-CARE

Self-Care Procedures

If you have TMJ, you may be able to minimize symptoms in the following ways:
- Don't chew gum.
- Try not to open your jaw wide (including yawning or taking big bites out of large sandwiches or other difficult-to-eat foods).
- Massage the jaw area several times a day, first with your mouth open, then with your mouth closed.
- To help reduce muscle spasms that can cause pain, apply moist heat to the jaw area.

(A washcloth soaked in warm water makes a convenient hot compress.)
- If stress is a factor, consider biofeedback and relaxation training.

Toothaches

The pain of a toothache can be felt in the tooth itself or in the region around the tooth. Most toothaches are usually the result of either a cavity or an infection beneath or around the gum of a tooth. Insufficient oxygen to the heart as experienced with angina or a heart attack can also cause a toothache. A toothache is common after having corrective dental work on a tooth, but should not last longer than a week. (If it does, inform the dentist.)

Generally, toothaches can be prevented with regular visits to the dentist and daily self-care measures. Self-care includes proper daily brushing and flossing, good nutrition and using fluoridated water, toothpastes, rinses and supplements (if prescribed).

Because these may lead to a toothache if left unchecked, tell your dentist if you notice any of the following:
- Sensitivity to hot, cold or sweet foods
- Brown spots or little holes on a tooth
- A change in your bite (the way your teeth fit together)
- Loose teeth in an adult

Questions to Ask

Do you have any of these problems with the tooth pain:
- Gnawing pain in the lower teeth or neck
- Chest discomfort beneath the breast bone
- Pain that travels to or is felt in the shoulder or arm
- Sweating

YES →

SEEK EMERGENCY CARE

NO ↓

flowchart continued on next page

Are any of the following symptoms present:

- Fever
- Red, swollen or bleeding gums
- Swollen face
- Foul breath even after thorough brushing and flossing
- Constant toothache even when sleeping at night
- Toothache only when eating or just after eating

YES

SEE DOCTOR

NO

PROVIDE SELF-CARE

Self-Care Procedures

- To reduce discomfort, take aspirin or another mild pain reliever. *Note: Do not give aspirin or any medication containing salicylates to anyone 19 years of age or younger, unless directed by a physician, due to its association with Reye's syndrome, a potentially fatal condition.*
- Hold an ice pack on the jaw. This will relieve some of the pain.
- Never place a crushed aspirin on the tooth. Aspirin burns the gums and destroys tooth enamel.
- Do not drink extremely hot or cold liquids.
- Do not chew gum.
- Avoid sweets, soft drinks and hot and spicy foods. (These can irritate cavities and increase pain.) It may be best not to eat at all until you see your doctor.
- Gargle with warm salt water every hour.
- For a cavity, pack it with a piece of sterile cotton soaked in oil of cloves (available at drugstores).
- See a dentist even if the pain subsides.

SECTION III

MAJOR MEDICAL CONDITIONS

About This Section

Section III presents 30 major medical conditions. Where applicable, the discussions of the conditions include the following:

- Information about the condition
- Signs and symptoms of the condition
- Treatment and care for the condition
- Strategies for prevention

Unlike the common health problems in Section II, which you may be able to treat with Self-Care Procedures alone, these 30 medical conditions need a doctor's diagnosis and medical treatment from health care professionals. However, there will be things you still need to do to take care of yourself if you have any of these conditions.

CHAPTER 22

CHRONIC ILLNESSES

AIDS

AIDS is an acronym for acquired immune deficiency syndrome. It is thought to be caused by the human immunodeficiency virus (HIV). This virus destroys the body's immune system, leaving the person unable to fight certain types of infection or cancer. The AIDS virus also attacks the central nervous system, causing mental and neurological problems.

The virus is carried in bodily fluids (semen, vaginal secretions, blood and breast milk).

Certain activities are likely to promote contracting the AIDS virus. High-risk activities include:

- Unprotected* anal, oral and/or vaginal sex except in a monogamous relationship in which neither partner is infected with HIV. Particularly high-risk situations are having sex:
  - When drunk or high
  - With multiple or casual sex partners
  - With a partner who has had multiple or casual sex partners
  - With a partner who has used drugs by injection or is bisexual
  - When you or your partner has signs and symptoms of a genital tract infection
- Sharing needles and/or "the works" when injecting any kind of drugs
- Pregnancy and delivery if the mother is infected with HIV. (This can put the child at risk.)
- Having had blood transfusions, especially before 1985, unless tested negative for HIV

* Unprotected sex means without condoms and other latex barriers. When used correctly, every time and for every sex act, they provide protection from HIV. Though not 100 percent effective, they will reduce the risk.

There is some concern about the risk of getting AIDS from an infected doctor, dentist or patient. There are almost no cases of health professionals passing HIV to a patient. Patient-to-health-professional transmission has been more noted. Measures are being proposed and required by medical and dental associations to decrease these possible risks, even though they are extremely low. AIDS, however, cannot be contracted by donating blood. Blood-screening tests are also done on donated blood which makes it extremely unlikely that AIDS will be passed along in current blood transfusions. You cannot get AIDS through casual contact such as:

- Touching, holding hands or hugging
- A cough, sneeze, tears or sweat
- An animal or insect bite
- A toilet seat
- Using a hot tub or swimming

Screening tests for AIDS are available through doctors' offices, clinics and health departments. A small sample of your blood is tested for antibodies to the HIV virus. If these antibodies are present, you test positive for and are considered infected with HIV. It could take as long as six months from exposure to the virus for these antibodies to show up. The most common reason for a false-negative test is when a person gets tested before HIV antibodies have formed. If you test positive for HIV, a second type of blood test is done to confirm it. HIV/AIDS symptoms may not show up for as long as eight to 11 years after a person is infected with the virus.

Signs and Symptoms

Early symptoms of AIDS include:
- Fatigue
- Loss of appetite
- Chronic diarrhea
- Weight loss
- Persistent dry cough
- White spots on the mouth
- Fever
- Night sweats
- Swollen lymph glands

Persons with full-blown AIDS fall prey to many diseases such as skin infections, fungal infections, tuberculosis, pneumonia and cancer. These "opportunistic" infections are what lead to death in an AIDS victim, not the AIDS virus itself. When the virus invades the brain cells, it leads to forgetfulness, impaired speech, trembling and seizures.

Prevention, Treatment and Care

Someday a cure for AIDS may exist. For now, prevention is the only protection. Take these steps to help avoid contracting the AIDS virus:
- Unless you are in a long-term, monogamous relationship, during sexual intercourse use latex condoms treated with, or along with, a spermicide containing Nonoxynol-9. (Studies suggest this spermicide may inactivate the AIDS virus.)
- Don't have sex with people who are at high risk for contracting AIDS. These have been noted to be:
  - Homosexual or bisexual men, especially those with multiple sex partners or who use illegal intravenous drugs
  - Heterosexual partners of persons infected or exposed to HIV
  - Persons who have had multiple blood transfusions, especially before 1985, unless tested negative
- Don't have sex with more than one person.
- Ask specific questions about your partner's sexual past (i.e., has he or she had many partners or unprotected [no-condom] sex?).

- Do not be afraid to ask if he or she has been tested for HIV and if the results were positive or negative.
- Don't have sex with anyone who you know or suspect has had multiple partners. (If you've had sex with someone you suspect is HIV-positive, see your doctor.)
- Don't share needles and/or "the works" with anyone. This includes not only illegal drugs such as heroin but also steroids, insulin, etc. Don't have sex with people who use or have used intravenous drugs.
- Don't share personal items that have blood on them (e.g., razors).

Current treatment for AIDS includes:
- The drugs AZT, DDI and DDC, approved for use in the United States to treat AIDS. They slow the virus, but do not destroy it. Hence, they may delay the onset and slow the progress of AIDS, but may have only short-term effects.
- Taking measures to reduce the risk of disease development such as adequate rest, proper nutrition and vitamin supplementation
- Emotional support
- Treating the "opportunistic" infections that occur
- Radiation therapy and surgery, which have been successful in treating some patients

AIDS is under intensive study and research. Better forms of treatment and a vaccine are being researched worldwide. A single vaccine to protect against AIDS is not very likely, though, because HIV quickly creates a new strain of the virus.

Alzheimer's Disease

Mysterious and frustrating, Alzheimer's disease afflicts nearly four million Americans, about 10 percent of the population over age 65, and over 45 percent of those over age of 85. (In rare instances, Alzheimer's strikes earlier than 65.)

No one knows what causes Alzheimer's disease. Some research hints that a virus or infectious agent is the culprit. Other research points to brain chemical deficits, a genetic predisposition and/or environmental toxins. Nevertheless, the end result is the death of brain cells that control intellect, the way your brain receives and processes information.

Signs and Symptoms

Alzheimer's disease has a gradual onset. The signs and symptoms may progress in stages. (The stages very often overlap.) How quickly they occur varies from person to person. The disease may, however, eventually leave its victims totally unable to care for themselves.

Stage one:
• Forgetfulness
• Disorientation of time and place
• Increasing inability to do routine tasks
• Impairment in judgment
• Lessening of initiative
• Lack of spontaneity
• Depression and fear

Stage two:
• Increasing forgetfulness
• Increasing disorientation
• Wandering
• Restlessness and agitation, especially at night
• Repetitive actions
• Possible muscle twitching and/or convulsive seizures

Stage three:
• Disorientation
• Inability to recognize either themselves or other people
• Speech impairment (may not be able to speak at all)
• Develop need to put everything into their mouths
• Develop need to touch everything in sight
• Become emaciated
• Complete loss of control of all body functions

Treatment and Care

If someone you care about shows signs of Alzheimer's disease, see that he or she gets medical attention to confirm (or rule out) the diagnosis. Not everything that looks like Alzheimer's is Alzheimer's. There are many diseases or other problems that can cause dementia—severe problems with memory and thinking. These include:
• Brain tumors
• Blood clots in the brain
• Severe vitamin B_{12} deficiency
• Hypothyroidism
• Depression
• Some medication side effects

Unlike Alzheimer's, these problems can be treated.

There is no known cure for Alzheimer's. Because no specific treatment or drug exists to slow the steady deterioration that typifies Alzheimer's, good planning or medical and social management are necessary to help both the victim and caregivers cope with the symptoms and maintain the quality of life for as long as possible. It's especially helpful to put structure in the life of someone who's in the early stages of Alzheimer's. Some suggestions include:
• Maintain daily routines.
• Post reminders on an oversized and prominently displayed calendar.
• Make "to do" lists of daily tasks for the person with Alzheimer's to complete, and ask him or her to check them off as they're completed.
• Put things in their proper places after use, to help the person with Alzheimer's find things when he or she needs them.
• Post safety reminders (like "turn off the stove") at appropriate places throughout the house.
• See that the person with Alzheimer's eats well-balanced meals, goes for walks with family members and otherwise continues to be as active as possible.

Most drug therapies currently being used are experimental. One prescription medication, tacrine (Cognex), which is no longer experimental, may help with memory in some persons with the early stage of Alzheimer's disease. Sometimes medications to treat depression, paranoia and agitation can minimize symptoms, but they will not necessarily improve memory.

At late stages, providing a safe environment is of utmost importance. Alzheimer's victims should wear identification bracelets or necklaces so they can be identified should they be separated from their home environment. Seeking adult foster care or nursing home care for those who require supervision or medical management may be necessary.

Caregivers of Alzheimer's victims should also be given "care." They must deal with a number of financial, social, physical and emotional issues. Care for caregivers can be provided by professionals of home care, day care, respite care, service programs and self-help groups.

Angina

Angina is a common term shortened from the medical term "angina pectoris." The word angina itself means pain; pectoris means chest. Angina is the chest pain or discomfort brought on by decreased circulation in the heart and heart muscle itself. It results from a shortage of oxygen and other nutrients to any part of the heart muscle.

Signs and Symptoms

- Squeezing pressure, heaviness or mild ache in the chest (usually behind the breastbone)
- Aching in a tooth accompanied by this squeezing pressure or heaviness in the chest
- Aching in the neck muscles or jaw
- Aching in one or both arms in whole or in part
- Backache

- A feeling of gas in the upper abdomen and lower chest
- A feeling that you're choking
- Paleness and sweating

These symptoms may not be extreme so they are often neglected. It is better to report an episode when these symptoms of angina occur than not to do so because you might feel foolish if something minor is causing them. Episodes of angina are usually associated with:

- Anger or excitement
- Emotional shock
- Physical work in which the discomfort goes away when the work is stopped
- Waking up at night with discomfort
- Arm use

In all of these situations, there is relief from the distress when the activity is stopped.

Many people who experience angina for the first time fear they're having a heart attack. Here's why angina and heart attack are mistaken for each other:

- Both can be caused by a buildup of fatty plaque (atherosclerosis) in the heart arteries (coronary arteries). These plaques cause a decrease in flow to the heart muscle beyond the partial obstruction.
- In both, the pain is felt in the chest and may spread to both arms, shoulders or neck.
- Both may be brought on by physical exertion.
- Both are most prevalent in men who are 50 and older and women who are past menopause.

But there are key differences, too:

- A heart attack results in a damaged or injured heart muscle, but angina does not. Rather, anginal pain is a warning sign of a potential heart attack. The pain indicates that the heart muscle isn't getting enough blood.
- Rest or nitroglycerin relieves angina, but not a heart attack.

A doctor can generally diagnose angina as stable or unstable, based on your description of the painful episode, but he or she may need to confirm it with a stress test (a measurement of heart function taken while you exercise on a treadmill). Unstable angina, a symptom of coronary artery disease, requires immediate attention. This serious medical condition affects many Americans, some of whom may not know they have heart disease. Although unstable angina can be a precursor to a heart attack, prompt treatment can lower the risk of death or serious cardiac events.

Contributing factors like high blood pressure, obesity, diabetes, high cholesterol, smoking or a family history of atherosclerotic heart disease increase the odds of experiencing episodes of atherosclerosis and, hence, episodes of angina.

Treatment and Care

Seek emergency care for any chest pain which is suspicious for angina. Contact your physician or a cardiologist, who should insist on close follow-up, appropriate studies to diagnose your condition and therapy to treat it. The keystones to treatment are:
- Take appropriate medicine such as one to control high blood pressure, nitroglycerin or other medication to temporarily dilate or widen the coronary arteries which eases blood flow to the heart. Nitroglycerin takes effect within a minute or two.
- Engage in daily physical exercise for endurance, preferably prescribed just for you by an exercise physiologist to whom a cardiologist has referred you. (Exercise must be maintained below the onset of any discomfort. It may not be applicable at all for some individuals.)
- Don't smoke. Nicotine in cigarettes constricts the arteries and prevents proper blood flow.
- Avoid large, heavy meals. Instead, eat lighter meals throughout the day.
- Rest after eating or engage in some quiet activity.
- Minimize exposure to cold, windy weather.
- Lower your cholesterol level, if high, by eating a low-saturated-fat diet and/or taking lipid-lowering medication, if necessary and prescribed.
- Avoid sudden engagement in rather severe exercise or other physical stress.
- Avoid anger and frustration whenever possible.

Arthritis

Arthritis robs some 40 million Americans of their freedom of movement by breaking down the protective cartilage in the joints. By destroying cartilage, arthritis results in pain and decreased movement.

Many forms of arthritis exist. Three of the most common are osteoarthritis, rheumatoid arthritis and ankylosing spondylitis.

Osteoarthritis is a painful degeneration of the cartilage in the weight-bearing and frequently used joints. As far as researchers can tell, this kind of arthritis is typically brought on by genetics and wear and tear on the joints. It can also follow an injury to the joint. Osteoarthritis usually affects older people and is the most common type of arthritis. Brief pain and stiffness at the beginning of the day are typical.

Rheumatoid arthritis (RA) is caused by a chronic inflammation of the fingers, wrists, ankles, elbows and/or knees, causing pain, swelling and tenderness. Morning stiffness lasting longer than an hour is very common. RA affects women more often than men, striking in their 30s and 40s.

Ankylosing spondylitis generally affects young men between the ages of 15 and 45 and is characterized by a stiff backbone, accompanied by low back pain.

Signs and Symptoms

Symptoms of arthritis, therefore, depend upon the type of arthritis that is present. Symptoms generally include:
- Stiffness
- Swelling in one or more joints
- Deep, aching pain in a joint
- Any pain associated with movement of a joint
- Tenderness, warmth or redness in afflicted joints

- Fever, weight loss or fatigue that accompanies joint pain

Treatment and Care

If your doctor does diagnose arthritis, he or she may prescribe medication (usually aspirin or another nonsteroidal anti-inflammatory medication), rest, heat or cold treatment and some physical therapy or exercise, depending on what kind of arthritis you have. The goal is to reduce pain and improve joint mobility.

Among those treatments, exercise is perhaps the most important, whether it be some form of stretching, isometrics or simple endurance exercise. Exercise seems to provide both physical relief and psychological benefits. For example, it prevents the muscles from shrinking, while inactivity encourages both loss of muscle tone and bone deterioration. Too much exercise, however, will cause more pain in those with rheumatoid arthritis. So if you have arthritis, consult your physician, a physical therapist or a physiatrist (a doctor who specializes in rehabilitative treatment) to assist you in developing an exercise program.

One effective and soothing form of exercise is hydrotherapy, or movement done in water. It allows freedom of movement and puts less stress on the joints because nearly all of the body weight is supported by the water. Doctors highly recommend swimming, too.

But remember, hydrotherapy or any form of exercise should never produce pain. One message that can't be emphasized enough is "Go easy." If you begin to hurt, stop and rest or apply ice packs.

The following exercise suggestions may provide relief:
- Choose exercise routines that use all affected joints.
- Keep movements gradual, slow and gentle.
- If a joint is inflamed, don't exercise it.
- Don't overdo it. Allow yourself sufficient rest.
- Concentrate on freedom of movement, especially in the water, and be patient.

Cancer

Cancer refers to a broad group of diseases in which body cells grow out of control and are or become malignant (harmful).

Cancer is the second leading cause of death in the United States (heart disease is first). Current estimates say that 30 percent of all Americans will develop some kind of cancer in their lifetimes. The most common forms are cancer of the skin, lungs, colon and rectum, breast, prostate, urinary tract and uterus.

Exactly what causes all cancers has not yet been found. Evidence suggests, however, that cancer could result from complex interactions of viruses, a person's genetic makeup, immune status and exposure to other risk factors that may promote cancer. These risk factors include:
- Exposure to the sun's ultraviolet rays, nuclear radiation, X-rays and radon
- Use of tobacco and/or alcohol (for some cancers)
- Use of certain drugs such as DES (a synthetic estrogen) or anabolic steroids
- Polluted air and water
- Dietary factors such as a high-fat diet, specific food preservatives (e.g., nitrates and nitrites), charbroiling and grilling meats
- Exposure to a variety of chemicals such as asbestos, benzenes, VC (vinyl chloride), wood dust and some ingredients of cigarette smoke

Signs and Symptoms

Symptoms of cancer depend on the type of cancer, the stage that it is in and whether or not it has spread to other parts of the body (metastasis). The following signs and symptoms should always be brought to your doctor's attention because they could be warning signals of cancer:
- Any change in bladder or bowel habits
- A lump or thickening in the breast, testicles or anywhere else
- Unusual vaginal bleeding or rectal discharge or any unusual bleeding

- Persistent hoarseness or nagging cough
- A sore throat that won't go away
- Noticeable change in a wart or mole
- Indigestion or difficulty swallowing

Treatment and Care

Cancer is not necessarily fatal and is, in many cases, curable. Early detection and proper treatment increase your chances for surviving cancer. Early detection is more likely if you:

- Know the warning signs for cancer and report any of these warning signs to your doctor if they occur.
- Do regular self-examination such as monthly breast self-examination if you are a woman (see page 162) and a testicular self-examination, monthly or as directed by your doctor, if you are a man (see page 181).
- Look at yourself in the mirror for any notice-able changes in warts or moles or for any wounds that have not healed.
- Ask your doctor to perform routine tests such as Pap tests, breast exams and mammograms, if you are a woman.

Other tests include one for colorectal abnor-malities (sigmoidoscopy) and one to check for blood in the stools. (See "Common Health Tests" on page 17.)

If and when cancer is diagnosed, treatment will depend on the type of cancer present, the stage it is in and your body's response to treatment. Cancer treatment generally includes one or more of the following:

- Surgery to remove the cancerous tumor(s) and clear any obstruction to vital passage-ways caused by the cancer
- Radiation therapy
- Chemotherapy
- Possibly immunotherapy

Prevention

Moreover, measures can be taken to lower the risk for certain forms of cancer:

Dietary:

- Reduce the intake of total dietary fat to no more than 30 percent of total calories, and reduce the intake of saturated fat to less than 10 percent of total calories.
- Eat more fruits, vegetables and whole grains, especially:
  - Broccoli, cabbage and other vegetables in the cabbage family, including brussels sprouts. These contain cancer-fighting chemicals such as sulforaphane and antioxidants.
  - Deep yellow-orange fruits and vegetables such as cantaloupe, peaches, tomatoes, carrots, sweet potatoes, squash and very dark green vegetables like spinach, greens and broccoli for their beta-carotene content
  - Strawberries, citrus fruits, broccoli and green peppers for vitamin C
  - Whole-grain breads, cereals, fresh fruits and vegetables and legumes for their dietary fiber content
- Consume salt-cured, salt-pickled and smoked foods only in moderation.
- Drink alcoholic beverages only in modera-tion, if at all.

Lifestyle:

- Do not smoke, use tobacco products or inhale secondhand smoke.
- Limit your exposure to known carcinogens such as asbestos, radon and other work-place chemicals, as well as pesticides and herbicides.
- Have X-rays only when necessary.
- Limit your exposure to the sun's ultraviolet (UV) rays, sunlamps and tanning booths. Protect your skin from the sun's UV rays with protective clothing (e.g., sun hats and long-sleeve shirts) and sunscreen. Be sure your sunscreen is applied frequently and contains a sun protection factor (SPF) of 15 or higher.
- Reduce stress. Emotional stress weakens the immune system, inhibiting its ability to fight off stray cancer cells.

Cataracts

A cataract is a cloudy area in the lens or lens capsule of the eye. A cataract blocks or distorts light entering the eye. This causes problems with glare from lamps or the sun, and vision gradually becomes dull and fuzzy, even in daylight. Most of the time, cataracts occur in both eyes, but only one eye may be affected. If they form in both eyes, one eye can be worse than the other, because each cataract develops at a different rate. During the time cataracts are forming, vision can be helped with frequent changes in eyeglass prescriptions.

Although there are several causes of cataracts, senile cataracts are the most common form. Cataracts can accompany aging, probably due to changes in the chemical state of lens proteins. About half of Americans ages 65 to 74 have cataracts. About 70 percent of those over 75 have this condition.

Traumatic cataracts develop after a foreign body enters the lens capsule with enough force to cause specific damage.

Complicated cataracts occur secondary to other diseases (e.g., diabetes mellitus) or other eye disorders (e.g., detached retinas, glaucoma and retinitis pigmentosa). Ionizing radiation or infrared rays can also lead to this type of cataract.

Toxic cataracts can result from medicine or chemical toxicity. Smokers have an increased risk for developing cataracts.

Signs and Symptoms

- Cloudy, fuzzy, foggy or filmy vision
- Sensitivity to light and glazed nighttime vision. This can cause problems when driving at night because headlights seem too bright.
- Double vision
- Normally black pupils that appear milky white
- Halos which may appear around lights
- Changes in the way you see colors
- Problems with glare from lamps or the sun
- Better vision for awhile, only in farsighted people. This is called "second sight."

Prevention

- Limit exposing your eyes to X-rays, microwaves and infrared radiation.
- Use sunglasses that block ultraviolet (UV) light.
- Wear a wide-brimmed hat or baseball cap to keep direct sunlight from your eyes while outdoors.
- Avoid overexposure to sunlight.
- Wear glasses or goggles that protect your eyes whenever you use strong chemicals, power tools or other instruments that could result in eye injury.
- Don't smoke.
- Avoid heavy drinking.
- Eat a lot of foods high in beta-carotene and/or vitamin C, which are thought to help prevent or delay cataracts. Carrots, cantaloupes, oranges and broccoli are examples of such foods.
- Follow your doctor's advice to keep other illnesses such as diabetes under control.

Treatment and Care

If the vision loss caused by a cataract is only slight, surgery may not be needed. A change in your glasses, stronger bifocals or the use of magnifying lenses, and taking measures to reduce glare may help improve your vision and be enough for treatment. To reduce glare, wear sunglasses that filter UV light when you are outdoors. When indoors, make sure your lighting is not too bright or pointed directly at you. Use soft, white light bulbs instead of clear ones, for example, and arrange to have light reflect off walls and ceilings. When cataracts interfere with your life, however, surgery should be considered.

Modern cataract surgery is safe and effective in restoring vision. Ninety-five percent of operations are successful. For the most part, surgery can be done on an outpatient basis or involve no more than an overnight hospital stay.

A person who has cataract surgery usually gets an artificial lens at the same time. A plastic disc called an intraocular lens is placed in the lens capsule inside the eye. Other choices are contact lenses and cataract glasses. Your doctor will help you to decide which choice is best for you.

It takes a couple of months for an eye to heal after cataract surgery. Experts say it is best to wait until your first eye heals before you have surgery on the second eye if it, too, has a cataract.

Following surgery, continue to protect your eyes from ultraviolet light by wearing UV-filtered sunglasses.

Chronic Fatigue Syndrome

Chronic fatigue syndrome has sometimes been called "yuppie flu" because its victims are often well-educated professionals in their 20s, 30s and 40s. Many are women. Until about 1983, doctors knew next to nothing about this malady, and even today its exact cause is unknown. Early on, some researchers believed it was caused by the Epstein-Barr virus, whereas others suggested its cause could be a virus that has not yet been identified. Most experts now lean toward a theory of multiple causes.

Signs and Symptoms

Symptoms of chronic fatigue syndrome are:
• Fatigue for at least six months
• Sore throat
• Swollen glands
• Low-grade fever
• Headaches
• Depression
• Muscle aches
• Mild weight loss
• Short-term memory problems

• Sleep disturbances (insomnia or hypersomnia)
• Confusion, difficulty thinking, inability to concentrate

Unfortunately, these symptoms could signal any one of many diseases, and chronic fatigue syndrome can be diagnosed, therefore, only after other illnesses, such as AIDS, tuberculosis, chronic inflammatory diseases, autoimmune diseases (e.g., lupus) or psychiatric illnesses have been ruled out. There are no specific laboratory tests as yet that can diagnose the syndrome. For some, the symptoms are so debilitating that a normal working life is impossible. Yet others experience only a vague sense of feeling ill. In some cases, symptoms never let up, while in others they come and go.

Treatment and Care

Until more is known, people with chronic fatigue syndrome are encouraged to do the following:
• Get plenty of rest.
• Learn to manage stress.
• Take good care of their general health.
• Try to lead as normal a life as possible.
• Join a support group of others who have this problem.

Medicines may be prescribed to relieve pain and muscle aches and control fever, such as acetaminophen, aspirin, ibuprofen or naproxen sodium, or prescribed nonsteroidal, anti-inflammatory medicine. Antidepressant medicine may also be prescribed. A gradual exercise program, if tolerated, may also be beneficial.

Cirrhosis

Cirrhosis is a chronic disease of the liver. It can be caused by any injury, infection or inflammation of the liver. With cirrhosis, normal healthy liver cells are replaced with scar tissue. This prevents the liver from performing its many functions.

The liver is probably the body's most versatile organ. Among its many tasks are the following:
- Makes bile (a substance that aids in the digestion of fats)
- Produces blood proteins
- Helps the blood to clot
- Metabolizes cholesterol
- Helps maintain normal blood sugar levels
- Forms and stores glycogen (the body's short-term energy source)
- Manufactures more than 1,000 enzymes necessary for various bodily functions
- Detoxifies substances (e.g., alcohol and certain drugs)

The liver is equipped to handle a certain amount of alcohol without much difficulty. But too much alcohol, too often and for too long causes the vital tissues in the liver to break down. Fatty deposits accumulate and scarring occurs. Cirrhosis is most commonly found in men over 45, yet the number of women developing cirrhosis is steadily increasing.

To make matters worse, people who regularly overindulge in alcohol generally have poor nutritional habits. When alcohol replaces food, essential vitamins and minerals can be missing from the diet. Malnutrition aggravates cirrhosis.

While alcohol abuse is the most common cause of cirrhosis, hepatitis, taking certain drugs, or exposure to certain chemicals can also produce this condition.

Signs and Symptoms

Early signs and symptoms are vague but generally include:
- Poor appetite
- Nausea
- Indigestion
- Vomiting
- Weight loss
- Constipation
- Dull abdominal ache
- Fatigue

Doctors recognize the following as signs of advanced cirrhosis:
- Enlarged liver
- Yellowish eyes and skin and tea-colored urine (indicating jaundice)
- Bleeding from the gastrointestinal tract
- Itching
- Hair loss
- Swelling in the legs and stomach
- Tendency to bruise easily
- Mental confusion
- Coma

Treatment and Care

Cirrhosis can be life-threatening, so get medical attention if you have any of the above symptoms. And needless to say, you (or anyone you suspect of having cirrhosis) should abstain from alcohol and get treatment for alcoholism. If you suspect some toxic substance (e.g., medicines and industrial poisons) has caused the cirrhosis, discuss the possibility with your doctor so that you can identify and eliminate the culprit.

Coronary Heart Disease

The coronary arteries supply blood to the heart muscle. When they become narrow or blocked (usually by fatty deposits and/or blood clots), the heart muscle can be damaged. This is coronary heart disease. Two conditions of coronary heart disease are angina pectoris (see "Angina" on page 197) and acute myocardial infarction (heart attacks). Every day, about 4,000 Americans have heart attacks, one every 20 seconds. And each year, nearly 600,000 people die of coronary artery disease, making it the nation's number-one killer. Fortunately, heart disease claims fewer and fewer lives each year, thanks to advances in medical treatment of heart disease and growing public awareness of the benefits of exercise and good nutrition. Prevention is of utmost importance.

Prevention

To avoid coronary heart disease, the American Heart Association suggests the following steps:

- Have your blood pressure checked regularly. High blood pressure can increase the risk of atherosclerosis. To control high blood pressure, follow your doctor's advice.
- If you smoke, quit. Nicotine constricts blood flow to the heart, decreases oxygen supply to the heart and seems to play a significant role in the development of coronary heart disease.
- Be aware of the signs and symptoms for diabetes (see page 205), which is associated with atherosclerosis. Follow your doctor's advice if you have diabetes.
- Maintain a normal body weight. (People who are obese are more prone to atherosclerosis, high blood pressure and diabetes, and therefore coronary heart disease.)
- Eat a diet low in saturated fats and cholesterol. (Saturated fats are found in meats, dairy products with fat, hydrogenated vegetable oils and some tropical oils such as coconut and palm kernel oils.) High-saturated-fat, high-cholesterol diets contribute to the fatty sludge that accumulates inside artery walls.
- Reduce your intake of salt if you are "salt-sensitive." Salt-sensitive people's blood pressure goes up if they eat too much salt.
- Get some form of aerobic exercise at least three times a week for 20 minutes at a time. Sitting around hour after hour, day after day, week in and week out with no regular physical activity may cause circulation problems later in life and contributes to atherosclerosis. Start any new exercise program gradually. Report symptoms of chest pain and/or shortness of breath to your doctor.
- Reduce the harmful effects of stress by practicing relaxation techniques and improving your outlook on daily events. Stress has been linked to elevated blood pressure, among other health problems.
- Get regular medical checkups.

- Know the signs and symptoms of a heart attack so you can get immediate medical attention if necessary, before it's too late. The signs of heart attack are:
  - Chest discomfort or pressure lasting several minutes or longer
  - Discomfort or pressure that spreads to the shoulder, neck, arm and jaw
  - Nausea or vomiting associated with chest pain
  - A cold sweat
  - Difficulty breathing
  - Faintness or dizziness.
  - Stomach upset
  - A sense of impending disaster

Treatment and Care

If you think you're having a heart attack, get to a hospital as quickly as possible. A clot-dissolving injection can be given to reduce the risk of mortality and severity of damage to the heart muscle if given within four hours. Other emergency procedures can also prevent damage to the heart muscle.

The type of care following a heart attack will depend on the amount of damage done to the heart muscle. This can be assessed by specific medical tests and procedures. Your doctor will determine the course of treatment, which could include any or many of the following:

- Medication (cardiac, blood pressure, cholesterol-lowering drugs, etc.)
- Hospitalization for treatment and recovery from the heart attack
- Cardiac rehabilitation for lifestyle changes including: smoking cessation; weight loss; low-fat, cholesterol-controlling diet; behavior modification; stress management; relaxation techniques
- Surgery, if indicated: angioplasty, coronary artery bypass grafts, etc.
- Long-term maintenance and medical follow-up

Diabetes

Diabetes is a condition that results when a person's body doesn't make any insulin, or enough insulin, or doesn't use insulin the right way. Insulin is a hormone made in the pancreas gland that helps your cells use blood sugar for energy. When insulin is in short supply, the glucose (sugar) in the blood can become dangerously high. That's why a person with diabetes may have to take insulin, by injection or oral medicine, to help the body secrete more of its own insulin or make better use of the insulin it does secrete.

Some people diagnosed with diabetes, however, require no medication. All persons with diabetes must follow a controlled diet and exercise regularly to prevent their blood sugar from getting too high.

There are two forms of diabetes:

Type 1 - Sometimes called insulin-dependent diabetes mellitus (IDDM) or juvenile diabetes. It is more severe and usually shows up before the age of 30 (but may occur at any age). Insulin injections, as well as dietary control and exercise, are essential.

Type 2 - Sometimes called non-insulin-dependent diabetes mellitus (NIDDM) or adult-onset diabetes). It is less severe, usually affecting persons 40 years of age or older who are overweight. This type is most often treated with diet and exercise and sometimes oral medicine. Occasional insulin injections may be required as well.

Diabetes can contribute to and accelerate hardening of the arteries, stroke, kidney failure, blindness and gangrene.

Signs and Symptoms

The American Diabetes Association uses the acronyms DIABETES and CAUTION to help identify the warning signs of diabetes:

- **D** Drowsiness
- **I** Itching
- **A** A family history of diabetes
- **B** Blurred vision
- **E** Excessive weight
- **T** Tingling, numbness or pain in extremities
- **E** Easy fatigue
- **S** Skin infection, slow healing of cuts and scratches, especially on the feet

Other signs are:
- **C** Constant urination
- **A** Abnormal thirst
- **U** Unusual hunger
- **T** The rapid loss of weight
- **I** Irritability
- **O** Obvious weakness and fatigue
- **N** Nausea and vomiting

You don't necessarily have to experience all of these warning signs to be diabetic; only one or two may be present. Some people show no warning signs whatsoever and find out they're diabetic only after a routine blood test. If you have a family history of diabetes, you should be especially watchful of the signs and symptoms mentioned before. If you notice any of these signs, report them to your doctor. Being overweight increases your risk significantly. A diet high in sugar and low in fiber may increase your risk as well. Pregnancy can trigger diabetes in some women.

Treatment and Care

Treatment for diabetes will depend on the type and severity of the disorder. Both forms, however, require a treatment plan that maintains normal, steady blood sugar levels. This can be accomplished by:

- Regulating diet with prescribed amounts of protein, fat and carbohydrates set up in regular meals, and promoting weight reduction (if necessary)
- Exercise
- Medicine, in the form of oral hypoglycemic agents or insulin injections (if necessary)

With either type of diabetes, routine care and follow-up treatment are important. Careful control of blood sugar levels can allow a person with diabetes to lead a normal, productive life. Persons who are genetically predisposed to diabetes should watch their weight, control their eating habits and exercise regularly to reduce their risk of getting the disease.

Diverticulosis

No one is sure why, but sometimes small sac-like pockets protrude from the wall of the colon. This is called diverticulosis. Increased pressure within the intestines seems to be responsible. The pockets (called diverticuli) can fill with intestinal waste.

Sometimes, though, the intestinal pouches become inflamed, in which case the condition is called diverticulitis.

Many older persons have diverticulosis. The digestive system becomes sluggish as a person ages. Things that increase the risk for diverticulosis include:
- Not eating enough dietary fiber. Diverticulosis is common in nations where fiber intake is low.
- Continual use of medicines that slow bowel action (e.g., painkillers, antidepressants)
- Overuse of laxatives
- Having family members who have diverticulosis
- Having gallbladder disease
- Being obese

Signs and Symptoms

In most cases, diverticulosis causes no discomfort. When there are symptoms they are usually:
- Tenderness, mild cramping or a bloated feeling usually on the lower left side of the abdomen
- Sometimes constipation or diarrhea
- Occasionally, bright-red blood in the stools

With diverticulitis you can experience severe abdominal pain, feel nauseated and have a fever. The pain is made worse with a bowel movement. If these things occur, you should see your doctor.

Treatment and Care

Diverticular disease can't be cured, but you can reduce the discomfort and prevent complications. Eat a diet high in fiber throughout life. You can add more fiber to your diet with fresh fruits and vegetables and whole-grain foods. Check with your doctor about adding wheat bran to your diet. These pass through the system quickly, decreasing pressure in the intestines. Do, however, avoid corn, seeds and foods with seeds (e.g., figs). These are easily trapped in the troublesome pouches.

You should also drink 1½ to two quarts of water every day. Avoid the regular use of laxatives (e.g., Ex-Lax) that make your bowel muscles contract. In fact, you should consult your doctor before taking any laxatives. If you are not able to eat a high-fiber diet, ask your doctor about taking bulk-producing laxatives like Metamucil. These are not habit-forming. Try, too, not to strain when you have bowel movements. Finally, get regular exercise.

Emphysema

Can you imagine what it would feel like to breathe with a plastic bag over your head? That's exactly what emphysema feels like. Over one million Americans are forced to lead restricted lives because they have this chronic lung condition. The air sacs (alveoli) in the lungs are destroyed, and the lung loses its elasticity, along with its ability to take in oxygen. Genetic factors are responsible for 3 to 5 percent of all cases of emphysema. Occupational and environmental exposure to irritants can also cause the disease, but the vast majority of people with emphysema are cigarette smokers aged 50 or older. In fact, emphysema is sometimes called the smoker's disease because of its strong link with cigarettes.

Signs and Symptoms

Emphysema takes a number of years to develop, and early symptoms can be easily missed. Symptoms to look out for include:
- Breathing through pursed lips
- Shortness of breath on exertion
- Wheezing
- Fatigue
- Slight body build with marked weight loss and barrel chest

(Note: Persons with emphysema having severe symptoms may need emergency care.)

Emphysema is often accompanied by chronic bronchitis. Together they are referred to as *chronic obstructive pulmonary disease* (COPD). Persons with chronic bronchitis have symptoms of coughing and production of excess sputum.

Treatment and Care

A doctor can diagnose emphysema based on your medical history, a physical exam, a chest X-ray and a lung-function test (spirometry). By the time emphysema is detected, however, anywhere from 50 to 70 percent of your lung tissue may already be destroyed. At that point, your doctor may recommend the following:
- A program to help you stop smoking
- Avoidance of secondhand smoke
- Avoidance of dust, fumes, pollutants and other irritating inhalants
- Physical therapy to help loosen mucus in your lungs (if chronic bronchitis accompanies the emphysema)
- Daily exercise
- A diet that includes adequate amounts of all essential nutrients
- Prescription medication which may include a bronchodilator, steroids and antibiotics
- Annual flu vaccinations
- A pneumonia vaccination given once as recommended by your doctor
- Supplemental oxygen as needed

Emphysema is irreversible, however, so prevention is the only real way to avoid permanent damage.

Epilepsy

Epilepsy is a disorder of the brain. For some reason, with epilepsy there is excessive electrical activity in nerve cells in the brain. Some of the known causes of epilepsy include:
- Brain damage, either at birth or from a severe head injury
- Alcohol or drug abuse
- Brain infection
- Brain tumor

More often than not, however, the cause is not known. Epilepsy affects people of all ages, male and female. It often begins in childhood or adolescence, and while the disorder tends to run in families, epilepsy is not contagious.

Signs and Symptoms

The most common symptom is a seizure, of which there are many types. The type depends on the part of the brain the seizure starts in, how fast it takes place and how wide an area of the brain it involves.

Types of seizures fall in two general groups: general and partial. Involvement is confined to small areas of the brain with a partial seizure. A general seizure affects the whole brain and can cause loss of consciousness and/or convulsions.

Types of general seizures are:
- **Nonconvulsive.** These are also called absence or petit mal seizures. Symptoms include staring into space and repeated blinking. The sufferer is unaware of the seizure, but someone else may think he or she is daydreaming or not paying attention. These types of seizures can occur once a day or more than a hundred times a day. They occur most often in children and can result in learning problems.

- **Convulsive.** These are also called tonic-clonic or grand mal seizures. There can be many symptoms including crying out, falling down, losing consciousness, entire body stiffening, then uncontrollable jerks and twitches. The sufferer's muscles relax after the seizure. He or she may lose bowel and bladder control and may be confused, sleepy and have a headache.

Types of partial seizures are:
- Simple ones in which symptoms include tingling feelings, twitching, seeing flashing lights, hallucination of smell and/or taste
- Complex ones involving episodes (e.g., sitting motionless or moving or behaving in strange or repetitive ways) called automatisms. Examples include lip smacking, chewing and fidgeting with the hands. There is usually no loss of consciousness, but the person who has this type of seizure may be confused and not remember details of it.

If a partial seizure spreads, it could lead to a general seizure.

Treatment and Care

A medical diagnosis is necessary and will include:
- Information about the attacks. This may need to be given by someone else because the sufferer is often not aware of what has happened.
- A complete neurological exam that includes a test to measure the electrical activity of the brain (EEG). Specialized imaging tests (e.g., computerized tomography [CAT] scans and magnetic resonance imaging [MRI] scans) and blood tests may also be done.

Persons with recurrent seizures are usually given anticonvulsant drugs to prevent or lessen the chance for future seizures. Epileptics can lead normal lives once the seizures are controlled by medicine or do not occur for several years. This, however, depends on the type of seizure. Persons with general convulsive seizures may have restrictions on driving and high-risk activities (e.g., certain jobs, sports, anything involving heights, using dangerous machinery or being in any potentially hazardous situation). If medication is not effective and the seizures are confined to a specific single area of the brain, in rare cases, surgery may be performed.

Gallstones

Gallstones are stone deposits of a mixture of cholesterol (the same fat-like substance that clogs arteries), bilirubin and protein that are found in the gallbladder or bile ducts. These stones can range in size from less than a pinhead to three inches across. Over 16 million Americans (most of them women) have gallstones. Depending on their size and location, gallstones may cause no symptoms or may require medical treatment.

Doctors aren't sure why gallstones form, but some people are clearly more susceptible than others. Factors that invite gallstones to form include:
- A family history of gallbladder disease
- Obesity
- Middle age
- Being female
- Pregnancy
- Taking estrogen
- Diabetes
- Eating a diet high in cholesterol-rich foods
- Diseases of the small intestine

Signs and Symptoms

Symptoms of gallstones include:
- Feeling bloated and gassy, especially after eating fried or fatty foods
- Steady pain in the upper right abdomen that lasts from 20 minutes to five hours
- Pain between the shoulder blades or in the right shoulder
- Indigestion, nausea, vomiting
- Severe abdominal pain with fever and sometimes yellow skin and/or eyes (jaundice)

Treatment and Care

Treatments for gallstones include:
- Dietary measures (e.g., a low-fat diet) to reduce contractions of the gallbladder, thus limiting pain
- Medications to dissolve the stones
- Lithotripsy (the use of shock waves to shatter the stones)
- Surgery to remove the gallbladder

Glaucoma

Glaucoma happens when the pressure of the liquid in the eye gets too high and causes damage. Glaucoma tends to run in families and is one of the most common major eye disorders in people over the age of 60. In fact, the risk of getting glaucoma increases with age, but it can also be triggered or aggravated by some medicines like antihistamines and antispasmodics.

Signs and Symptoms

There are two types of glaucoma:

- **Chronic or open-angle glaucoma.** This type takes place gradually and usually causes no pain and no symptoms early on. When signs and symptoms begin, they include:
  - Loss of side (peripheral) vision
  - Blurred vision

  In the late stages, symptoms include:
  - Vision loss in larger areas (side and central vision), usually in both eyes
  - Blind spots
  - Seeing halos around lights
  - Poor night vision
  - Blindness if not treated early enough

- **Acute or angle-closure glaucoma.** This type can occur suddenly and is a medical emergency! Signs and symptoms include:
  - Severe pain in and above the eye
  - Severe throbbing headache
  - Fogginess of vision, halos around lights
  - Redness in the eye, swollen upper eyelid
  - Dilated pupil
  - Nausea, vomiting, weakness

Treatment and Care

Glaucoma may not be preventable, but the blindness that may result from it is. Ask to be tested for glaucoma whenever you get a regular vision checkup. It's a simple, painless procedure. If pressure inside the eyeball is high, an eye specialist (ophthalmologist) will probably give you eye drops and perhaps oral medicines. The aim of both is to reduce the pressure inside the eye.

Medicines given for acute glaucoma are prescribed for life. If you have glaucoma, let your doctor know or remind him or her of any medicines you take.

Also, do not take any medicine—even a nonprescription one—without first checking with your doctor or pharmacist. Most cold medications and sleeping pills, for example, can cause the pupil in the eye to dilate. This can lead to increased eye pressure, which is not recommended with glaucoma.

If medicines do not control the pressure, other options exist:
- Ultrasound, which uses sound waves to reduce the pressure in the eye. This is usually done as a short, outpatient procedure.
- Laser beam surgery and other surgical procedures that can widen the drainage channels within the eye. These relieve fluid buildup.

There are also some things you can do on your own:
- Avoid getting upset and fatigued. This can increase pressure in the eye.
- Don't smoke cigarettes. It causes blood vessels to constrict, which reduces blood supply to the eye.

Gout

Gout is a form of arthritis most common in men older than 30 and in postmenopausal women and is caused by increased blood levels of uric acid, produced by the breakdown of protein in the body. When blood levels of uric acid rise above a critical level, thousands of hard, tiny uric acid crystals collect in the joints. These crystals act like tiny, hot, jagged shards of glass, resulting in pain and inflammation. Crystals can collect in the tendons and cartilage, in the kidneys (as kidney stones) and in the fatty tissues beneath the skin. Gout can strike any joint, but often affects those in the feet, such as the big toe, and those in the legs.

A gout attack can last several hours to a few days. Persons who have gout can be symptom-free for years between attacks. Gout can be triggered by:
- Mild trauma or blow to the joint
- Drinking alcohol (beer and wine more so than distilled alcohol)
- Eating a diet rich in red meat (especially organ meats such as liver, kidney or tongue)
- Eating sardines or anchovies
- Taking certain medications (e.g., diuretics)

Signs and Symptoms
- Excruciating pain and inflammation in a joint or joints that strike suddenly and peak quickly
- Affected area that is swollen, red, feels warm and is very tender to the touch
- Feeling of agonizing pain after even the slightest pressure such as rubbing a sheet against the affected area
- Sometimes a low-grade fever
- Sometimes chills and fever

Treatment and Care

Never assume you have gout without consulting a physician. Many conditions can mimic an acute attack of gout, including infection, injury or rheumatoid arthritis. Only a doctor can accurately diagnose your problem.

If you do have gout, treatment will depend on the reasons behind your high levels of uric acid. Your doctor can conduct a simple test to determine if your kidneys aren't clearing uric acid from the blood the way they should or to determine whether your body simply produces too much uric acid.

The first goal is to relieve the acute gout attack. The second goal is to prevent a recurrence.
- For immediate relief, your doctor will prescribe a nonsteroidal anti-inflammatory medication or other pain reliever and tell you to rest the affected joint.
- For long-term relief, your doctor will probably recommend that you lose excess weight, limit your intake of alcohol, drink lots of liquids and take medication, if necessary. One type of medication (allopurinol) decreases uric acid production. Another (probenecid) increases the excretion of uric acid from the kidneys.

High Blood Pressure

High blood pressure (hypertension) isn't like a toothache, a bruise or constipation. Nothing hurts, looks discolored or fails to work. Usually, people with high blood pressure experience no discomfort or outward signs of trouble. Yet high blood pressure is a killer, a silent killer. Directly or indirectly, high blood pressure accounts for nearly a million deaths a year. Uncontrolled, high blood pressure increases the odds that you'll have a heart attack, stroke, kidney failure or loss of vision.

High blood pressure happens when your blood moves through your arteries at a higher pressure than normal. The heart is actually straining to pump blood through the arteries. This isn't healthy because:
- It promotes hardening of the arteries (atherosclerosis). Hardened, narrowed arteries may not be able to carry the amount of blood the body's organs need.

- Blood clots can form or lodge in a narrowed artery. (This could cause a stroke or heart attack.)
- The heart can become enlarged. (This could result in congestive heart failure.)

More than half of all older adults have high blood pressure. About 50 percent of all people who have it don't know it. Worse yet, many people who know their blood pressure is dangerously high are doing nothing to try to control it. And for 90 percent of those affected, there is no known cause. When this is the case, it is called primary or essential hypertension. When high blood pressure results from another medical disorder or a drug, it is referred to as secondary hypertension. In these cases (about 10 percent of total), when the root cause is corrected, blood pressure usually goes back to normal.

Detection

How's your blood pressure? Blood pressure is normally measured with a blood-pressure cuff placed on the arm. The numbers on the gauge measure your blood pressure in millimeters of mercury (mmHg). The first (higher) number measures the systolic pressure. This is the maximum pressure exerted against the arterial walls while the heart is beating. The second (lower) number records the diastolic pressure, the pressure between heart beats, when the heart is resting. The results are then recorded as systolic/diastolic pressure (120/80 mmHg, for example). Blood pressure is considered high in adults if it is consistently a reading of 140 mmHg systolic and/or 90 mmHg diastolic or higher.

To accurately determine your blood pressure, an average of two or more readings should be taken on two or more separate occasions. If your blood pressure is generally pretty good and suddenly registers high, don't be alarmed. Anxiety and other strong emotions, physical exertion, drinking a large amount of coffee or digesting a recently consumed meal can temporarily elevate normal blood pressure with no lasting effects. If, after several readings, your

doctor is convinced you do indeed have high blood pressure, follow his or her advice. The risk of stroke, heart attack and kidney disease increases when blood pressure is in the mild to severe range.

Treatment and Care

The amazing part is, blood pressure is one of the easiest health problems to control. Here's a multifaceted plan to control high blood pressure:
- If you're overweight, lose weight.
- Don't smoke.
- Limit alcohol to two drinks or less a day.
- Reduce your salt intake. (This is helpful for many people).
- Use salt substitutes if your physician says it's okay.
- Get regular exercise at least three times a week.
- Learn to handle stress by practicing relaxation techniques and rethinking stressful situations.
- Take any prescribed blood pressure medicine as directed.
- Don't skip your pills because you feel fine or because you don't like the side effects. Tell your doctor if you have any side effects of the medicine such as dizziness, faintness, skin rash or even a dry cough in the absence of a cold. Another medicine can be prescribed.
- Talk to your physician or pharmacist before you take antihistamines and decongestants. An ingredient in some of these can raise your blood pressure.
- Don't eat black licorice.

Kidney Stones

Kidney stones are hard masses of mineral deposits (e.g., calcium) or other organic substances (e.g., uric acid) that form in the kidneys or urinary tract. They can be found in the kidney itself or anywhere in the duct (ureter) that carries urine from the kidney to the bladder.

Kidney stones can be as small as a tiny pebble or an inch or more in diameter. They are more common in men (especially between 30 and 50 years old) than in women or children.

Signs and Symptoms

Kidney stones can be present for many years without causing symptoms. When a stone becomes large enough to produce problems, the following symptoms may occur:
• Blocked flow of urine
• Frequent and painful urination
• Blood in the urine
• Nausea and vomiting
• Fever, chills
• Severe pain and tenderness over the affected area
• Pain that can be agonizing and radiate down the side of the abdomen and into the groin area when the stone becomes lodged in the ureter

(Note: If these symptoms are severe, emergency care may be needed.)

Treatment and Care

Treatment will depend on the size, symptoms, location and cause of the kidney stone(s). The doctor will take blood and urine samples and ultrasound and/or X-rays to determine the location and type of stone present. If the stone is small and can be passed, treatment consists of drinking plenty of fluids. For kidney stones too large to be passed, a procedure known as lithotripsy is used in most cases.

Lithotripsy causes little or no pain and costs less than invasive surgery. In lithotripsy, which is usually performed as an outpatient procedure, shock waves are directed to the areas where the stone is located. The shock waves break it into fragments. After the treatment, the patient drinks lots of water to flush the stone fragments from his or her system.

Kidney stones can and do recur, though. If you're prone to developing stones, heed these guidelines:

• Save any stones you pass so your doctor can have them analyzed. (Treatment varies with the type of stones you form.)
• Follow your doctor's dietary advice. If you tend to form calcium stones, he or she will probably advise you not to take calcium in excess. If you form uric acid stones, your doctor may recommend that you eat less protein and take sodium bicarbonate.
• Drink plenty of fluids—preferably six to eight eight-ounce glasses of water daily.
• See your doctor frequently to be sure your kidneys are functioning as they should.

Lung Cancer

Today lung cancer is the leading cause of death from cancer in men and women. About 150,000 people develop lung cancer each year, and 85 percent of them can thank cigarettes for the disease. In less than a decade, lung cancer deaths for white females have increased an incredible 60 percent, replacing breast cancer as the most common cause of cancer-related death in women. Besides cigarette smoke, the risk for getting lung cancer increases with exposure to radon, asbestos or other environmental pollutants.

Lung cancer is especially deadly because the rich network of blood vessels that deliver oxygen from the lungs to the rest of the body can also spread cancer very quickly. By the time it's diagnosed, other organs may be affected.

Signs and Symptoms

Symptoms of lung cancer include:
• Chronic cough
• Blood-streaked sputum
• Shortness of breath
• Wheezing
• Chest discomfort with each breath
• Weight loss
• Fatigue

Treatment, Care and Prevention

Lung cancer is difficult to detect in its early, more treatable stages, so the best way to combat the disease is to prevent it. As you might guess, the first step is to eliminate the single greatest cause of lung cancer—smoking cigarettes.

The risk of developing lung cancer is proportional to the number of cigarettes smoked per day. Also, the longer a person smokes and the more deeply the smoke is inhaled, the greater the risk of getting lung cancer.

You should also avoid or limit exposure to environmental pollutants. Have your home tested for radon. This can be done professionally or with home testing kits.

Depending on the type of lung cancer and how far it has spread, the diseased portions of the lung will be surgically removed; radiation treatment or chemotherapy (or both) will follow.

Macular Degeneration

Macular degeneration is a common cause of blindness for those over 55 years of age. The central part of the retina (the macula) deteriorates, leading to loss of central, or straight-ahead, vision. One or both eyes may be affected.

The exact cause is not known. In many cases, though, the small vessels of the eye can become narrowed and hardened due to atherosclerosis. When this happens, the macula doesn't get the blood supply it needs, which in turn causes it to degenerate, or waste away. This is called the dry form. In the wet form (which is less common than the dry), tiny blood vessels leak blood or fluid around the macula.

Signs and Symptoms

Macular degeneration is painless. It usually develops gradually, especially the dry form. With the wet form, symptoms can occur more rapidly. Symptoms for both forms are:
- Blurred or cloudy vision
- Seeing a dark or blind spot at the center of vision
- Distorted vision such as straight lines that look wavy
- Difficulty reading or doing other close-up work
- Difficulty doing any activity that requires sharp vision (e.g., driving)
- Complete loss of central vision. Peripheral, or side, vision is not affected.

Treatment and Care

If you notice any of the signs and symptoms of macular degeneration, you should see your doctor or ophthalmologist right away. Laser-beam therapy, if performed before a lot of damage is done to the eyesight, may help to slow the progress of this condition if you have the wet form. Most dry form cases are not treatable. Even still, vision can be helped by special powerful eyeglasses if begun in the early course of the condition.

Multiple Sclerosis

The nervous system carries messages to and from the rest of your body. Normally, delicate nerves are encased in a protective covering called myelin. With multiple sclerosis, the myelin becomes inflamed and eventually dissolves. Over time, scar tissue (sclerosis) accumulates where the myelin used to be, in scattered locations in the brain and spinal cord. Nerve impulses, which normally travel at a speed of 225 miles per hour, either slow down considerably or come to a complete halt. People most susceptible to MS are:
- White adults between 20 and 40 years of age

- Those whose siblings or parents already have the disease
- Women (at a ratio of three women to every two men)
- Residents of the northern United States, Canada and northern Europe

No one knows what causes MS, but infection and other immunity factors are possibilities. Some theories point to toxins, trauma, nutritional deficiencies and other factors that lead to the destruction of myelin as possible causes. Overwork, fatigue, the postpartum period for women, acute infections and fevers have been known to precede the onset of multiple sclerosis.

Signs and Symptoms

Early signs and symptoms may be mild and present for years before the diagnosis is made for multiple sclerosis. Once diagnosed, the symptoms may last for hours or weeks, vary from day to day, and come and go with no predictable pattern. Symptoms include:
- Fatigue
- Weakness
- Numbness
- Muscle spasticity
- Poor coordination (trembling of the hand, for example)
- Bladder problems (frequent urination, urgency, infection, as well as incontinence)
- Blurred vision or double vision
- Transient blindness in one eye
- Emotional mood swings, irritability, depression, anxiety, euphoria

Treatment and Care

While no cure exists for multiple sclerosis, several steps can be taken to make living with the disease easier. These include:
- Getting plenty of rest
- Treating bacterial infections and fever as soon as they occur
- Minimizing stressful situations, especially physically demanding ones, since physical stress may aggravate the symptoms

- Staying out of the heat and sun since an increased body temperature can aggravate MS symptoms
- Avoiding hot showers or baths, since they, too, can aggravate symptoms. In fact, cool baths or swimming in a pool may improve symptoms by lowering body temperature.
- Maintaining a normal routine at work and at home if activities aren't physically demanding
- Getting regular exercise (physical therapy may be helpful)
- Having body massages to help maintain muscle tone
- Getting professional, supportive psychological counseling
- Taking prescribed medication. This may include:
  - Interferon beta I-B (Betaseron)
  - Short-term courses of cortisone-like drugs such as intravenous (IV) or oral steroids
  - Antispasmodics
  - Muscle relaxants
  - Antidepressants
  - Antianxiety drugs
  - Antibiotics (to treat any bacterial infections)
  - Medications to control urinary function

Osteoporosis

Osteoporosis is a major health problem that affects more than 25 million Americans. Persons with osteoporosis suffer from a loss in bone mass and bone strength. Their bones become weak and brittle, which makes them more prone to fracture. Any bone can be affected by osteoporosis, but the hips, wrists and spine are the most common sites. Peak bone mass is reached between the ages of 25 and 35 years. After 35, everyone's bones lose density.

The actual causes of osteoporosis are unknown. Certain risk factors, however, increase the likelihood of developing osteoporosis. Women are four times more likely to develop osteoporosis than men. The reasons are as follows:
- Their bones are generally thinner and lighter.

- They live longer than men.
- They have rapid bone loss at menopause due to a sharp decline of estrogen. (The risk also increases for women who experience menopause before age 45 naturally or as a result of surgery which removes the ovaries and for women who experience a lack of or irregular menstrual flow.)

Risk factors for women and men:
- Having a thin, small-framed body
- Race. Caucasians and Asians are at a higher risk than African Americans are. Having red or blond hair or freckles may also increase the risk.
- Lack of physical activity, especially walking, running, tennis and other weight-bearing exercises.
- Lack of calcium. Adequate calcium intake throughout life helps to prevent calcium deficiency that contributes to a weakening of bone mass.
- Heredity. The risk increases if there is a history of osteoporosis and/or bone fractures in your family.
- Cigarette smoking
- Alcohol. Regularly consuming alcoholic beverages, even as little as two to three ounces per day, may be damaging to bones. Heavy drinkers often have poor nutrition and may be more prone to fractures due to their predisposition to falls.
- Taking certain medications such as corticosteroids (anti-inflammatory drugs used to treat a variety of conditions such as asthma, arthritis and lupus), which can lead to bone-tissue loss. Some antiseizure medications and inappropriate overuse of thyroid hormones may also increase the risk.
- Other disorders such as hyperthyroidism, hyperparathyroidism and certain forms of bone cancer, which can also increase the risk

Signs and Symptoms

Osteoporosis is a "silent disease" because it can progress without any noticeable signs or symptoms. Often the first sign is when a bone fracture occurs. Symptoms include:

- A gradual loss of height
- A rounding of the shoulders
- Gum inflammation and loosening of the teeth
- Acute lower backache
- Swelling of a wrist after a fall

Treatment and Care

Medical tests such as the dual-energy X-ray absorptiometry (DEXA) and densitometry can measure bone mass in various sites of the body. They are safe and painless. These tests can help doctors decide if and what kind of treatment is needed. Treatment for osteoporosis includes:

- Dietary measures: a balanced diet rich in calcium and calcium supplementation if necessary
- Daily exercises approved by your doctor
- Fall prevention strategies:
  - Use grab bars and safety mats or nonskid tape in your tub or shower.
  - Use handrails on stairways.
  - Don't stoop to pick up things. Pick things up by bending your knees and keeping your back straight.
  - Wear flat, sturdy, nonskid shoes.
  - If you use throw rugs, make sure they have nonskid backs.
  - Use a cane or walker if necessary.
  - See that halls, stairways and entrances are well-lit. Put a night-light in your bathroom.
- Proper posture
- Medical management. Two medications have been approved by the Food and Drug Administration to treat osteoporosis. They are hormone replacement therapy and calcitonin.
- Surgery (such as hip replacement) if necessary

Prevention

To prevent or slow osteoporosis, take these steps now:
- Be sure to eat a balanced diet including adequate daily intakes of calcium. The National Osteoporosis Foundation recommends 1,000 milligrams (mg) a day for adults; 1,500 milligrams a day for postmenopausal women

not on hormone replacement therapy. The Recommended Dietary Allowance (RDA) is 800 mg a day for adults over 24 years of age.

Other age groups should get the following RDAs:

Birth-six months - 400 mg calcium a day

Six months-one year - 600 mg calcium a day

One year-10 years - 800 mg calcium a day

11-24 years - 1,200 mg calcium a day

- To get your recommended calcium, choose these high-calcium foods daily:
  - Skim and low-fat milks, yogurts and cheeses. (If you are lactose-intolerant, you may need to use dairy products that are treated with the enzyme lactase or you can add this enzyme in over-the-counter drops or tablets.)
  - Soft-boned fish and shellfish such as salmon, sardines, shrimp
  - Vegetables, especially broccoli, kale, collards
  - Beans and bean sprouts, as well as tofu (soy bean curd), if processed with calcium
  - Calcium-fortified foods such as some orange juices, apple juices and ready-to-eat cereals
- Check with your doctor before taking calcium supplements.
- Follow a program of regular, weight-bearing exercise (e.g., walking, jogging, low-impact or nonimpact aerobics) at least three or four times a week.
- Do not smoke. Smoking makes osteoporosis worse and may negate the beneficial effects of estrogen replacement therapy.
- Limit alcohol consumption.
- Check with your doctor regarding medical management to prevent and treat osteoporosis especially if you are at a high risk of getting the disorder. He or she may prescribe hormone replacement therapy (HRT). If you are female, this can prevent fractures from osteoporosis if started during or soon after menopause and taken for several years. There are risks with HRT, though, so you need to check with your doctor to see how they apply to you.

Parkinson's Disease

Parkinson's disease is a nervous system disorder. It causes tremors in which there is involuntary shaking in the limbs and head, a shuffling gait and stiffness. With it comes a gradual, progressive stiffness of muscles. Parkinson's disease is common only in older adults.

It most often strikes people over 60 years of age. The exact cause of Parkinson's disease is not known, but what is known is that it results from the degeneration of cells in the part of the brain that produces dopamine, a substance nerves need to function properly.

Signs and Symptoms

The signs and symptoms of Parkinson's disease include:
- Slow or stiff movement
- Stooped posture
- Shuffling or dragging of the feet
- Tremors and shaking of the head
- Monotonic voice, weak and high-pitched
- Blinking less frequently than normal
- Lack of spontaneity in facial expression
- Problems in swallowing
- Difficulty in adjusting positions
- Depression and anxiety
- Dementia (in advanced stages)

Treatment and Care

Parkinson's disease is not yet curable. Great strides, however, have been made in treatment, offering new hope for the nearly one million middle-aged and older people who are affected. For the most part, symptoms can be relieved or controlled. Parkinson's disease does not significantly lower life expectancy.

Medications such as Levodopa and Sinemet increase the dopamine level in the brain. For many people, these medicines control symptoms. Another medicine, Eldepryl, is sometimes used with Levodopa or Carbidopa to enhance its effects and may help to slow the progression of the disease.

Other treatments try to make the person with Parkinson's more comfortable. Warm baths and massages, for example, can help prevent muscle rigidity. Here are some other helpful hints:
- Take care to maintain a safe home environment. For example, replace razor blades with electric shavers, use nonskid rugs and handrails to prevent falls.
- Simplify tasks. Replace tie shoes with loafers, for instance, or wear clothing that can be pulled on or that has zippers or velcro closures instead of buttons.
- Include high-fiber foods in the diet and drink lots of fluids to prevent constipation.
- Get expert physical therapy.
- Remain as active as possible.
- Get professional help to relieve depression, if necessary.

Peptic Ulcers

Ulcers located in the stomach (gastric ulcers) and ulcers in the first section of the small intestine (duodenal ulcers) are grouped under the label peptic ulcers. They afflict men, women and children. No one knows exactly what causes ulcers, but doctors think they're a combination of excess stomach acid and failure of the stomach's inner lining to protect it from the acid. Also, bacteria called *Heliobacter pylori* may help cause some ulcers.

Tests can be done by your doctor to find out if you have this bacteria by doing a blood test, breath test and a biopsy of stomach tissue during an endoscopy. If *Heliobacter pylori* bacteria are present, antibiotics should be prescribed.

One study has shown that treating ulcers of this type protected nearly 90 percent of those affected from future ulcer attacks. Another showed that only 15 percent of persons with ulcers that were treated for *Heliobacter pylori* had recurrent ulcers after two years. People with a family history of ulcers tend to be at

greater risk for developing an ulcer as do people with type O blood. Eighty to 90 percent of the time, peptic ulcers recur within two years of the initial attack.

Certain things increase the risk of peptic ulcers in susceptible individuals:
- Stress and anxiety
- Irregular meal times and improper diet or skipping meals
- Excess alcohol, drugs and caffeine, which irritate the stomach

Signs and Symptoms

Peptic ulcers are characterized by:
- A gnawing or burning just above the navel within 1½ to 3 hours after eating
- Pain that frequently awakens the person at night
- Food or antacids that generally relieve the pain within minutes
- Pain that recurs, with each cluster of attacks lasting from several days to several months
- Pain that feels like indigestion, heartburn or hunger
- Nausea
- Unintentional weight loss or loss of appetite
- Anemia

Treatment and Care

Doctors can diagnose gastric and duodenal ulcers on the basis of X-rays or endoscopy (looking at your stomach through a tube that's inserted via your mouth).

Notify your doctor if:
- Your stools are ever bloody, black or tarry-looking. (Take a specimen to your doctor's office.)
- You vomit blood or material that looks like coffee grounds.
- You become unusually pale and weak.
- You have diarrhea with intolerable pain.

For treatment, your doctor may prescribe:
- Over-the-counter antacids
- Antibiotics and bismuth (Pepto-Bismol) if he or she thinks that *Heliobacter pylori* bacteria is

contributing to your ulcer. *Note: Do not give aspirin or any medication containing salicylates such as Pepto-Bismol to anyone 19 years of age or younger, unless directed by a physician, due to its association with Reye's syndrome, a potentially fatal condition.*

- Medicines to decrease or stop the stomach's production of hydrochloric acid or medicine to coat the ulcer, protecting it from the acid so it has time to heal
- Surgery to cut the nerves that stimulate acid production or to remove part of the stomach. This may be needed if other treatment methods fail.

If you have an ulcer, you can soothe the pain in various ways. Some suggestions are:

- Eat smaller, lighter, more frequent meals for a couple of weeks. Big, heavy lunches and dinners can spell trouble for people with ulcers. Frequent meals tend to take the edge off pain.
- Avoid anything that will stimulate excess stomach acid. That includes coffee, tea, alcohol and soft drinks containing caffeine. Even decaffeinated coffee should be avoided because it can cause heartburn.
- Discontinue use of aspirin and other non-steroidal anti-inflammatory medicine, which irritate the stomach lining. Try antacids (with your physician's okay) on a short-term basis. (Don't try to self-medicate an ulcer. You may soothe the symptoms without treating the problem itself.)
- Don't smoke. Smokers get ulcers more frequently than nonsmokers do. No one is sure why.
- Try to minimize stress in your life. Stress doesn't cause ulcers. But for some people, stress triggers the release of stomach acid—and subsequent ulcer flare-ups.

Phlebitis

The medical term for this condition is thrombophlebitis. In it, small blood clots form in a vein of the legs and the vein becomes inflamed. This is usually caused by infection or injury. Phlebitis is more common in women than in men.

Signs and Symptoms

Symptoms of phlebitis depend on its type:
- Superficial phlebitis affects the veins visible just beneath the skin surface. People who have varicose veins are susceptible, and the affected area will be red and swollen and feel warm, hard and tender to the touch. Usually amenable to home treatment, this type seldom results in clots that break loose and flow into the bloodstream.
- Deep vein thrombophlebitis, on the other hand, can result in a blood clot that breaks away from the wall of a vein forming an embolism. The clot can interfere with the circulation to the limb or cause death if it reaches the lung. This type of phlebitis may occur after prolonged bed rest, major surgery, a heart attack or a stroke. The only symptom may be an aching pain in the limb, but half of persons with deep vein thrombophlebitis have no symptoms. Others may have severe leg pain with swelling of the lower leg.

Other conditions that can lead to phlebitis of either kind include:
- General inactivity (from a sedentary job, after a prolonged trip by car or plane, or following surgery)
- Smoking or chewing tobacco
- Being overweight
- Trauma to the leg (from a blow or fall)
- Injury to the vein (from injections or intravenous needles)
- Some malignancies
- Advancing age

Treatment and Care

Only a medical professional can tell the difference between superficial and deep vein types.

If you're diagnosed as having superficial phlebitis, you'll probably be told to:

- Rest the affected limb and elevate it above the level of your heart until the pain and swelling subside.
- Apply moist heat to the affected area for 20 minutes on and 20 minutes off.
- Take aspirin or nonsteroidal anti-inflammatory medications (e.g., ibuprofen or naproxen sodium). *Note: Do not give aspirin or any medication containing salicylates to anyone 19 years of age or younger, unless directed by a physician, due to its association with Reye's syndrome, a potentially fatal condition.*

Deep vein thrombophlebitis requires hospitalization and treatment with blood-thinning medicine to prevent an embolism from forming. If you notice any symptoms of this type, especially severe leg pain and swelling of the lower leg, see your doctor.

Prevention

- Avoid prolonged periods of uninterrupted sitting or standing.
- Avoid smoking if you take birth control pills or estrogen medication.
- Never sit with your legs crossed.
- Avoid wearing garters, knee-high hosiery or other stockings that restrict blood flow in the legs.
- Wear properly fitting elastic stockings made to help blood flow in the legs.
- Exercise your legs at least every hour or two on long auto or airplane trips.
- Try this if you're confined to bed: With your feet against a pillow, pretend you're pressing on a gas pedal and then releasing it. Alternate with one foot, then the other.

Pneumonia

Pneumonia is lung inflammation. It is the sixth leading cause of death in the United States.

Pneumonia can develop when the lungs are infected by either bacteria, viruses, fungi or toxins, causing inflammation. Certain people are at a greater risk for pneumonia than others. They include:

- Elderly people, because the body's ability to fight off disease diminishes with age
- People who are hospitalized for other conditions
- Individuals with suppressed cough reflex following a stroke
- Smokers, because tobacco smoke paralyzes the tiny hairs that otherwise help to expel germ-ridden mucus from the lungs
- People who suffer from malnutrition, alcoholism or viral infections
- Anyone with a recent respiratory viral infection
- People with emphysema or chronic bronchitis
- People with sickle-cell anemia
- Cancer patients undergoing radiation treatments or chemotherapy, both of which wear down the immune system
- People with HIV (human immunodeficiency virus)

Signs and Symptoms

Pneumonia symptoms include:

- Chest pain (may worsen when inhaling)
- Fever and chills
- Coughing with little or no sputum or sometimes with bloody, dark yellow or rust-colored sputum
- Difficulty in breathing, rapid breathing
- General fatigue, headache, nausea, vomiting
- Bluish lips and fingertips

Treatment, Care and Prevention

Treatment for pneumonia will depend on its type (viral, bacterial or chemical, for example) and location. X-rays, sputum analysis and blood tests can help identify these. Treatment includes:

- Getting plenty of bed rest
- Using a cool-mist humidifier in the room or rooms in which you spend most of your time

- Drinking plenty of fluids
- Taking acetaminophen to relieve minor discomfort and reduce fever
- Taking any medications your doctor prescribes: antibiotics to treat bacterial pneumonia or to fight a secondary bacterial infection; antiviral medicines, if indicated; nose drops, sprays or oral decongestants to treat congestion in the upper respiratory tract
- Cough medicines as needed: a cough suppressant for a dry, nonproductive cough; a nonsuppressant expectorant type for a mucus-producing cough
- Removing fluid from the lungs by suction. Anti-inflammatory medications and oxygen therapy may be used for chemically induced pneumonias.
- Also, vaccines against influenza and pneumonococcus (pneumonia bacteria). They are recommended in persons aged 65 and older. They may also be recommended sooner than age 65 for persons with chronic diseases. Ask your doctor about them. (See "Immunization Schedule" on page 18.)

Scoliosis

Scoliosis generally shows up between the ages of 10 and 15 and affects girls seven to nine times more often than boys. In most cases, no one knows the cause.

In the beginning, scoliosis isn't painful. But it slowly twists the upper portion of the spine. One shoulder may curve one way while the lower back twists another, so that the chest and back are distorted. The spine begins to rotate, and one side of the rib cage becomes more prominent. This is more obvious if the person bends forward at the waist, with the arms hanging freely. In fact, a doctor can detect scoliosis by asking the patient to assume that position during a routine physical or screening for scoliosis.

Signs and Symptoms

The appearance of any of the following may mean scoliosis:
- An uneven hemline or unequal pant leg
- One hip higher than the other
- One shoulder higher than the other or one shoulder blade sticks out (noticeable when the shirt is off)
- One arm hanging farther away from the body than the other when the child's arms hang loosely at his or her sides
- Tilting to one side when standing
- A hump on the back at the ribs or near the waist when bending forward

Parents should report any of these signs to their child's doctor. The doctor's exam and X-rays will determine or rule out scoliosis.

Treatment and Care

Sometimes the only treatment needed for scoliosis is doing exercises that stretch the spine and strengthen the muscles of the trunk. In some cases, though, other treatments are necessary to prevent heart and lung problems or back pain later in life. There are several treatment options:
- Wearing a molded body brace, hidden by clothing, is the most conservative approach. This brace is typically worn most of the day and night for several years. Because the spine grows rapidly during adolescence, wearing a brace at this time can arrest further abnormal curving.
- A special form of mild electrical stimulation to the spine is sometimes as effective as brace treatment.
- Surgery to straighten the spine is a more radical alternative, used when the spine is severely curved. A thin steel rod is implanted alongside the spine.

In most instances, scoliosis can be sufficiently treated so that the adolescent doesn't suffer any complications as an adult.

Sickle-Cell Anemia

If you're an African American, you should know about sickle-cell anemia. About one in 12 African Americans carries the gene for the sickle-cell trait (i.e., they have the ability to produce children with sickle-cell anemia but have no symptoms of the disease). If both parents carry the trait, the chance of having a child with sickle-cell anemia is one out of four, or 25 percent. (This trait occurs only in the African-American population.)

Red blood cells are normally round. In sickle-cell anemia, the red blood cells take on a sickle-cell shape. This makes the blood thicker and affects the red blood cells' ability to carry oxygen to the body's tissues. The disease usually doesn't become apparent until the end of the child's first year. As many as one out of four affected children will die, usually before they're five years old.

Signs and Symptoms

A blood test can detect sickle-cell anemia, but signs and symptoms include the following:
- Pain, ranging from mild to severe, in the chest, joints, back or abdomen
- Swollen hands and feet
- Jaundice
- Repeated infections, particularly pneumonia or meningitis
- Kidney failure
- Gallstones (at an early age)
- Strokes (at an early age)

Treatment, Care and Prevention

For now, no drugs exist to effectively treat sickle-cell anemia. At best, treatment is geared toward preventing complications. Painful episodes are treated with painkillers, fluids and oxygen. The diet is supplemented with folate. Because people with sickle-cell anemia are prone to developing pneumonia, they should be vaccinated against pneumonia.

The only possible way to prevent sickle-cell anemia and to avoid giving birth to children with the disease is to find out whether or not you carry the genes for the disease before you get pregnant. African-American couples should have a blood test to determine if either one is a carrier. After conception, sickle-cell anemia can be diagnosed by amniocentesis in the second trimester of pregnancy.

Stroke

Strokes (also called cerebrovascular accidents) are the third leading cause of death in the United States. A stroke can be caused by lack of blood (and therefore lack of oxygen) to the brain, usually due to either atherosclerosis or rupture of a blood vessel in the brain. In either case, the end result is brain damage (and possible death). Persons who suffer from both high blood pressure and hardening of the arteries are most susceptible to having a stroke. A stroke can happen suddenly, but it often follows years of the slow buildup of fatty deposits inside the blood vessels.

Some people experience a temporary mini-stroke, or a transient ischemic attack (TIA). The symptoms mimic a stroke (see Signs and Symptoms) but clear within 24 hours. TIAs are a warning that a real stroke may follow.

Prevention

Measures can be taken to prevent a stroke. Here's what to do to reduce your risks:
- Control your blood pressure. Have it checked regularly and, if necessary, take medication prescribed by your physician.
- Reduce blood levels of cholesterol to below 200 mg/dl (measured by a blood test).
- Get regular exercise.
- Keep your weight down.
- Don't smoke.
- Keep blood-sugar levels under control if you're diabetic.
- Use alcohol in moderation, if at all.

- Avoid taking oral contraceptive pills, if possible. (If you must use them, don't smoke.)
- Learn to manage stress.
- Ask your doctor about taking aspirin (low-dose, such as a daily baby aspirin).
- Ask your doctor to evaluate you for a surgical procedure that scrapes away fatty deposits from inside one or both of the main arteries in the neck.

Signs and Symptoms

To minimize the damage of a stroke, it's important to know the warning signals of a stroke and get immediate medical attention. To help you remember what to look out for, the initials of the signs and symptoms spell DANGER.
- **D** Dizziness
- **A** Absent-mindedness, or temporary loss of memory or mental ability
- **N** Numbness or weakness in the face, arm or leg
- **G** Garbled speech
- **E** Eye problems, including temporary loss of sight in one eye or double vision
- **R** Recent onset of severe headaches

Treatment and Care

Tests can be done to locate the obstruction of blood flow to the brain. The doctor may then prescribe appropriate medicines and/or surgery.

When an actual stroke occurs, it is crucial to get immediate treatment. Treatment often includes:
- Medications that reduce brain-tissue swelling, control blood pressure and inhibit the normal clotting of the blood or prevent existing clots from getting bigger
- Surgery if warranted
- Rehabilitation as needed by speech, physical and occupational therapists

Thyroid Problems

The thyroid is a small, butterfly-shaped gland located just in front of the windpipe (trachea) in your throat. Its normal function is to produce L-thyroxine and L-thyronine, hormones that influence a variety of metabolic processes in the body. These include converting food to energy, regulating growth and fertility and maintaining body temperature. Thyroid problems occur when conditions exist that cause too much or too few thyroid hormones.

Signs and Symptoms

Hyperthyroidism (two common forms of which are Graves' disease and toxic multinodular goiter) occurs when the thyroid produces too much thyroid hormone. Some signs and symptoms are:
- Tremors
- Mood swings
- Weakness
- Diarrhea
- Heart palpitations
- Heat intolerance
- Shortened menstrual periods
- Unexplained weight loss
- Fine hair (or hair loss)
- Rapid pulse
- Nervousness
- Bulging eyes
- Enlarged thyroid gland

Hypothyroidism occurs when the thyroid gland does not make enough thyroid hormone to meet the body's needs. Some signs and symptoms are:
- Fatigue and excessive sleeping
- Dry, pale skin
- Deepening of the voice
- Weight gain
- Dry hair that tends to fall out
- Decrease in appetite
- Frequently feeling cold
- Puffy face (especially around the eyes)

- Heavy and/or irregular menstrual periods
- Poor memory
- Constipation
- Enlarged thyroid gland (in some cases)

Treatment, Care and Prevention

Treatment for thyroid problems depends on which condition is present. Hypothyroidism is generally treated with medicine to supplement thyroid hormones. A person may require life-long supplementation and follow-up care to monitor treatment. Hyperthyroidism treatment varies with its cause, but generally involves one or more of the following:

- Surgical removal of the thyroid
- Radioactive iodine
- Medicine to stop overproduction of thyroid hormones

Surgical removal and radioactive iodine treatments frequently result in the need to take thyroid supplementation thereafter.

SECTION IV

EMERGENCY PROCEDURES AND CONDITIONS

About This Section

This section contains information on several emergency situations.

- Chapter 23 provides information and drawings to illustrate cardiopulmonary resuscitation (CPR) and first aid for choking. Take an emergency/first aid course to learn and become certified in these and other first aid procedures. Knowing when and how to do these procedures correctly can save a person's life.
- Chapter 24 presents six conditions for which emergency care and/or first aid is vital. Read about any emergency condition, and ask yourself the "Questions to Ask." Start at the top of the flowchart and answer yes or no to each question. Follow the arrows until you get to one of these answers:
  - Seek Emergency Care
  - See Doctor
  - Call Doctor
  - Provide Self-Care

In addition, "Provide First Aid Procedures for Non-Emergencies" is sometimes given as an answer. A list of first aid procedures for these non-emergencies is provided.

The "Seek Emergency Care" symbol may direct you to do one of the following:
- Perform CPR, rescue breathing or the Heimlich Maneuver.
- Give first aid before emergency care. A list of first aid procedures is given.
- Call the Poison Control Center.
- Give shot from and follow other instructions in emergency kit that some highly allergic people carry with them.

If you are alone with a victim, you may need to start first aid before you seek emergency care (as is the case with CPR, rescue breathing and the Heimlich Maneuver), but you should yell for help. If you are not alone, let the person who is best trained to give first aid stay with and help the victim. Have someone else seek emergency care.

When you see the phrase "And perform first aid before Emergency Care," seek emergency care first and then do the first aid measures listed while you wait for emergency care.

CHAPTER 23

EMERGENCY PROCEDURES

Cardiopulmonary Resuscitation (CPR)

CPR Techniques

Early CPR is an important link in the chain of survival for a victim of sudden cardiac or respiratory arrest. CPR involves a combination of mouth-to-mouth rescue breathing (or other artificial ventilation techniques) and chest compressions. It keeps some oxygenated blood flowing to the brain and other vital organs until appropriate medical treatment can restore normal heart action.

Cardiac arrest causes the victim to lose consciousness within seconds. *If there is early access to the EMS system (Phone First! Phone Fast!), early CPR, early defibrillation and early advanced care, the person has a chance to survive.*

CPR techniques include three basic rescue skills, the ABCs of CPR: **A**irway, **B**reathing and **C**irculation.

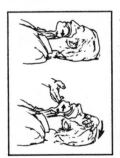

Airway - A key action for successful resuscitation is immediate opening of the airway by positioning the head properly. It is important to remember that the back of the tongue and the epiglottis are the most common causes of airway obstruction in the unconscious victim. Since the tongue, directly, and the epiglottis, indirectly, are attached to the lower jaw, tilting the head back and moving the lower jaw (chin) forward lifts the tongue and the epiglottis from the back of the throat and usually opens the airway.

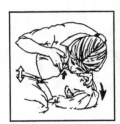

Breathing - When breathing stops, the body has only the oxygen remaining in the lungs and bloodstream. Therefore, when breathing stops, cardiac arrest and death quickly follow. Mouth-to-mouth rescue breathing is the quickest way to get oxygen into the victim's lungs. There is more than enough oxygen in the air you breathe into the victim to supply the victim's needs.

Rescue breathing should be performed until the victim can breathe on his or her own or until trained professionals take over.

- If the victim is unconscious and breathing and there is no evidence of trauma, you should place the victim on his or her side in the recovery position.
- If the victim's heart is beating, you should:
  - Maintain an open airway.
  - Breathe for the victim.
- If the victim's heart is not beating, you should perform rescue breathing plus chest compressions.

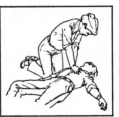

Circulation - Chest compressions can maintain some blood flow to the lungs, brain, coronary arteries and other major organs. When chest compressions are performed, rescue breathing should also be performed.

Reproduced with permission.
Basic Life Support Heartsaver Guide, 1993
Copyright American Heart Association.

Recovery position - If the victim resumes breathing and regains a pulse during or following resuscitation, you should place the victim in the recovery position.

To perform CPR correctly, you need some expert training. It takes just three hours to learn, and anyone strong enough to compress the sternum (breastbone) one-half inch is capable of learning CPR.

Call your local chapter of the American Heart Association, Red Cross or local hospital to find out where you can learn CPR.

First Aid for Choking

Performance Guidelines Obstructed Airway: Conscious Adult

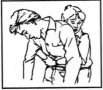

Determine if the victim is able to speak or cough. Rescuer can ask "Are you choking?" Victim may be using the "universal distress signal" of choking: clutching the neck between thumb and index finger.

Abdominal Thrust

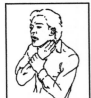

Perform the Heimlich maneuver until the foreign body is expelled or the victim becomes unconscious. Stand behind victim and wrap your arms around victim's waist. Press your fist into victim's abdomen with quick inward and upward thrusts.

Chest Thrust

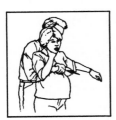

For victims who are in advanced pregnancy or who are obese:
Chest thrusts: Stand behind victim and place your arms under victim's armpits to encircle the chest. Press with quick backward thrusts.

Performance Guidelines Obstructed Airway: If Victim Is or Becomes Unconscious

Activate EMS - Call for medical assistance.

Check for foreign body - Sweep deeply into mouth with hooked finger to remove foreign body.

Attempt rescue breathing - Open airway. Try to give two breaths. If needed, reposition the head and try again.

If airway is obstructed, perform the Heimlich maneuver. Kneel astride the victim's thighs. Place the heel of one of your hands on the victim's abdomen, in the midline slightly above the navel and well below the tip of the xiphoid (the lowest part of the breastbone). Place the second hand on top of the first. Press into abdomen with quick upward thrusts.

Repeat sequence until successful. Alternate these maneuvers in rapid sequence:
• Finger sweep
• Rescue breathing attempt
• Abdominal thrusts

Reproduced with permission.
Basic Life Support Heartsaver Guide, 1993
Copyright American Heart Association.

CHAPTER 24

EMERGENCY CONDITIONS

Accidental Poisoning and Poisoning First Aid

Each year millions of cases of accidental poisoning occur. Most of them are in children, particularly those ages one to six.

The kitchen, between 4 p.m. and 6 p.m., is the time and place when most accidental poisonings occur. The bathroom is the next most likely site.

The most common poisons include:
- Medicines (e.g., aspirin, tranquilizers, sleeping pills)
- Household cleaners (e.g., bleach, dishwasher detergent, floor and furniture polishes and waxes, drain cleaners)
- Ammonia, lye
- Insecticides and rat poison
- Vitamins
- Alcoholic beverages
- Rubbing alcohol, iodine, hair dye, mouthwash and mothballs
- Some indoor plants
- Some outdoor plants and berries
- Gasoline, antifreeze, oil and other chemicals for the car
- Lighter fluid
- Paint thinner

Most of the damage done by accidental poisons occurs from swallowing. Strong lyes like drain cleaners quickly destroy tissue as they slide down the throat. Some substances that are toxic can cause serious medical problems when they are inhaled or absorbed through the skin. Some examples are:

- Airplane glue
- Gasoline
- Auto exhaust
- Formaldehyde and other chemicals

Prevention

To prevent poisoning:
- Keep all potentially poisonous products out of children's reach. Better yet, keep the products locked up.
- Buy and install easy-to-attach, plastic, child-proof latches on cabinet doors.
- Do not store hazardous materials or medications in food containers. It's best to keep these items in their original containers, out of reach and out of sight.
- Place plants where children cannot reach a leaf or berry for tasting.
- Store all medications and vitamins in containers with child-resistant tops. Even vitamins with iron can be deadly to a small child.
- Read warning labels on pesticides, household cleaners and other potentially poisonous products so you know what to do in the event of an accidental poisoning. Some label instructions may be outdated, so always call the Poison Control Center when poisoning occurs.
- Flush unused medications down the toilet and rinse the containers before discarding them.
- Buy a one-ounce bottle of syrup of ipecac and replace it with a new one each year. Syrup of ipecac is used to induce vomiting after certain poisons have been swallowed.
- Also keep activated charcoal on hand. This may be necessary to give when certain chemicals are swallowed.

- Teach your child never to touch anything with a skull and crossbones on it. This is the standard symbol of a poisonous product.
- Never refer to medications or vitamins as "candy" in front of a child.
- Wear protective clothing, masks and gloves when using chemicals that could cause harm if inhaled or absorbed by the skin.
- Use potentially dangerous volatile substances only in areas that are well-ventilated. Product labels tell you if ventilation is necessary.
- Post the phone number of your local poison control center next to the phone. And keep the numbers of the closest hospital emergency room, your doctor and ambulance service near the phone as well.

Poison Control Center Telephone Number:

_____

If and when you need to call the Poison Control Center, your doctor or nearby hospital, be prepared to give as much information as possible. This includes:
- The name of the substance taken
- The amount
- The list of ingredients on the product label
- Information about the person who took the poison:
  - His or her age, gender and weight
  - How he or she is feeling and reacting
  - Any medical problems he or she has

Questions to Ask

Is the person not breathing, and does he or she have no pulse?

SEEK EMERGENCY CARE

 NO And perform CPR. (See "CPR" on page 226.)

Is the person not breathing, but he or she has a pulse?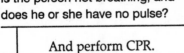

SEEK EMERGENCY CARE

NO And perform rescue breathing. (See "Airway and Breathing" on page 226.)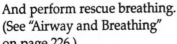

flowchart continued in next column

flowchart continued

Is the person unconscious or having convulsions? **YES**

SEEK EMERGENCY CARE

And give first aid before Emergency Care:
Lie the victim down on his or her left side and check airway, breathing and pulse often before Emergency Care. Perform CPR (see page 226) or rescue breathing (see "Airway and Breathing" on page 226) if needed.

NO

Has any substance been swallowed, inhaled or absorbed by the skin that:
- Has a "harmful or fatal if swallowed" warning on the label **YES**
- A skull and crossbones sign on the container
- You are unsure whether or not it is poisonous

SEEK EMERGENCY CARE

And call Poison Control Center. Remain calm. Follow the Poison Control Center instructions promptly and correctly.

The Poison Control Center may tell you to:
- Give the victim a large glass of water or milk. This will help dilute the poison.
- Induce vomiting:
  - Give a specific dose of syrup of ipecac, followed by 12 or more ounces of water. This will likely induce vomiting within 20 to 25 minutes. If not, give one more dose of the syrup of ipecac. *Note: Syrup of ipecac should not be given to a child younger than one year because ipecac-induced vomiting can become violent.*
  - Walk the person around to help the syrup of ipecac work faster and to keep the person awake.
  - Keep the victim's head lower than the chest to prevent the vomit from entering the lungs.

- Place a spoon or finger in the back of the throat to induce vomiting if you do not have syrup of ipecac.
- Save the vomit for the doctor to examine.

The Poison Control Center may also tell you:
- Do not induce vomiting if the victim is:
  - Having convulsions
  - Unconscious
  - In the late stages of pregnancy
  - Experiencing a burning sensation in the mouth or throat
  - Likely to have swallowed:
    - A corrosive agent like lye, dishwater detergent, bleach or drain opener
    - A petroleum product like kerosene or gasoline
    - Pills that can cause rapid loss of consciousness such as antidepressants, sedatives, antipsychotic medication
- Give activated charcoal if you have some on hand and only if you are told to do so. This comes in liquid and powder forms. The powder form has to be mixed with liquid before given. Activated charcoal absorbs some poisons. Like syrup of ipecac, it is available without a prescription. *Note: Do not give syrup of ipecac and activated charcoal at the same time.*

Breathing Difficulties

Some 44 million Americans suffer from allergies and asthma and have trouble breathing during an attack. What's more, there are millions of people who have breathing difficulties because of grey, gritty smog and air polluted by poorly tuned engines and cigarette smoke.

Breathing difficulties also plague people who are very allergic to some types of shellfish, nuts, medications and insect bites. These people can suffer a life-threatening allergic reaction called anaphylactic shock. This reaction begins within minutes of exposure to the substance causing the allergy. During this type of allergic reaction, the airways narrow, making it difficult to breathe. Soon the heartbeat races and blood pressure drops. Anaphylactic shock can kill if a person is not treated within 15 minutes.

Breathing difficulties from some things may require emergency care. In children they include:
- Wheezing
- Croup
- Epiglottitis, which is inflammation of the flap of tissue at the back of the throat that closes off the windpipe
- Diphtheria, which is a very contagious throat infection
- Congenital heart defects

Breathing difficulties in children and adults that may require emergency care include:
- Severe allergic reactions
- A face, head, nose or lung injury
- Carbon monoxide poisoning
- Harsh chemical burns in the air passages
- Choking
- Drug overdose
- Poisoning
- Asthma
- Bronchitis and pneumonia

In adults they include:
- Emphysema
- Congestive heart failure
- Heart attack
- Blood clot in lungs

Prevention

- Avoid allergic substances or agents that induce asthma, if you have it.
- Do not walk, run or jog on roads with heavy automobile traffic.
- If you have a gas furnace, have it checked periodically for carbon monoxide leaks.
- Never leave your car running in a closed garage.
- Make sure immunizations against childhood diseases, especially diphtheria, are up-to-date.
- If you smoke, quit.

- Keep small objects a child could choke on out of reach and do not give gum—especially bubble gum—nuts, hard candy or popcorn to children under five years old.
- Lock up all medications and poisonous substances so small children can't get to them.

Questions to Ask

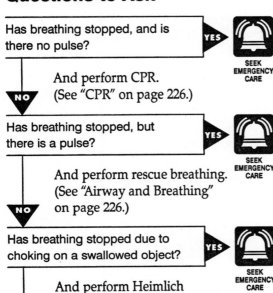

Has breathing stopped, and is there no pulse? **YES** → SEEK EMERGENCY CARE

NO ↓

And perform CPR. (See "CPR" on page 226.)

Has breathing stopped, but there is a pulse? **YES** → SEEK EMERGENCY CARE

NO ↓

And perform rescue breathing. (See "Airway and Breathing" on page 226.)

Has breathing stopped due to choking on a swallowed object? **YES** → SEEK EMERGENCY CARE

NO ↓

And perform Heimlich maneuver. (See "First Aid for Choking" on page 227.)

Are there signs of anaphylactic shock:
- Difficult breathing
- Swollen tongue, eyes or face
- Unconsciousness
- Difficulty in swallowing
- Dizziness, weakness
- Pounding heart
- Itching, hives

YES → SEEK EMERGENCY CARE

Inject the substance from the emergency kit that some very allergic people carry with them, if available. Follow all the instructions in the kit. *Note: You can get this kit only with a doctor's prescription.*

NO ↓

flowchart continued in next column

---

flowchart continued

Are any of these problems present with difficulty in breathing:
- Signs of a heart attack (e.g., chest pain, pressure or tightness, pain that spreads to the arm, neck or jaw, irregular pulse)
- Serious injury to the face, head or chest
- Signs of a stroke (e.g., blurred or double vision, slurred speech, one-sided body weakness or paralysis)
- Signs of drug overdose (e.g., drunklike behavior, slurred speech, slow or rapid pulse, heavy sweating, enlarged or very small eye pupils)

YES → SEEK EMERGENCY CARE

NO ↓

Is it so hard to breathe that you or someone else can't talk (say four or five words between breaths) and/or is there wheezing that doesn't go away? **YES** → SEEK EMERGENCY CARE

NO ↓

Is bloody sputum being coughed up? **YES** → SEEK EMERGENCY CARE

NO ↓

Does the difficulty in breathing occur with a cough in a baby and make the baby unable to eat or take a bottle? **YES** → SEEK EMERGENCY CARE

NO ↓

Is there:
- Breathlessness at night or at rest
- Pink or frothy phlegm being coughed up and/or
- A high fever along with the rapid and labored breathing

YES → SEEK EMERGENCY CARE

NO ↓

flowchart continued on next page

| Is a greenish-yellow or grey phlegm being coughed up? | **YES** | ☎ CALL DOCTOR |

NO

🏠 PROVIDE SELF-CARE

Self-Care Procedures

For people affected by air pollution or pollen:
- Put on a face mask that covers the nose and mouth. Most hardware stores carry inexpensive ones.
- Don't smoke. Avoid secondhand smoke. *Note: This applies to anyone with breathing difficulties.*
- Install an air-filtering system in your home or an air purifier in the room. Tests show that air filters effectively clear the air of air-carried allergy-causing agents.

For people allergic to molds, breathing problems can be avoided or lessened if you:
- Do not rake leaves that have sat on the ground for awhile. Molds and mildew grow on leaves after they've been on the ground for a few days.
- Keep your basement dry, well-ventilated and well-lighted. Use dehumidifiers and exhaust fans to reduce moisture in the air.
- Get rid of house plants.

If you or anyone in your family has severe allergies, it is a good idea to wear a medical identification tag such as those available at drugstores or custom-made by the Medic Alert Foundation. For more information, contact Medic Alert Foundation International at 800-344-3226.

See Chapter 11 for Self-Care Procedures for asthma, bronchitis, common cold, coughs and flu. See Chapter 17 for Self-Care Procedures for croup.

Drug Overdose

Drug overdoses can be accidental or intentional. The amount of a certain drug needed to cause an overdose varies with the type of drug and the person taking it. Overdoses from prescription and over-the-counter (OTC) medicines, "street" drugs and/or alcohol can be life-threatening. Know, too, that mixing certain medications or "street" drugs with alcohol can also kill.

Physical symptoms of a drug overdose vary with the type of drug(s) taken. They include:
- Abnormal breathing
- Slurred speech
- Lack of coordination
- Slow or rapid pulse
- Low or elevated body temperature
- Enlarged or small eye pupils
- Reddish face
- Heavy sweating
- Delusions and/or hallucinations
- Drowsiness, sleep which may lead to coma

Parents need to watch for signs of illegal drug and alcohol use in their children. Morning hangovers, the odor of alcohol and red streaks in the whites of the eyes are obvious signs of alcohol use. Items such as pipes, rolling papers, eye droppers and butane lighters may be the first telling clues that someone is abusing drugs. Another clue is behavior changes such as:
- Lack of appetite
- Insomnia
- Hostility
- Mental confusion
- Depression
- Mood swings
- Secretive behavior
- Social isolation
- Hallucinations
- Deep sleep

Prevention

Accidental prescription and over-the-counter medication overdoses may be prevented by asking your doctor or pharmacist:
- What is the medication and why is it being prescribed?
- How and when should the medication be taken and for how long? (Follow the instructions exactly as given.)
- Can the medication be taken with other medicines or alcohol, or should it not be?
- Are there any foods to avoid while taking this medication?
- What are the possible side effects?
- What are the symptoms of an overdose and what should be done if it occurs?
- Should any activities be avoided (e.g., operating heavy machinery, driving and exposure to sun)?
- Should the medicine still be taken even if there is a preexisting medical condition?

Medication overdoses can be avoided by observing the following:
- Never take a medicine prescribed for someone else.
- Never give or take medication in the dark. Before each dose, always read the label on the bottle to be certain it is the correct medication.
- Always tell the doctor of any previous side effects or adverse reactions to medication as well as new and unusual symptoms that occur after taking the medicine.
- Always store medications in bottles with childproof lids and place those bottles on high shelves, out of a child's reach, or in locked cabinets.
- Take the prescribed dose, not more.
- Keep medications in their original containers.

Illicit drug use among children can be discouraged by observing the following:
- Set a good example for your children by not using drugs yourself.
- Teach your child to say no to drugs and alcohol. Explain the dangers of drug use, including the risk of AIDS.

- Get to know your children's friends and their parents.
- Know where your children are and who they are with.
- Listen to your children and help them express their feelings and fears.
- Encourage your children to engage in healthy activities such as sports, scouting, community-based youth programs and volunteer work.
- Learn to recognize the signs of drug and alcohol abuse.

Questions to Ask

Is the person not breathing, and does he or she have no pulse? **YES**
SEEK EMERGENCY CARE

NO And perform CPR. (See "CPR" on page 226.)

Is the person not breathing, but has a pulse? **YES**
SEEK EMERGENCY CARE

NO And perform rescue breathing. (See "CPR" on page 226.)

Is the person unconscious? **YES**
SEEK EMERGENCY CARE

NO And give first aid before Emergency Care:
Lie the victim down on his or her left side and check airway, breathing and pulse often before Emergency Care. Perform CPR (see page 226) or rescue breathing (see "Airway and Breathing" on page 226) as needed.

Is the person hallucinating, confused, convulsing, breathing slowly and shallowly and/or slurring words? **YES**
SEEK EMERGENCY CARE

 NO

flowchart continued on next page

Do you suspect the person has taken an overdose of drugs? **YES**

SEEK EMERGENCY CARE

And call Poison Control Center.

Give the Poison Control Center the following information:

- The name of the medication or drug, if known
- The amount taken, if known (e.g., the number of pills or amount of liquid you suspect was swallowed)
- When the medication or drug was taken
- The person's age, gender and weight
- How the person is feeling and reacting
- Any medical problems the person has

Follow the Poison Control Center's instructions. If poison control tells you to induce vomiting:

- Approach the victim calmly and carefully.
- Give the person syrup of ipecac as instructed. General guidelines are:
  - One tablespoon to children one to six years and two tablespoons to those older than six years followed by a large glass of water or milk.
  - Walk the person around to help the ipecac work faster and to keep him or her awake.
  - Give syrup of ipecac again in 20 minutes if the person has not yet vomited.
  - Touch the back of the person's throat with a finger or spoon, if syrup of ipecac is not available.
  - After vomiting begins, continue giving clear fluids until the vomited material is clear.
  - When the vomiting has stopped, give nothing by mouth for two hours to give the stomach a chance to rest.

flowchart continued in next column

Note: If after taking two doses of syrup of ipecac the person has not vomited, seek emergency care.

See "Accidental Poisoning and Poisoning First Aid" on page 228.

NO

Is the person's personality suddenly hostile, violent and aggressive? **YES**

SEEK EMERGENCY CARE

Note: Use caution. Protect yourself. Do not turn your back to the victim or move suddenly in front of him or her. If you can, see that the victim does not harm you, himself or herself. Remember, the victim is under the influence of a drug. Call the police to assist you if you cannot handle the situation. Leave and find a safe place to stay until the police arrive.

NO

Have you or someone else accidentally taken more than the prescribed dose of a prescription or over-the-counter medicine? **YES**

CALL DOCTOR

If doctor is not available, call Poison Control Center. Follow instructions given.

Eye Injuries

There are many causes of eye injuries. These include:

- Physical blow to the eye
- Harsh chemicals like lye, bleach and acids, which can burn eye tissue and permanently damage the eyes
- A grain of sand, fleck of paint, sliver of metal or splinter of wood, which can scratch the cornea and induce infection
- Excessive exposure to the sun, very low humidity or a strong wind, which may dry the eyes so much they feel like sandpaper rubbing against your lids
- Insect bites

Prevention

- Wear protective plastic glasses during sports and other potentially dangerous activities.
- Be careful when using harsh chemicals. Wear rubber gloves and protective glasses. Don't rub your eyes if you've touched harsh chemicals. Wash your hands. Turn your head away from chemical vapors so as not to let any get into your eyes.
- Don't allow a child to stick his or her head out of the window of a moving vehicle. Sand, insects and other flying objects can strike the eye like a flying missile, irritating or damaging the cornea.
- Avoid alcohol, use a humidifier and limit exposure to smoke, dust and wind to help prevent dry eyes.
- Use artificial teardrops if recommended by your doctor.
- Never stare directly at the sun, especially during a solar eclipse.
- Wear sunglasses that block UV rays anytime you're in the sun.

All eye injuries should be taken seriously and all should be checked by a physician.

Questions to Ask

Is there a foreign body sticking into the eye? **YES**
SEEK EMERGENCY CARE

And perform first aid procedures before Emergency Care:
- Do not try to remove object.
- Do not press on, touch or rub eye(s).
- Wash hands with soap and water.
- Cover the affected eye with a paper cup or other clean object that will not touch the eye or the foreign object. Hold covering in place with tape without putting pressure on the eye.

flowchart continued in next column

flowchart continued

- Gently cover unaffected eye with a clean bandage and tape. This will help to keep the affected eye from moving. *Note: If you are alone, do not cover the unaffected eye, but try to keep it from moving side to side or up and down. Phone for or yell for help.*

NO

Is there a severe blow to the eye, with or without a broken bone of the face? **YES**
SEEK EMERGENCY CARE

And perform first aid procedures before Emergency Care:
- Close the eye.
- Put a cold compress over the injured area, not directly on, the eye. You can use ice in a plastic bag or wrapped in a cloth or a bag of frozen vegetables.
- Do not use firm pressure.
- Keep the victim lying down with eyes closed, if possible. *Note: If you are alone, phone for or yell for help.*

NO

Is there a cut to the eye or eyelid? **YES**
SEEK EMERGENCY CARE

And perform first aid procedures before Emergency Care:
- Loosely cover both eyes with a sterile cloth or pad and gently tape in place.
- Keep the victim lying flat on his or her back when seeking emergency care. *Note: If you are alone, phone for help. Loosely cover only the affected eye with a sterile cloth or pad and try to keep your other eye from moving side to side or up and down.*

NO

flowchart continued on next page

Have harmful chemicals gotten into the eye(s)? **YES**

SEEK EMERGENCY CARE

Flush the eye(s) with water immediately!
Then seek Emergency Care

How to flush the eyes with water:
• Have the victim lie down and turn his or her head to the side with the affected eye lower than the other eye.
• Hold the affected eye open with your thumb and forefinger.
• Pour large quantities of warm water, not hot, from a pitcher or other clean container, over the entire eye starting at the inside corner and downward to the outside corner. This lets the water drain away from the body and keeps it from getting in the other eye. Continue pouring the water for at least 10 minutes—30 minutes is better.
• Loosely bandage the eye with sterile cloth and tape.
• Do not touch the eye.
• If both eyes are affected, pour water over both eyes at the same time or quickly alternate the above procedure from one eye to another.
• Or place the victim's face in a sink or container filled with warm water. Have the person move his or her eyelids up and down. *Note: Do this procedure if you are alone.*
• You can also use industrial eye solutions, if available.

NO

flowchart continued in next column

Has a bee sting or insect bite to the eye caused a severe allergic reaction with these symptoms:
• Wheezing, shortness of breath and breathing difficulties
• Severe swelling the eye and in other parts of the body such as the tongue, lips and throat
• Bluish lips and skin
• Collapse

YES

SEEK EMERGENCY CARE

Give shot from and follow other instructions in emergency insect kit, if available. *Note: You can get this kit only with a doctor's prescription.*

NO

Do any of these problems occur after an eye injury:
• Blurred or double vision
• Blood in the pupil

YES

SEEK EMERGENCY CARE

NO

Does eye pain last longer than two days? **YES**

SEE DOCTOR

NO

PROVIDE FIRST AID PROCEDURES FOR NON-EMERGENCIES

First Aid Procedures for Non-Emergencies:

To remove a foreign object in the eye:
• Wash your hands.
• Twist a piece of tissue, moisten the tip with tap water, not saliva, and gently try to touch the speck with the tip. As you carefully pass the tissue over the speck, it should cling to the tip.
• If the foreign object is under the upper lid, look down and pull the upper lid away from the eyeball by gently grabbing the eyelashes. Try to touch the debris with the tip of a moistened tissue until it is caught on the tissue.
• Do not rub the eye. And never use tweezers or anything sharp to remove a foreign object. Doing so can scratch the cornea.

- Gently wash the eye with cool water.
- Cover the eye with a patch and leave it on for at least 24 hours. This helps to relieve the pain.

To treat a black eye from a minor injury:
- Immediately put a cold compress over the injured area. This helps to slow the bleeding under the skin and lessens swelling and discoloration.
- Take aspirin, ibuprofen or naproxen sodium for the pain and inflammation. Acetaminophen will help the pain, but not the inflammation. *Note: Do not give aspirin or any medication containing salicylates to anyone 19 years of age or younger, due to the association with Reye's syndrome, a potentially fatal condition.*
- Later, put a warm compress over the injured area.
- Seek medical attention if these measures do not help.

To ease the discomfort of dry eyes:
- Try an over-the-counter artificial tear product (e.g., Ocu-Lube, Refresh and Liquifilm). Check the label. If there are no preservatives, keep the solution refrigerated. Always wash your hands before putting drops in the eyes.

To ease the discomfort of an insect bite that has not caused a severe allergic reaction:
- Gently wash the eye(s) with warm water.
- Ask your doctor whether or not you should take an antihistamine and have him or her recommend one.

Heat Exhaustion and Heat Stroke

Perspiration acts like our natural air-conditioning. As perspiration evaporates from our skin, it cools us off, especially on hot, sweltering days. But, like a room air conditioner, our personal cooling system can fail if we overexert ourselves on hot and humid days.

When this happens, our body heat climbs to dangerous levels causing heat exhaustion or a life-threatening heat stroke.

Heat exhaustion takes time to develop. Fluids and salt so vital for maintaining good health are lost as children and adults perspire heavily during exercise or other strenuous activity. That's why it is very important to drink lots of liquids before, during and after exercise in hot weather. As strange as it seems, people suffering from heat exhaustion have low, normal or only slightly elevated body temperatures.

Signs and symptoms of heat exhaustion include:
- Cool, clammy, pale skin
- Sweating
- Dry mouth
- Fatigue, weakness
- Dizziness
- Headache
- Nausea, sometimes vomiting
- Muscle cramps
- Weak and rapid pulse

Heat stroke, unlike heat exhaustion, strikes suddenly, with little warning. When the body's cooling system fails, the body's temperature rapidly rises, creating an emergency condition.

Signs of heat stroke include:
- Very high temperature (104°F or higher)
- Hot, dry, red skin
- No sweating
- Deep breathing and fast pulse, followed by shallow breathing and weak pulse
- Dilated pupils
- Confusion, delirium, hallucinations
- Convulsions
- Loss of consciousness

Chronic medical conditions such as diabetes, use of alcohol, and vomiting or diarrhea can put children and adults at risk for a heat stroke during very hot weather. Heat stroke in children is not only due to high temperatures and humidity, but also to not drinking enough fluids.

Prevention

Heat exhaustion and heat stroke can be prevented by following this advice:

- Do not stay in or leave anyone in closed, parked cars during hot weather.
- Take caution when you must be in the sun. At the first signs of heat exhaustion, get out of the sun or your body temperature will continue to rise.
- Do not exercise vigorously during the hottest times of the day. Instead, run, jog or exercise closer to sunrise or sunset. If the outside temperature is 82°F or above and the humidity is high, consider shortening your activity session.
- Wear light, loose-fitting clothing (preferably cotton), so sweat can evaporate. Also wear a well-ventilated, wide-brimmed hat.
- Drink lots of liquids, especially if your urine is a very dark yellow or amber, to replace the fluids you lose from perspiring. Thirst is not a reliable sign that your body needs fluids. When you exercise, it is better to sip rather than gulp the liquids.
- Drink water or water with salt added if you sweat a lot. (Use ½ teaspoon salt in a quart of water.) Sport drinks such as Gatorade, All Sport and PowerAde are good too.
- If you feel very hot, try to cool off by opening a window, using a fan or turning on an air conditioner.
- Limit your stay in hot tubs or heated whirlpools to 15 minutes. Never use them when you are alone.
- Do not drink alcohol or beverages with caffeine because they speed up fluid loss.
- Stay out of the sun if you are taking diuretics, mood-altering drugs or antispasmodic medications. Check which ones are safe with your doctor.
- Do not bundle a baby in blankets or heavy clothing. Infants don't tolerate heat well because their sweat glands are not well developed.
- Some people perspire more than others. Those who do should drink as much fluid as they can during hot, humid days.
- Know the signs of heat stroke and heat exhaustion and don't ignore them.

Questions to Ask

Are any signs of heat stroke present:
- Body temperature 104°F or higher
- Skin that is red, dry and/or hot
- Pulse that is rapid and then gets weak
- No sweating
- Confusion, hallucinations or loss of consciousness or convulsions

YES →

SEEK EMERGENCY CARE

Give first aid for heat stroke before Emergency Care:

- Do CPR if the person is not breathing and has no pulse. (See "CPR" on page 226.)
- Do rescue breathing if the person is not breathing, but does have a pulse. (See "Airway and Breathing" on page 226.) Until emergency care arrives, it is important to lower the body temperature. To do this:
  - Move the person to a cool place indoors or under a shady tree. Place the feet higher than the head.
  - Remove the clothing and either wrap the person in a cold, wet sheet; sponge the person with towels or sheets that are soaked in very cold water; or spray the person with cool water. Fan the person. If using an electric fan, use caution. Make sure your hands are dry when you plug the fan in and turn it on. Keep the person with wet items far enough away from the fan so as not to cause electric shock.
  - Put ice packs or cold compresses to the neck, under the armpits and to the groin area.
  - Immerse a child in cold water if he or she is unconscious.

flowchart continued on next page

- Place the person in the recovery position once his or her temperature reaches 101°F. To do this:
  - Kneel at the side of the person. Straighten the victim's arm that is closest to you and raise it above his or her head.
  - Cross his or her other arm over his or her chest. Bend the victim's far leg and cross it over his or her near leg.
  - Hold the victim's clothing at the hip and gently pull the person toward you, moving the head with the body.
  - Bend the victim's upper arm and leg until each forms a right angle to the body. Cover the person with a wet sheet. If the temperature starts to climb, repeat all of the above.
- Give as much cold water as the person can drink until he or she feels better.

NO

Is the person too dizzy or weak to stand, or does he or she have persistent vomiting?

YES

SEEK
EMERGENCY
CARE

Perform first aid procedures for heat stroke before Emergency Care (see page 238).

NO

Are two or more of these signs of heat exhaustion present:
- Pale, cool and clammy skin
- Sweating
- Dry mouth
- Dizziness
- Fatigue and weakness
- Headache
- Nausea, vomiting
- Weak and rapid pulse
- Muscle cramps

YES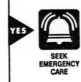

SEEK
EMERGENCY
CARE

And perform first aid procedures for heat exhaustion.

First Aid Procedures for Heat Exhaustion:

(These apply to you or anyone else who has heat exhaustion symptoms.)
- Move to a cool place indoors or in the shade.
- Loosen clothing.
- Take fluids such as cool or cold water. If available, add ½ teaspoon of salt to a quart of water and sip it or drink sport drinks such as Gatorade, All Sport or PowerAde.
- Have salty foods like saltine crackers, if tolerated.
- Lie down in a cool, breezy place.

Neck and Spine Injuries

Anything that puts too much pressure or force on the neck or back can result in a neck and/or spinal injury. Suspect a neck injury, too, if a head injury has occurred. Common causes are:
- Accidents involving cars, motorcycles, snowmobiles, toboggans, roller blades and the like
- Falls, especially from high places
- Diving mishaps (e.g., diving into water that is too shallow)
- A hard blow to the neck or back while playing a contact sport such as football
- Violent acts (e.g., a gunshot wound that penetrates the head, neck or trunk)

Some neck and spinal injuries can be serious because of their potential for causing paralysis. These need emergency medical care. Others (e.g., whiplash) can be temporary, minor injuries.

A mild whiplash typically causes neck pain and stiffness the following day. Some people, though, have trouble raising their heads off the pillow the next morning. Physical therapy and a collar to support the neck are the most common types of treatment. It often takes three to four months for all symptoms to disappear.

Prevention

- Use padded headrests in your car to prevent whiplash.
- Drive carefully and defensively.
- Wear seatbelts, both lap belts and shoulder harnesses.
- Buckle children into approved car seats appropriate for their ages.
- Wear a helmet whenever riding bicycles or motorcycles or when roller-skating or roller-blading.
- Wear the recommended safety equipment for contact sports.
- Be careful when jumping up and down on a trampoline, climbing a ladder or checking a roof.
- Check the depth before diving into water. Do not dive into water that is less that nine feet deep. Never dive into an above-ground pool.

Note: If you suspect a neck or back injury in you or someone else, it is imperative to keep the neck and/or back perfectly still until an emergency crew arrives. Do not move someone with a suspected neck or spine injury unless the person must be moved because his or her safety is in danger. Any movement of the head, neck or back could result in paralysis or death. Immobilize the neck by holding the head, neck and shoulders perfectly still. Use both hands, one on each side of the head.

Questions to Ask

Is the injured person not breathing, and does he or she have no pulse? **YES**

SEEK EMERGENCY CARE

And perform CPR, but without moving the neck or spine. (See "CPR" on page 000.) But when you do the "Airway and Breathing" part of CPR, do not tilt the head back or move the head or neck. Instead, pull the lower jaw (chin) forward to open the airway.

 NO

flowchart continued in next column

---

flowchart continued

Is the injured person not breathing, but he or she has a pulse? **YES**

SEEK EMERGENCY CARE

And perform rescue breathing without moving the neck or spine. (See "CPR" on page 226.) But do not tilt the head back or move the head or neck. Instead, pull the lower jaw (chin) forward to open the airway.

Additional first aid procedures before Emergency Care:

- Tell the victim to lie still and not move his or her head, neck, back, etc.
- Immobilize the neck and/or spine. Place rolled towels, articles of clothing, etc. on both sides of the neck and/or body. Tie and wrap in place, but don't interfere with the victim's breathing. If necessary, use both of your hands, one on each side of the victim's head, to keep the head from moving.

If you must move someone with a suspected neck or spinal injury, follow the above procedures and:

- Select a stretcher, door or other rigid board.
- Use several people to carefully lift and move the person onto the board, being very careful to align the head and neck in a straight line with the spine. The head should not rotate or bend forward or backward.
- Make sure one person uses both of his or her hands, one on each side of the victim's head, to keep the head from moving. If you can, immobilize the neck and/or spine by placing rolled towels, articles of clothing, etc. on both sides of the neck and/or body. Tie and wrap in place, but don't interfere with the victim's breathing.

flowchart continued on next page

240

If you suspect someone has injured his or her neck in a diving or other water accident:

- Protect the neck and/or spine from bending or twisting. Place your hands on both sides of the neck and keep in place until help arrives.
- If the person is still in the water, help the person float until a rigid board can be slipped under the head and body, at least as far down as the buttocks.
- If no board is available, several people should take the person out of the water, supporting the head and body as one unit, making sure the head does not rotate or bend in any direction.

NO

Does the injured person have any of these signs or symptoms:
- Paralysis
- Inability to open and close his or her fingers or move his or her toes
- Feelings of numbness in the legs, arms, shoulders or any other part of the body
- Appearance that the head, neck or back is in an odd position

YES

SEEK EMERGENCY CARE

NO

Are any of these present following a recent injury to the neck and/or spine that did not get treated with emergency care at the time of the injury?
- Severe pain
- Numbness, tingling or weakness in the face, arms or legs
- Loss of bladder control

YES

SEEK EMERGENCY CARE

NO

flowchart continued in next column

Do you suspect a whiplash injury or has pain from any injury to the neck or back lasted longer than one week?

YES

SEE DOCTOR

NO

PROVIDE SELF-CARE

Self-Care Procedures

If you suspect a whiplash injury:
- See your doctor as soon as you can so he or she can assess the extent of injury.
- For the first 24 hours, apply ice packs to the injured area for up to 20 minutes an hour.
  - To make an ice pack, wrap ice in a face towel or cloth.
  - After 24 hours, use ice packs or heat to relieve the pain.
  - Take a hot shower for 20 minutes a few times a day. This is a good source of heat to the neck.
  - Use a hot water bottle, heating pad (set on low) or a heat lamp directed to the neck for 10 minutes several times a day.
- Use a cervical pillow or a small rolled towel positioned behind your neck instead of a regular pillow.
- Wrap a folded towel around the neck to help hold the head in one position during the night.
- If you arm or hand is numb, buy or rent a cervical-traction device. Ask your doctor how to use it.
- Take aspirin, acetaminophen or ibuprofen for minor pain. *Note: Do not give aspirin or any medication containing salicylates to anyone 19 years of age or younger, due to the association with Reye's syndrome, a potentially fatal condition.*
- Get plenty of rest.

APPENDIX A

Family Medical Records

DISEASE HISTORY

(Fill in dates for each one, if applicable.)

Name	Chicken Pox	Measles/Mumps	German Measles	Whooping Cough	Meningitis	Hepatitis	Tuberculosis	Scarlet Fever	Mononucleosis	Pneumonia
1.										
2.										
3.										
4.										
5.										

HEALTH INFORMATION

Name	Blood Type	Drug Sensitivities	Allergies
1.			
2.			
3.			
4.			
5.			

HOSPITAL RECORDS

Name	Hospitalization, Surgery/Injury	Date(s)	Method of Treatment	Doctor/Hospital	Comments
1.					
2.					
3.					
4.					
5.					

APPENDIX B
Your Home Pharmacy

Listed are medications and supplies that should be kept at home for self-care procedures. Be sure to store them in a convenient dry place, but out of children's reach. Check the expiration dates periodically and discard and replace as needed.

MEDICATIONS	USE
Acetaminophen (e.g., Aspirin-Free Anacin, Tylenol)	Pain relief, fever reduction
Antacids, liquid or tablets (e.g., Tums, Rolaids, Mylanta, Amphojel)	Stomach upset, heartburn
Antidiarrheal medicine (e.g., Kaopectate, Immodium A-D, Donnagel)	Diarrhea
Antihistamines (e.g., Dristan, Triaminic, Benadryl)	Allergies, cold symptoms relief
Antimotion sickness (e.g., Dramamine)	Motion sickness
Antiseptic preparation (e.g., Betadine)	Abrasions, cuts
Aspirin* (e.g., Anacin, Bayer, Bufferin)	Pain relief, fever reduction, swelling reduction
Cough suppressant without expectorant (e.g., Robitussin Max Strength, Robitussin)	Dry cough without mucus
Decongestant (tablets, nose spray, etc.) (e.g., Dristan Nasal Spray, Sudafed, Dimetapp)	Stuffy and runny nose, postnasal drip from colds, allergies
Expectorant with Dextromethorphan (e.g., Robitussin DM)	Cough with mucus
Ibuprofen (adult) (e.g., Advil)	Pain relief, fever reduction, swelling reduction
Laxatives (e.g., Ex-Lax, Correctol, Milk of Magnesia)	Constipation

*Note: Do not give aspirin or any medication containing salicylates to anyone 19 years of age or younger, unless directed by a physician, due to its association with Reye's syndrome, a potentially fatal condition.

SUPPLIES	USE
Activated charcoal (binds certain chemicals when swallowed)	Oral poisoning for some poisons (Note: Call Poison Control Center first.)
Adhesive bandages	Minor wounds
Adhesive tape, sterile gauze pads, roll of sterile gauze and scissors	To dress minor wounds
Antibiotic cream or ointment (e.g., Bacitracin)	Minor skin infection, wounds
Antifungal preparations (e.g., Tinactin)	Fungal infections such as athlete's foot
Cotton balls, cotton tipped applicators	Minor wounds
Ear wax dissolver (e.g., Debrox)	Ear wax
Elastic bandages and clips	Minor strains and sprains
Eye drops and artificial tears (e.g., Murine, Visine)	Minor eye irritations
Heating pad/hot water bottle	Minor pains, strains, menstrual cramps
Hemorrhoid preparations (e.g., Preparation H)	Hemorrhoids
Humidifier, vaporizer (cool-mist)	Add moisture to the air
Hydrocortisone cream (e.g., Cortaid, Lanacort)	Minor skin irritations, itching and rashes
Ice pack/Heat pack	Minor pain and injuries
Petroleum jelly (e.g., Vaseline)	Chafing, diaper rash, dry skin
Rubbing alcohol	Topical antiseptic, cleans thermometer
Sunscreen (look for one with SPF, or sun protection factor, of 15 or more)	Prevent sunburn, protect against skin cancer
Syrup of ipecac (Note: Call Poison Control Center first.)	To induce vomiting for some poisons
Thermometer (mercury-containing, digital, etc.)	To measure temperature
Throat anesthetic preparations (e.g., Sucret throat lozenges, Chloraseptic spray)	Minor sore throat
Tongue depressor, flashlight	Check for redness or infection in throat
Toothache-relief preparation (e.g., Anbesol)	Toothache, teething
Tweezers	Remove splinters

APPENDIX C
Health Hotlines

Free health information is just a phone call away. The toll-free numbers listed here correspond to organizations (listed alphabetically by subject). Most organizations staff their hotlines from 9:00 a.m. to 5:00 p.m. local time, Monday through Friday.

To find a toll-free number not listed in this directory, call the toll-free information operator at 800-555-1212 and explain what kind of information you need.

Inclusion in this directory does not indicate endorsement of the organization by the American Institute for Preventive Medicine or the People's Medical Society.

Alcohol and Drug Abuse

"Just Say No" International
2101 Webster St., Suite 1300
Oakland, CA 94612
800-258-2766
Assists parents, children and schools in setting up "Just Say No" clubs to prevent drug abuse.

National Cocaine Hotline
c/o Phoenix House
164 W. 74th St.
New York, NY 10023
800-COCAINE or 800-662-HELP
Answers questions, makes referrals to local programs and offers counseling on cocaine use and other drug problems.

National Council on Alcoholism
12 W. 21st St.
New York, NY 10010
800-622-2255
Offers various kinds of information on alcoholism.

Children's Diseases

Cystic Fibrosis Foundation
6931 Arlington Rd.
Bethesda, MD 20814
800-344-4823 or 800-CF-FIGHT
Provides information and local physician referrals for children with cystic fibrosis.

Juvenile Diabetes Foundation International
432 Park Ave. South
New York, NY 10016
800-223-1138
Provides information and answers questions about juvenile diabetes.

National Reye's Syndrome Foundation
P.O. Box 829
Bryan, OH 43506
800-233-7393
Distributes information to the public and the medical community on Reye's syndrome.

General Health Information

American Academy of Family Physicians
8880 Ward Pkwy.
Kansas City, MO 64114
800-274-2237
A national association of family doctors who govern and maintain high standards in such areas as patient care and continuing education.

American Osteopathic Association
142 E. Ontario St.
Chicago, IL 60611
800-621-1773
Provides information on osteopathic medicine and makes local referrals to osteopathic centers.

National Health Information Center
P.O. Box 1133
Washington, DC 20013-1133
800-336-4797
Provides information and referrals for consumers looking for various types of health information.

Health Problems

Acquired Immune Deficiency Syndrome (AIDS)

AIDS Information Hotline
U.S. Public Health Service
American Social Health Association
P.O. Box 13827
Research Triangle Park, NC 27709
800-342-AIDS
800-344-7432 (in Spanish)
800-243-7889 (for hearing impaired)
Provides information on AIDS and makes local referrals for medical assistance.

Alzheimer's Disease

Alzheimer's Association
919 N. Michigan Ave., Suite 1000
Chicago, IL 60601-1676
800-272-3900
Provides information to the public and health care professionals and makes referrals to local chapters and support groups.

Anemia

Cooley's Anemia Foundation
129-09 26th Ave.
Flushing, NY 11354
800-522-7222
Provides information on patient care, support groups and research on Cooley's anemia.

Cancer

Cancer Information Service
National Cancer Institute
900 Rockville Pike
Bethesda, MD 20892
800-4-CANCER
Provides information on cancer to both the public and the medical community.

Diabetes

American Diabetes Association
1660 Duke St.
Alexandria, VA 22314
800-232-3472
Provides health education information, supports research and offers assistance in forming diabetes support groups.

Disabilities

National Rehabilitation Information Center
8455 Colesville Rd., Suite 935
Silver Spring, MD 20910
800-34-NARIC
Provides current information and referrals for people with disabilities.

Dyslexia

Orton Dyslexia
Chester Bldg., Suite 382
8600 LaSalle Rd.
Baltimore, MD 21204-6020
800-ABCD-123
Provides information, supports research and makes referrals for people suffering from this learning disability.

Epilepsy

Epilepsy Foundation of America
4351 Garden City Dr., 4th Floor
Landover, MD 20785
800-332-1000
Provides information about epilepsy and makes referrals to local resources.

Headaches

National Headache Foundation
5252 N. Western Ave.
Chicago, IL 60625
800-843-2256
Provides information on headaches and their treatment and gives physician member list and headache clinic list.

Hearing and Speech Problems

Better Hearing Institute Hearing Help Line
P.O. Box 1840
Washington, DC 20013
800-327-9355
Offers information and help for hearing problems and prevention of deafness.

National Hearing Aid Helpline
20361 Middlebelt Rd.
Livonia, MI 48152
800-521-5247
Provides information on hearing loss and referrals to those in need of hearing aids. Serves both the general public and health professionals.

Heart Disease

American Heart Association
7272 Greenville Ave.
Dallas, TX 75231-4596
800-242-8721
Supports research and public education and offers multiple services focusing on the prevention and treatment of heart disease.

Kidney Diseases

American Kidney Fund
6110 Executive Blvd., Suite 1010
Rockville, MD 20852
800-638-8299
Provides information on kidney disease and organ donations and grants financial assistance to needy kidney patients.

Liver Diseases

American Liver Foundation
1425 Pompton Ave.
Cedar Grove, NJ 07009
800-223-0179
Makes referrals to local self-help support groups and offers educational information for people with liver ailments. Also publishes a newsletter for physicians and the general public.

Lung Diseases

National Jewish Center for Immunology and Respiratory Medicine Lung Line
1400 Jackson St.
Denver, CO 80206
800-222-LUNG
Answers questions and provides information on respiratory problems, including asthma, emphysema and chronic bronchitis.

Lupus

Lupus Foundation of America
4 Research Place, Suite 180
Rockville, MD 20850-3226
800-558-0121*
Provides patient education, support groups, and public and professional services to people with lupus.

*Not available in Washington, D.C.

Parkinson's Disease

National Parkinson Foundation
1501 N.W. 9th Ave.
Bob Hope Rd.
Miami, FL 33136
800-327-4545
Answers questions, furnishes information and makes physician referrals for people with Parkinson's disease.

Sickle-Cell Anemia

National Association for Sickle-Cell Disease
200 Corporate Pointe
Culver, CA 90230
800-421-8453
Prepares and distributes educational materials,
trains counselors and conducts educational
programs for the public and health care
professionals. Also supports research and
conducts diagnostic screenings.

Vision Problems

American Council for the Blind
1155 15th St., N.W., Suite 720
Washington, DC 20005
800-424-8666
Provides information and cassettes and makes
referrals to local agencies and vision-care
professionals.

Prevent Blindness America
500 E. Remington Rd.
Schaumberg, IL 60173
800-221-3004
Sponsors research and glaucoma screenings.
Also offers educational materials, consultations
and professional education programs.

Hospital and Hospice Care

Hill-Burton Hospital Free or Reduced-Cost
Health Care Program
U.S. Public Health Service
Parklawn Bldg.
5600 Fishers Ln., Room 1125
Rockville, MD 20857
800-638-0742
800-492-0359 (for Maryland only)
Furnishes information and referrals to
participating hospitals.

Insurance

Inspector General's Hotline
P.O. Box 17303
Baltimore, MD 21203-7303
800-368-5779
Handles Medicare and Social Security fraud,
abuse and waste.

Medical Identification

Medic Alert Foundation International
P.O. Box 1009
Turlock, CA 95381
800-344-3226
Dispenses medical identification bracelets or
cards to individuals who have chronic medical
conditions.

Mental Health

American Mental Health Fund
800-433-5959
Provides booklets on various mental health
problems.

National Adolescent Suicide Hotline
3080 N. Lincoln Ave.
Chicago, IL 60657
800-621-4000
Makes referrals and provides counseling to
troubled and/or runaway teenagers.

National Mental Health Association
1021 Prince St.
Alexandria, VA 22314-2971
800-969-NMHA (6642)
Provides information on a variety of mental
health issues. Can also give location of local
community mental health centers.

Nutrition

National Center for Nutrition and Dietetics
American Dietetic Association
216 W. Jackson Blvd., Suite 800
Chicago, IL 60606
Consumer Nutrition Information Hotline:
800-366-1655
Provides general information on nutrition.
Can also give referral to a registered dietitian
in your area.

Organ Donation

The Living Bank
P.O. Box 6725
Houston, TX 77265
800-528-2971
Registers people who wish to donate their
organs or tissues after death. Offers printed
materials and encourages public education
for both health care professionals and organ
donors.

Pregnancy

International Childbirth Education
Association (ICEA)
P.O. Box 20048
Minneapolis, MN 55420
800-624-4934
Furnishes information on pregnancy-related
concerns through its book center.

ASPO-LaMaze
1200 19th St., N.W., Suite 300
Washington, DC 20036
800-368-4404
Provides information and makes local
referrals for childbirth preparation classes
and instruction in breathing techniques used
during delivery.

Safety

National Highway Traffic Safety Administration
Auto Safety Hotline
400 7th St., S.W.
Washington, DC 20590
800-424-9393
Provides information on passenger safety,
auto recalls and child safety seats. Also
handles consumer questions about auto-safety
regulations.

National Safety Council
1121 Spring Lake Drive
Itasca, IL 60143-3201
800-621-7619
Provides information on accident prevention
and general safety guidelines.

U.S. Consumer Product Safety Commission
Washington, DC 20207
800-638-2772
Takes calls from consumers with product
complaints. Also works to protect consumers
from injury in and around their homes caused
by products, including children's toys.

Senior Citizen Health

Healthy Older People
National Health Information Center
P.O. Box 1133
Washington, DC 20013-1133
800-336-4797
Supplies public education materials on health
promotion for older Americans.

National Council on Aging
409 3rd St., S.W., Suite 200
Washington, DC 20024
800-424-9046
Provides information on aging and makes
referrals to local agencies.

Sports

Aerobics and Fitness Association of America
15250 Ventura Blvd., Suite 200
Sherman Oaks, CA 91403
800-445-5950
Answers questions about safe exercise practices
and aerobic fitness programs.

Surgery

American Society of Plastic and
Reconstructive Surgeons, Inc.
444 E. Algonquin Rd.
Arlington Heights, IL 60005
800-635-0635
Provides information on aesthetic and
reconstructive surgical procedures and makes
physician referrals.

Medicare Telephone Hotline
200 Independence Ave., S.W.
Washington, DC 20201
800-638-6833
Provides referrals to local surgeons who can
provide second opinions regarding a
recommended surgery.

SOURCE: Adapted from *Toll-Free Hotlines to Health*
(Farmington Hills, Mich.: American Institute for
Preventive Medicine, 1994).

Other Books by the American Institute for Preventive Medicine

Self-Care: Your Family Guide to Symptoms and How to Treat Them is one of a series of publications offered by the American Institute for Preventive Medicine. It is designed to help consumers reduce health care costs and improve the quality of their lives. Other publications in the series include:

365 Health Hints

(Published by Simon & Schuster)

This best selling, tip-a-day book offers the latest ideas on how to make your health last a lifetime.

HealthyLife® Self-Care Guides

Each booklet addresses 25 of the most common health problems and teaches when to see the doctor or provide self-care. Adult, children's, senior and women's editions are available.

HealthyLife® Emergency/First Aid

From insect bites to frostbite and from splinters to sunburn, this reference will be an important part of your medicine cabinet.

HealthyLife® Mental Fitness Guide

Using this book, readers can review 25 psychological conditions and determine the best course for treatment.

All the Right Questions™

This reference guides individuals in making wise medical decisions.

Being a Wise Health Care Consumer™

This book teaches people to be more knowledgeable about the health care system.

Healthy Savings™

Readers can review 101 tips on how to save money on medical care.

Toll-Free Hotlines to Health™

This guide allows your fingers to do the walking to more than 150 health organizations that provide free advice, referrals and/or information.

Minding Your Mental Health™

This publication provides consumers with a guide to the mental health care field.

For more information about the institute's programs, products and services, call or write:

American Institute for Preventive Medicine
30445 Northwestern Hwy., Suite 350
Farmington Hills, MI 48334
810-539-1800
810-539-1808 FAX

INDEX

Family problems, for medical history, 14

Famvir, shingles, 88

Fat, 44

Fatigue, 119-120. *See also* Chronic fatigue syndrome

Fever, 120-121, 151-153, 243

Fiber, 44

Fibroids, 166-168

Fifth disease, 92

Finasteride, benign prostatic hypertrophy, 178

Flatulence, 98

Flu, 74-75

Food Guide Pyramid, 42-43, 46

Frostbite, 79, 83-84

Functional incontinence, 128

Fungus
  athlete's foot, 77
  jock itch, 180

G

Gallstones, 208-209

Gamma globulin, measles prevention, 150

Gas. *See* Flatulence

Gastroenterologist, 13

Generic medications, 21

Glaucoma, 16, 17, 209

Gonorrhea, 182, 185-186

Gout, 210

Graves' disease, 222

Gum disease, 189-190

Gynecologist, 13

H

H. influenzae type b vaccine, 18

Hair loss, 84-85

Hay fever, 58-59

HB. *See* Hepatitis B

Headaches, 122-123, 247

Health-care proxy, 27

Health hotlines, 245-250

Health maintenance organization (HMO), doctor selection, 12

Health tests
  insurance coverage, 17
  recommendations, 17

Hearing aids, 59, 61

Hearing loss, 59-61, 247

Heart attack, 16, 115, 117, 197, 230-231

Heart disease, 16, 18, 36, 79, 203-204, 247

Heartburn, 99-100, 116

Heat exhaustion/stroke, 237-239

Heat rash, 90, 92

Heat treatment
  arthritis, 199
  back pain, 105
  menstrual cramps, 171, 244
  minor pains/strains, 244
  neck/spine injuries, 241
  phlebitis, 219
  shoulder and neck pain, 109-110

Heimlich maneuver, 227, 231

Hemorrhoids, 94, 100-101, 244

Hepatitis B immunization, 18

Hernia, hiatal, 99, 116

Herpes, genital, 16, 182, 184-185

Herpes zoster. *See* Shingles

Hiccups, 61

Phobias, 33, 35, 135

Physiatrist, 13

Physical exam, 16-17

Physical fitness. *See* Exercise

Pinched nerve, 107, 109-110

Pinkeye, 63-64

PMS, 119, 173-174

Pneumococcal vaccine, 18, 207, 220

Pneumonia, 18, 143, 158, 207, 219-220, 230

Podiatrist, 80

Poison ivy, 87-88, 90, 92, 154-155

Poison oak. *See* Poison ivy

Poison sumac. *See* Poison ivy

Poisoning, accidental, 23, 228-230

Polio, oral vaccine, 18

Pollen, 59, 63, 70, 85, 159

Post-traumatic stress disorder, 35, 135

Pregnancy
    fainting during, 117-118
    information, 249
    precautions/guidelines, 50-52
    premature labor, 51-52
    self-testing kits, 19
    smoking and, 36

Premenstrual syndrome (PMS). *See* PMS

Presbycusis, 59-60

Prescriptions. *See also* Medications
    abbreviations, 20-21

Preventive care
    alcohol, 47-49
    exercise, 40-42
    generally, 36
    nutrition, 42-45
    pregnancy, 50-52
    publication listing, 251
    safety at home, 49-50
    smoking cessation, 36-37

stress, 38-40
    weight control, 46-47

Prickly heat. *See* Heat rash

Probenecid, gout, 210

Prostate, enlarged, 131, 178-179

Prostate-specific antigen test. *See* PSA test

Prosthodontics, 32

PSA test, benign prostatic hypertrophy and, 178

Psychiatrist, 13

Public health dentistry, 32

Punctures, 81-82

Q

Quinine, 60

R

Race
    glaucoma, 17
    sickle-cell anemia, 221

Radiation, 160, 162

Radioactive iodine for thyroid problems, 223

Radiologist, 13

Rashes, skin. *See* Skin rashes

Raynaud's disease, 79

Rectal exam. *See* Digital rectal exam

Repetitive motion injuries, 125-127

Respiratory disease, immunization and, 18

Retirement, for medical history, 14

Reye's syndrome
    aspirin/salicylates and, 56, 62, 65-66, 75, 78,
        81-82, 87, 91, 93, 97, 105, 107, 109-111, 113,
        116, 121, 123, 126-127, 132, 145, 151-152,
        158, 166, 171, 173, 185, 188-189, 192, 218,
        241, 243
    information, 245

NOTES

NOTES

NOTES

NOTES